Midbrain Mutiny: The Picoeconomics and Neuroeconomics of Disordered Gambling

Midbrain Mutiny: The Picoeconomics and Neuroeconomics of Disordered Gambling

Economic Theory and Cognitive Science

Don Ross, Carla Sharp, Rudy Vuchinich, and David Spurrett

A Bradford Book
The MIT Press
Cambridge, Massachusetts
London, England

MIT Press books may be purchased at special quantity discounts for business or sales promotional use. For information, please e-mail special_sales@mitpress.mit.edu or write to Special Sales Department, The MIT Press, 55 Hayward Street, Cambridge, MA 02142.

This book was set in Palatino by SNP Best-set Typesetter Ltd., Hong Kong, and was printed and bound in the United States of America.

Library of Congress Cataloging-in-Publication Data

Midbrain mutiny : the picoeconomics and neuroeconomics of disordered gambling : economic theory and cognitive science / Don Ross . . . [et al.].
    p. ; cm.
Includes bibliographical references and index.
ISBN 978-0-262-18265-2 (hardcover : alk. paper)
1. Compulsive gambling. 2. Motivation (Psychology). 3. Reward (Psychology). 4. Choice (Psychology). 5. Neuroeconomics. 6. Economics. 7. Cognitive science. I. Ross, Don, 1962–.
[DNLM: 1. Gambling. 2. Behavior, Addictive. 3. Cognitive Science. 4. Economics. WM 190 M627   2008]
RC569.5.G35M53   2008
616.85'841—dc22   2007034671

10 9 8 7 6 5 4 3 2 1

Contents

Note to Readers about
Economic Theory and Cognitive Science

This book is a case study application of a highly abstract thesis about the relationship between microeconomic theory and related cognitive and behavioral sciences defended in a 2005 book, *Economic Theory and Cognitive Science: Microexplanation*, by one of the present authors, Don Ross.

Despite this relationship between the present book and Ross's earlier one, we don't intend this volume to be merely, or even mainly, read for the sake of illustrating by example a philosophical view on economics and neighboring sciences. This is a book about disordered (problem and pathological) gambling, and about the significance of this subject to our general scientific understanding of phenomena thought of as "addictions." We intend it to be of interest not only to theoretical psychologists and other behavioral scientists with mainly research interests, but also to clinicians and policy makers concerned with gambling and addiction problems. We don't want to address these readers in a way that first *requires* them to master the conceptual foundations of microeconomics (though we *encourage* everyone to do that).

On the other hand, Ross's perspective on the relationships among behavioral sciences is, in its 2005 presentation, crucially incomplete in the absence of an extended application. The present book is thus meant to flesh out the account of microexplanation, in advance of the continuation of Ross's project extending it to explanation of social-behavioral phenomena by macroeconomics and neighboring social sciences. So we also intend that some readers of the 2005 book whose main interest is in the foundations of economic theory, rather than in gambling or addiction per se, will be motivated to read this one.

Is it not eccentric of us to have written two books, with two orthogonal purposes, in one? Perhaps. Let us then add just a bit more here by way of explanation. Two of us (Ross and Spurrett) were trained (though not exclusively) as philosophers of science. We hold the metaphilosophical opinion, defended at length elsewhere (Ladyman and Ross 2007), that there is no such thing as a justifiable *purely* philosophical conclusion about any empirical phenomenon (and there are no such things as "non-empirical phenomena"). Therefore, anyone who wants to defend a philosophical thesis had better be prepared to defend it as, in large part, a scientific proposition based on scientific evidence. Once one gets to that point, though, surely one should try to make the science in question independently interesting *as* science, even (indeed, especially) to people whose tastes don't run to philosophy. Ross 2005 is mainly a project in applied philosophy of science. Thus, by our intellectual rules just described, it must underwrite some science that a person needn't be a philosopher, or be particularly interested in philosophy, to appreciate. Both sets of readers for whom this book is intended will, in their different ways, be the judges of whether this test is passed here.

We conclude this note with a bare summary of the main conclusions defended in *Economic Theory and Cognitive Science: Microexplanation*.

(1) There is a thesis commonly taken to be central to mainstream (neoclassical) economics that is in no way part of or implied by the mathematics of that framework. This is that the paradigmatic model of an economic agent is an individual human being. In fact, the *empirical* paradigm cases of economic agency are simple, consistent pursuers of low-dimensional goals; insects and neurons are examples. Whole human beings *approximate* economic agency, usefully enough for many practical modeling purposes, in the same way that countries and corporations do.

(2) The way in which whole humans, countries, and corporations approximate economic agency is made theoretically precise by *picoeconomics*, a branch of behavioral economics. A country's approximate economic agency is a consequence of strategic interactions among its citizens, who are compelled by exogenous pressures and their own aims to try to coordinate their behavior (up to a point). A country's approximate economic agency, to whatever extent it holds in a given case at a given time, is thus a dynamic equilibrium in a dynamic n-person game among its citizens. Similarly, a person's economic agency, to whatever extent it holds in a given case at a given time, is a dynamic equilibrium in a dynamic game among n *subpersonal interests*.

(3) The subpersonal interests above are *virtual* objects—that is, they are theoretically inferred from the economic model of personal behavior. They describe what psychologists call *molar scale* patterns in behavior, not anatomical or functional *parts* of people's brains.

(4) At the same time, the view of *neuroeconomists* that neurons and groups of neurons fit the model of economic agency is true. These agents influence a person's behavior on what psychologists call the *molecular* scale. (This does not refer to literal chemical molecules; it merely means "small *and* isolable from context.") Molar-scale descriptions don't reduce to and aren't entailed by molecular-scale ones, because molar-scale accounts index behavioral patterns to environmental contexts and molecular-scale accounts don't.

(5) Therefore, there are *two* non-identical kinds of subpersonal economic agents: picoeconomic interests and neurons. An account of a given person's two subpersonal economies at a given time must be *compatible* (in the sense of non-contradictory), and should ideally be *complementary* (in the sense of informing one another), but molecular-scale accounts don't generally render the molar-scale accounts redundant (except in cases of occasional "local reductions" that are empirical discoveries and can't be predicted by philosophical speculation).

(6) All of the varieties of models described above are built using the resources of standard postwar neoclassical microeconomic theory. These models can be used to explain and predict the many ways in which individual human behavior systematically differs from the behavior of true economic agents. Therefore, claims by behavioral economists that observed systematic "irrationality" in human behavior "refutes" standard neoclassical theory should be rejected. (Claims that "predictions of game theory" are refuted by observations of human behavior should be dismissed out of hand. Game theory is a body of mathematics; it thus makes no empirical predictions, and so cannot be "refuted" by observation of anything.)

Acknowledgments

All four authors thank Tom Stone of MIT Press for supporting the project, Nelleke Bak for careful proofreading and formatting of the manuscript, and Peter Collins of the South African Responsible Gambling Foundation and National Responsible Gambling Programme for arranging funding of our research into gambling and freeing some of our time from other duties.

Don Ross additionally thanks his four heads of department(s) during the period of writing—Melvin Ayogu, Johannes Fedderke, Harold Kincaid, and Lance Nail—for their support in researching the book. For assistance in managing scientific budgets and research staff he thanks Jacques Rousseau, and for administrative assistance Gadija Allison, Paula Bassingthwaite, Carol Knoetzer, Minnie Randle, and Pam Williams. For comments on parts of the manuscript he thanks George Ainslie, Paul Glimcher, and James MacKillop. For research assistance he thanks Andrew Dellis, Andre Hofmeyr, and Peter Schwardmann.

Carla Sharp additionally thanks Brie Linkenhoker, Norma Clarke, Thom Kosten, Read Montague, Mike Beauchamp, Phil Burton, and Christian Emden for valuable discussions about some of the ideas contained in this book; Carolyn Ha for essential administrative assistance; and heads of departments or divisions Stuart Yudofsky, Efrain Bleiberg, Peter Fonagy, and Mindi Stanley for their generous support.

Rudy Vuchinich additionally thanks E. Lanette Milligan for keeping the grant project going, and Rachel Vuchinich and Jason Vuchinich for their continued love and support.

David Spurrett additionally thanks Ben Murrell and Hugh Pastoll for research assistance.

1   Is There Such a Thing as Addiction?

To some extent, everyone engages in the same activities repeatedly over time. Chaos would reign if we did not show such behavioral regularities. Much of this behavior is constructive and healthy, such as work, physical exercise, and social interactions, while some of it is destructive and unhealthy, such as excessive drinking, drug use, or gambling. Given current understanding, however, we cannot distinguish good from bad repetitive behavior simply by reference to type, since some people drink, use drugs, or gamble in moderation and therefore avoid the destructiveness of excess, while others work or exercise too much and turn an otherwise healthy repetitive pattern into an unhealthy one. A scientific issue of immediate relevance to the clinical professions is to develop a theoretical framework that allows a clear empirical demarcation of the boundary between normal/healthy and excessive/ unhealthy repetitive behavior patterns. Although there is now no consensus on what form such a theory would take, most professionals would agree that excessive and unhealthy repetitive behavior patterns are characterized by (1) experiences of craving prior to engagement, (2) impaired control over engagement, and (3) repeated engagement despite negative consequences (Potenza 2006).

"Habit," "addiction," and "compulsion" are popular terms used by both lay persons and scientists to describe these phenomena. A crude gauge of the extent of their use is provided by the Internet, with Google searches for "habit," "addiction," and "compulsion" yielding 46, 48, and 6 million hits respectively. This indicates that repetitive behavior patterns are very interesting to a lot of people. This interest is certainly warranted, as the costs of unhealthy excessive behavior patterns are high by any reasonable standard. Alcohol abuse, drug abuse, and smoking annually cost the United States $176 billion, $114 billion, and $137 billion respectively (Rice 1999), in terms of lost productivity, health care costs, and damage from accidents. The indirect costs in terms of crime fueled by addiction—and in terms of emotional suffering, which is difficult to shadow price—must be many times larger.

Psychiatric syndrome definitions and classification systems provide a sort of official history of the development of terms used to describe repetitious behavior patterns. "Addiction" was professionally respectable in the mid-twentieth century, as it was included in the first edition of the *Diagnostic and Statistical Manual of Mental Disorders* (*DSM*), or *DSM-I* (American Psychiatric Association 1952), as a diagnostic label under the more general category of "sociopathic personality disturbances." The meaning of the term addiction was not defined, however, and the label applied only to "alcoholism" and "drug addiction" as subtypes. In 1957 the World Health Organization distinguished between drug "addiction" and "habituation" (World Health Organization 1957). An "addiction" was characterized by (1) an overpowering desire (compulsion) to continue taking the drug and to obtain it by any means, (2) a tendency to increase the dose, (3) a psychic and generally a physical dependence on the effects of the drug, and (4) a detrimental effect on the individual and on society. A "habituation," on the other hand, was characterized by (1) a desire (but not compulsion) to continue taking the drug, (2) little or no tendency to increase the dose, (3) some degree of psychic dependence on the effect of the drug, and (4) detrimental effects primarily on the individual.

Subsequent classification systems moved away from use of the term "addiction." A 1982 World Health Organization report recommended that the term "dependence" replace the term "addiction" (World Health Organization 1982). This recommendation was based on concern over the stigma arising from the negative social connotations of "addiction," and on the hope that the term "dependence" would allow for more objectivity and precision in definition (Henningfield, Cohen, and Pickworth 1993). In keeping with this sentiment, *DSM-II* (American Psychiatric Association 1968) no longer used "addiction" as the overarching label for consumption disorders, but instead included "alcoholism" and "drug dependence" as separate diagnoses under the category of "personality disorders" and "certain other non-psychotic mental disorders." "Alcohol addiction" was separate from "episodic excessive drinking" and "habitual excessive drinking," with presumptive evidence (i.e., withdrawal symptoms) of physical dependence necessary for the "alcohol addiction" diagnosis. Interestingly, the description of the "drug dependence" diagnosis distinguished between addiction and dependence, although the basis of the distinction was not explained. *DSM-II* contained no mention of gambling.

DSM-III (American Psychiatric Association 1980) included "substance use disorders" as its own overarching diagnostic category, and distinguished between "substance abuse" (pattern of pathological use, impairment in social or occupational functioning due to substance use, and minimal duration of one month) and "substance dependence" (presence of physiological dependence as manifested by tolerance and/or withdrawal), but did not use the term "addiction" to refer to either.

DSM-III featured "pathological gambling" (PG) for the first time, among "disorders of impulse control not elsewhere classified" along with "kleptomania," "pyromania," and "intermittent" and "isolated explosive disorders." PG was defined as: "Gambling that compromises, disrupts, or damages family, personal, and vocational pursuits, as indicated by at least three of the following: (1) arrest for forgery, fraud, embezzlement, or income tax evasion due to attempts to obtain money for gambling, (2) default on debts or other financial responsibilities, (3) disrupted family or spouse relationship due to gambling, (4) borrowing of money from illegal sources (loan sharks), (5) inability to account for loss of money or to produce evidence of winning money, if this is claimed, (6) loss of work due to absenteeism in order to pursue gambling activity, and (7) necessity for another person to provide money to relieve a desperate financial situation."

DSM-III-R (American Psychiatric Association 1987) provided a significant revision of the "substance use disorders" diagnostic criteria. Unlike *DSM-III*, evidence of tolerance or withdrawal was no longer required for a diagnosis of "psychoactive substance dependence." Any three of the following nine symptoms was sufficient for a "dependence" diagnosis: (1) substance taken in larger amounts or for longer period than intended, (2) persistent desire or one or more unsuccessful efforts to cut down or control substance use, (3) a great deal of time spent obtaining or consuming the substance or recovering from its effects, (4) frequent intoxication or withdrawal when expected to fulfill major role obligations, (5) important social, occupational, or recreational activities given up because of use, (6) continued use despite recurrent problems related to use, (7) tolerance, (8) withdrawal, and (9) use in order to avoid withdrawal.

In *DSM-IV* (American Psychiatric Association 2000), the current diagnostic system, the criteria for "substance-related disorders" remained essentially unchanged from *DSM-III-R*. Again, PG was included among "disorders of impulse control not elsewhere classified," along with "kleptomania," "pyromania," and "intermittent and isolated explosive disorders." The diagnostic criteria for PG (see chapter 2) were modified to focus less on financial/criminal aspects and more on psychological/behavioral aspects.

Two general points are relevant regarding these diagnostic systems. First, the evolution of *DSM* demonstrates how syndrome definitions, classification systems, and criteria are not pure scientific concepts, and do not develop on the basis of new scientific evidence alone. Rather, these systems and criteria are heavily influenced by wider cultural, political, and economic forces. Babor (1990, p. 33) notes that "The primary issue with regard to definitions of dependence [or addiction] thus becomes who or which group controls the defining process, and how they use definitions to promote their own ends, be they medical, legal, scientific, or moral."

Second, there is the question of whether one can explain a person's excessive engagement in an activity by appealing to their "addiction" or "dependence." Historically, the term "addiction" has been used to attempt to explain the excessive consumption of alcohol for well over 300 years (e.g., Warner 1994), of opiates and other now-illicit drugs for about 100 years (e.g., Levine 1978), of tobacco for several decades (e.g., Henningfield, Cohen, and Pickworth 1993), and, more recently, of gambling (Marks 1990). British clergy in the early seventeenth century initiated the use of the term "addiction" to describe substance use in reference to excessive alcohol consumption (Warner 1994). At that time, "addiction" meant an obligation or devotion to something. Thus, the term "addiction" became a metaphor describing a person's pathological preference for a given activity, which leads him or her to behave "as if addicted" (i.e., obligated) to the activity. There is a standing tendency for metaphors of this sort to be reified, internalized, and attributed causal significance (Sarbin 1968). This appears to have happened over the years with the term "addiction," which has gone from being a metaphorical description of devotion to a particular activity, to being an hypothesized internal state, the existence of which is revealed by that devotion, and, finally, to being the cause of that devotion.

Definitions and diagnostic criteria for addiction or dependence have generally been descriptive and not explanatory (Akers 1991); that is, they have denoted behavioral, cognitive, and emotional patterns and associated consequences that have proven useful in reliably placing individuals into categories based on similarities. The traditional diagnostic criteria and category labels do not explain why individuals engage in those patterns, however. It may be a useful description to say that an individual's excessive engagement meets the diagnostic criteria for addiction or dependence, or that some activity is addictive, but this does not mean that it is useful to say that an individual's excessive engagement occurs *because* of addiction or dependence. Akers (1991, p. 779) makes this point as follows:

The problem is that there is no independent way to confirm that the addict cannot help himself, and therefore the label is often used as a tautological explanation of the addiction. The habit is called an addiction because it is not under control, but there is no way to distinguish between a habit that is uncontrollable from one that is simply not controlled. However precisely it is defined, addiction is a label, a term applied to behavior. It cannot, itself, provide an explanation for that behavior. We label excessive involvement in drugs which a person cannot seem to give up as addictions, and we think we have explained the excessive, hard-to-stop behavior by saying that the person is suffering from an addiction. The label of addiction is attached to the behavior because the person is assumed to have lost control of the substance use; when asked why the person has lost control, the answer is that he is addicted. In other words, addiction causes addiction.

A key issue is whether activity engagement becomes controlled by something other than the individual's choice to continue that use. Advocates of explaining excessive engagement by appealing to the individual's "addiction" believe that in addicts use becomes something other than a choice. For example, the 1988 Surgeon General's report (US Department of Health and Human Services 1988, pp. 248–249) asserted that "the term 'drug dependence' or 'drug addiction' refers to self-administration of a psychoactive drug in a manner that demonstrates that the drug controls or strongly influences behavior. In other words, the individual is no longer entirely free to use or not use the substance." Alterations in some aspect of brain function as a result of substance use typically are thought to override the individual's choice. This argument is made forcefully by Henningfield, Schuh, and Jarvik (1995, p. 1715) in relation to tobacco use: "The pathophysiological consequences of tobacco smoke exposure include tissue destruction contributing to lung disease, cellular changes contributing to cancer, and the cellular and molecular reinforcing effects leading to dependence. Once the pathophysiological consequences of tobacco use have occurred, it may be no more a matter of personal choice to abstain from tobacco than to reverse metastasizing lung cells."

An alternative view was expressed by Heyman (1998, p. 807), who argued that "neuroadaptation could just as likely influence preference as preclude it. The difference is important. An addict who takes drugs voluntarily can be persuaded by contingencies or new information to stop using them. An addict who takes drugs involuntarily cannot be persuaded by costs and incentives to stop using them." Studies have shown systematic inverse relations between price and consumption of a variety of "addictive" substances, and between the availability of alternative activities and substance consumption (see Vuchinich and Heather 2003 for an overview). Such work by behavioral economists builds a picture of excessive engagement as the outcome of a reinforcement or utility maximization process. In this view, the activity is chosen to the extent that the reinforcement or utility gained from it exceeds the reinforcement or utility gained from engagement in other activities. Importantly, models of excessive consumption (i.e., "addiction") in this literature (e.g., Becker and Murphy 1988; Heyman 1996; Rachlin 1997) describe how substance use over time could change the utility or reinforcement gained from that use relative to the utility or reinforcement gained from other sources, rendering the former relatively more attractive. Thus, according to many behavioral economists, an individual's current choice to use a substance is influenced by their prior consumption, but both now and in the past the individual is choosing to consume the substance. The implications of this literature are that "(i) drug use in addicts can be altered by the proper arrangement of costs and benefits, (ii) addictive drugs reduce options but do not eliminate choice, and (iii) the biology of addiction is the biology of voluntary behavior" (Heyman 1998, p. 808). It is important to point out that in the behavioral economics (BE) literature, concepts of "voluntariness" and "choice" are not used so as to take a side in philosophers' debates over the existence of free will, or to morally convict excessive consumers of bad character. Rather, the intended emphasis is on the way in which the classical "addictions" are sensitive to positive and negative incentives in the same sense as non-excessive consumption; thus, they are cast as fit explananda for economics.

In the chapters to come, we will argue that current science appears to vindicate the insights of *both* behavioral economists and proponents of internal state (or, less accurately, "disease") models of addiction, dissolving the traditional tension between these views. We regard this as a surprising development. Unlike the dominant intellectual tradition in psychiatry, which prefers to trace the roots of all pathology to a mechanical or chemical condition in the brain, our thinking begins at the molar scale, in economics. From this perspective, prospects for reduction to strictly molecular scales look prima facie doubtful; however, the view to which we have been led by consideration of empirical evidence fits neither the neat model of addiction as an endogenous disease nor the clinically defeatist model of addiction as an irredeemably complex social syndrome enmeshed in so many layers of cultural and moral construction that it is better handed over from scientists to novelists and oral historians. We are convinced that addiction is complicated but comprehensible, subject to some robust generalizations, and potentially much more effectively treatable than is usually assumed in popular discussions.

Let us first say a bit more about the complications our perspective urges on psychiatry. Given the growing volume of basic and clinical research using neuroscientific tools to study psychiatric disorders, one might naively assume that psychiatry is in the process of transforming itself through full and fearless exposure to these new investigative technologies. In fact, strong methodological and conceptual conservatism largely continues to hold sway. For the most part, only conditions that psychiatrists have already modeled as "organic disorders" are investigated under the rubric of neuropsychiatry, so their defining properties are treated as fixed in advance of the new research. Organic disorders are individuated by their "psychiatric presentations" (Agrawal 2004)—that is, their manifestations in degenerative disorders like dementia, head injury, strokes, or epilepsy, in movement disorders like Parkinson's disease, intracranial tumors or infections, and in nutritional, toxic or endocrine disorders. It is only more recently that psychiatric disorders such as schizophrenia and autism have tentatively been added to the investigative domain of neuropsychiatry. In the 1960s autism was thought to be caused by a "refrigerator mother." Evidence in the last two decades now provides overwhelming support for the notion that autism is very much a brain disorder.

Historically, the division of psychiatric disorders into organic and non-organic types was based partly on the fear that reducing them to underlying brain pathologies would imply disregard for environmental influences. In most of the behavioral sciences, decades of heated "nature–nurture" controversy have given way to a general acknowledgment of bidirectional feedback relationships between biological and environmental influences as the norm in behavioral ontogenesis and regulation. For instance, thanks to the successful integration of neuroscience into parenting research, we now understand how sensitive caregiving affects the developing brain of an infant (Sharp and Fonagy forthcoming; Fonagy et al. 2002). As an example of causal influence in the other direction, it has recently been appreciated that reduced amygdala functioning in psychopaths affects their ability to recognize fear in others, leading to behavior that is inadequately governed by societal norms (Blair 2001, 2003; Blair et al. 2006).

In this general context of opening new windows between psychiatry and neuroscience, our perspective from an economics standpoint leads us to ask how neuroeconomics (NE) can best contribute. In chapter 5 we will make extended use of the new neuroeconomic model of valuation in the brain's so-called reward circuit. Valuation is the process by which reinforcement signals provide feedback to an organism regarding the predicted value of a stimulus. To cite an evocative example, the mysterious pleasure one feels when one "clicks" with another person (a "meeting of minds"), a key contributor to the sense of connectedness humans share, can be captured by a positive valuation assigned to the experience by the brain. As the neuroeconomist Read Montague puts it in his recent popular book (2006, p. 20), "valuations put meaning back into computations."

It is also the case, however, that many humans do not receive the same positive reinforcement signals from stimuli that typical people do. For instance, some individuals, notably psychopaths, rarely experience a sense of connectedness or a meeting of minds. Psychopathy is characterized by a combination of antisocial behavior, proneness to boredom, impulsivity, a callous interpersonal style, superficial charm, and a diminished capacity for remorse (Cleckley 1941; Hare 1991). Within a reinforcement learning framework, experimental paradigms derived from NE, such as economic exchange games, can be usefully applied to understand psychiatric disorders such as psychopathy. For example, Rilling et al. (2007) used an iterated version of the prisoner's dilemma to probe the neural correlates of interpersonal deficits associated with psychopathy. Results showed that subjects scoring higher on psychopathy, particularly males, defected more often and were less likely to continue cooperating after establishing mutual cooperation with a partner. Further, they experienced more outcomes in which their cooperation was not reciprocated. After such outcomes, subjects scoring high in psychopathy showed less amygdala activation, suggesting weaker aversive conditioning to those outcomes. Compared with low-psychopathy subjects, subjects higher in psychopathy also showed weaker activation within the orbitofrontal cortex when choosing to cooperate and showed weaker activation within the dorsolateral prefrontal and rostral anterior cingulate cortices when choosing to defect.

By applying NE and computational models of reinforcement learning to disorders such as psychopathy, in the same way that we will do in this book to PG, we may begin to describe how computational valuation may go awry in a variety of different psychiatric disorders. While a significant literature exists that applies computational neuroscience approaches to probe psychiatric disorders (see Williams and Dayan 2005; Williams and Taylor 2004; Dayan and Williams 2006), it is only recently that studies are conducted under the umbrella of an emerging new field called computational psychiatry (Dayan and Williams 2006; Montague 2006). This is founded on the fact that most psychiatric disorders involve neuromodulators and that an established literature exists on the normative function of these neuromodulators through work in computational neuroscience.

In retrospect, it is clear that one of the half-dozen most momentous scientific breakthroughs of the past century was McCulloch and Pitts's 1943 demonstration that neurons are computers, transformers of informational input into informational output, in a precise and generalizable mathematical sense. This insight was extensively developed by artificial intelligence researchers and philosophers of cognitive science during the succeeding decades, in consequence of which it gradually became clear that the mysterious relationship between mind and brain had at last been decisively illuminated by the concept of computation. That concept allows us to understand how the mind can be more than a metaphorical residue of nonphysical Cartesian spirit, while nevertheless not simply being equivalent to the anatomical matter of the brain. Like software that is "real enough" to make its designers wealthy, the mind exists "virtually," as patterns of information processing and computations that the brain specifically implements in the electrodynamics and molecular chemistry of its enormous neural network. Amit (1989) and Churchland and Sejnowski (1992) mark the earliest consolidation of the mature conceptual synthesis.

Cognitive information processing initially modeled in the abstract frameworks of artificial intelligence (e.g., universal Turing machines, von Neumann architectures, or generic parallel distributed processing nets) is now increasingly being grounded in biological information processing. The detailed interanimation of molecular biology and cognitive science is putting testable, exact structure on the idea, articulated decades ago by a few philosophers such as Daniel Dennett (1969), that the algorithms of mental function (in philosophical jargon, the inferential patterns constituting "intentionality") are based on brain structure, as interpreted in the context of social interaction. Montague (2006) now articulates the significance of these developments for neuropsychiatrists. "Structure and function," he tells them, "are really information processing being implemented by the physical and chemical properties made available by biological molecules, cells, networks of cells, and so forth" (Montague 2006, p. 15).

Despite our appreciation of the importance of neurocomputational modeling, our perspective remains fundamentally behaviorist.[1] Contrary to stereotype, behaviorists need not and should not deny that brains perform computational processes or generate representational content for other brain processes to use as inputs. Nor need they or should they deny that (many) animals have subjective experiences: some of the representations that brains produce are accessible to second-order awareness. Sensible behaviorism as we understand and endorse it consists in the following philosophical convictions (explained and defended at length in Ross 2005, chapter 1):

(1) Computational models (including neurocomputational models) of the brain are functionally parsed by reference to the contributions of specific modules and processes to behavior. Of course, neuroanatomy puts strong constraints on such parsing; if a computational model says that functional module a is realized in neural area x, that functional module b is realized in neural area y, and that a sends output to b, then either x and y had better turn out to be synaptically connected in the right direction, or x had better produce changes in neurotransmitter levels that demonstrably modulate the activity of y. But to say that, for example, cells in the superior colliculus process retinal information is to say that those cells make a contribution of a certain sort to the behavior of extracting and using information about the distribution of light in the ambient environment—that is, seeing.

(2) Behavioral patterns are not individuated by reference to computational processes or representations in the brain. They are individuated by reference to the roles they play in organisms' ecological interactions. In the case of the peculiar hyper-social mammal *H. sapiens*, the over-

whelmingly most salient such interactions are social, and are culturally mediated (see Sterelny 2003 for an account of cultural mediation); thus, what counts as behavioral pattern p in one ecological context might not count as another instance of p in a different ecological context. What we are affirming here is the view philosophers call "externalism about mental content," which is the dominant perspective among philosophers of mind at present. Philosophers defending this view whose names are most likely to be familiar to behavioral scientists include Ludwig Wittgenstein, W. V. Quine, Wilfrid Sellars, Gilbert Ryle, Daniel Dennett, and Andy Clark.

(3) Because functional brain processes and types of representations are (ultimately) individuated by reference to their roles in behavior, and because types of behavior are individuated ecologically, it would be very surprising if brain processes and types of representations individuated only by reference to neurophysiological properties lined up neatly with functional brain processes and types of representation. That outcome would imply extraordinary success by past behavioral sciences in inferring invisible brain structures entirely on the basis of observing complex behavioral patterns.

(4) Therefore, in general, neuroscientific explanations of psychological processes will take the following logical form. A neuroanatomical–neurophysiological–neurochemical–neurodynamic account will explain a neurocomputational account. The neuroanatomical (etc.) facts that do the explaining will use different—noncognitive—concepts from the neurocomputational account. The neurocomputational account will in turn combine behavioral and nonbehavioral concepts to partly (sometimes mainly) explain psychological phenomena described in behavioral terms. Full explanations of behavioral regularities will more often combine neurocomputational, developmental, social, and cultural facts.

Among the behavioral sciences, economics begins at further logical distance from the brain than any other. This is because, its practitioners' frequent commitment to *normative* individualism notwithstanding, economics since the mid-1930s has been mainly concerned with *aggregate* social phenomena—for example, constructing community indifference curves for representing aggregate demand. These curves cannot be decomposed into the behavior of individual members of the community in question, let alone into contributions of the brains of individuals. If the terms in which microeconomic phenomena were individuated mapped neatly onto the terms in which neurochemical processes are described, this would be doubly miraculous, since it would rely on an improbable mapping from the microeconomic to the psychological, and then on another improbable mapping from the psychological to the neurochemical.[2]

Despite this, we are not skeptics about the thriving science of BE and its exciting new collaborator NE (Glimcher 2003; Montague and Berns 2002). From the fact that microeconomic processes do not *reduce* to psychological ones, it does not follow that psychology isn't relevant to explaining some microeconomic regularities. Similarly, from the fact that behavioral processes don't reduce to neurocomputational ones, it doesn't follow that neuroscience isn't relevant to explaining behavior. (In the second case, if this *did* follow, it would constitute a reductio ad absurdum of the antireductionist claim. We expect neuroscience to swamp all other sources of behavioral explanation in importance; we just don't expect it to completely *replace* them.)

NE finds useful purchase because the brain, like an economy, is a parallel processor of information in which units compete and cooperate for scarce resources. Viewed "from the bottom up," the scarce resource for which neurons compete is blood hemoglobin. Functional magnetic resonance imaging (fMRI) monitors the tussle over this asset. Viewed "from the top down," the scarce resource for which neurons compete is influence over behavior. (This is the "neural Darwinian" perspective of Edelman 1987.) We do not expect BE (or, to anticipate ideas we will introduce in chapter 3, "picoeconomics") to reduce to NE (Ross 2005, forthcoming), but we expect a steady parade of fruitful insights as the top-down and bottom-up perspectives are adjusted to accommodate and shed light on one another—that is, as NE partly explains picoeconomic phenomena in neurochemical and neurodynamic terms, and picoeconomics (PE) partly explains neuroeconomic phenomena in functional–behavioral terms.

Now let us come back to addiction. As we reviewed above, the history of this concept is rooted in behavioral observation, and scientifically shallow observation at that; thus, it might have been expected that, at best, addiction would not project usefully into the brain or, at worst, addiction would not have even stood the test of rigor as an organizing concept for behavioral science (including BE). No philosophical presupposition is ever a guarantor of scientific experience, however. In any case, philosophical externalism does not deny that ecologically centered observation does not *sometimes* detect underlying internal mechanisms and then successfully track them across ecological contexts. (So, for example, we take it that popular observation picked up on strokes and successfully tracked them; on the other hand, it was not so successful at distinguishing the internal correlates of anxiety and depression.) We think that recent neuroscience strongly suggests that addiction is an internally governed kind of state that, in addicts, sufficiently dominates ecological variables as to be behaviorally stable and salient across ecological (including social) contexts. We argue that this is particularly evident when one understands addictive responses by reference to the neuroeconomic model of the dopaminergic reward system.

This general thesis emerges from our *assuming* a strong working hypothesis. This hypothesis is that if there is a core manifestation of addiction at the neural level of analysis, this should be gambling addiction. Behaviorally, as we will discuss in the next chapter, pathological gamblers resemble substance abusers very closely. We would expect (rightly, as it turns out) that *if* there is a common neural process underlying all behavioral addictions, this will be accompanied by different neurochemical aspects in the case of different drugs on which people get hooked. These differences are likely to constitute noise through which the hypothetical core neural process of addiction is obscured. By contrast, *if* there really is a distinctive neural phenomenon of addiction, and *if* some people who gamble more than they aim to are addicted to gambling, then gambling is an ideal candidate to serve as the basic model of addiction in general. If there are gambling addicts, and if it is a neurochemical process of a certain sort that makes these individuals so, then in gambling addiction the brain develops the pathology using only endogenous chemical resources. If one could identify these, the obvious next step would be to examine how exogenously introduced chemicals on which people become dependent bring about, by multiple pathways, the same endogenous disorder displayed in shining causal isolation in the case of gambling addicts.

We will argue in chapters 6 and 7 that our hypothesis above is well supported by the evidence; thus, where addictive gambling is concerned, our position will closely match the expectations of the reductive neuroeconomist. We doubt very much, however, that all people who have gambling problems according to *DSM* criteria are gambling addicts. The problem of the non-addicts, insofar as they *share* a common problem, is ecological rather than neurological. We do not thereby

mean to suggest that non-addicted problem gambling behavior is causally independent of all brain processes; no behavior is, of course. Our
point is that non-addicted problem gamblers may not—probably do
not—share any *common* neurochemical syndrome that explains what
they have in common behaviorally. For understanding and treatment
of the behavior of people falling into this category we will recommend
appeal to a picoeconomic model.

This book thus constitutes, as indicated in the "Note to Readers
about *Economic Theory and Cognitive Science*," an application to a particular phenomenon of Ross's hybrid picoeconomic–neuroeconomic
framework for relating economic theory to the cognitive and behavioral sciences. At the same time we intend the work to stand on its own
as an account of addiction and of the varieties of gambling disorders,
demanding neither understanding of nor agreement with Ross's general
explanatory program. (Thus, for example, a reader might decide that
the program works well enough in application to disordered gambling,
but fails with respect to other phenomena.)

The book is organized as follows. Chapter 2 provides a general
introduction to the scientific study of disordered gambling (DG). This
study has naturally been motivated chiefly by clinical and policy concerns, which crucially interact with basic scientific issues throughout
the book. In this respect, DG, and impulsive consumption in general,
resemble all problems in applied economics. Like most scientific disciplines, economics is partly driven by philosophical curiosity and partly
by our needs for successful engineering.

We think it useful to remind ourselves, and readers, of this practical
side of the issue before chapter 3 wades into foundational problems
around the *kind* of theory that best captures both scientific and
clinical objectives. The chapter first presents our view of the relationship between standard ("neoclassical") microeconomic theory and
BE. In particular, it explains why we view the latter as complementary to the former rather than as a challenge to it (as much
recently fashionable literature urges). We then explain the foundations
of, and principal models and variations in, the subdivision of BE
that we apply to DG. George Ainslie has dubbed this subfamily
"picoeconomics," and this is usage we embrace in the subtitle of the
book. The picoeconomic perspective explains impulsive consumption in such a way as to shift the principal puzzle before us from the
question "Why do some people suffer from chronic consumption
impulsivity?" to the question "How do most people avoid such behav-

ior?" We explain the principal mechanism to which PE appeals in addressing this second question: establishment of "personal rules" as equilibria in negotiations among virtual subpersonal interests with divergent preferences over reward scheduling and reward types. Chapter 3 concludes with a review of leading criticisms of the picoeconomic model that have recently been articulated by other scientists. We provide partial responses to some of these, completion of which is deferred until the end of the book following mustering of relevant empirical evidence.

Chapter 4 begins that review. It surveys experimental investigations, first into consumption impulsivity in general and then into DG in particular, that test the predictions of the picoeconomic model. As we will see, the model has proven to be a fruitful organizing framework for designing empirical research and consolidating its results; this cannot be regarded as having proven conclusive, however, and we believe there is a principled reason for this. Most disordered gamblers do not *merely* have difficulty establishing and maintaining personal rules, though such difficulties are indeed a necessary condition for their problem. Subjects recruited for comparative studies of disordered gamblers and controls are selected using instruments, discussed in chapter 2, that attempt to diagnose people who are thought to suffer from a psychiatric pathology of the old-fashioned sort as characterized earlier in this chapter. Evidence strongly indicates that PE, as a molar-scale account of behavioral patterns, is a partial and essential, but incomplete, account of what goes wrong for severely disordered gamblers—so-called "pathological gamblers." To describe the situation in terms of the concepts discussed above, pathological gamblers indeed suffer from what traditionally minded psychiatrists might have called an "organic disorder." This neuropsychiatric condition, we maintain, has empirically turned out to meet the core criteria for true addiction, and conceptual confusion is best minimized if we regard addiction as reduced to it.

Though addiction may be "organic" in the sense of being identifiable by neuroscientific (in this case, neurochemical) properties, it is a neurocomputational model that allows us to identify it and systematically connect these properties to the behavioral patterns classically regarded as addictive. More specifically, the model is neuroeconomic. This newest subdiscipline of neuroscience, which appeals to economic theory and modeling techniques to understand the relationship between valuation and behavioral control at the scale of brain processes, is given a general introduction in chapter 5. That chapter then presents the structure of and empirical evidence for the emerging neuro-economic model of addiction as a distinctive pathology afflicting a functionally and chemically specifiable part of the brain known as the dopamine reward system. In consequence (probably) of interacting contributions from genetically inherited vulnerability and developmental contingencies, this system can usurp control of the motivational, attentional, and even cognitive and conscious aspects of the whole person. In effect, this midbrain circuit commits mutiny against the normal personal control apparatus. For reasons explained by the neuroeconomic model, the dopamine mutineer, considered as an economic agent, then maximizes its utility by relent-lessly pursuing goods with certain properties that the targets of addic-tion all share.

It is often supposed that these properties must be, or must reside in, exogenous chemicals that addicts introduce into their bodies by ingest-ing substances. The best evidence that this is not the case comes from empirical application of the neuroeconomic model of addiction to PG. In chapter 6 we review this empirical work, pausing at various stages to consolidate its theoretical significance. PG, we conclude, is not only genuine addiction in the neuropsychiatric sense that previous parts of the book have identified; it is *the* variety of addiction which, by involv-ing minimal incidental effects on other brain processes of the sort brought about by exogenous chemicals, provides the cleanest window on addiction as an endogenous neuroeconomic–neurochemical phe-nomenon. Simply put, pathological gambling is the basic form of addic-tion, the form on which drug addictions are then special complications for purposes of general understanding.

Only part of the evidence for this involves what philosophers of science think of as "theory (or model) testing." We would not be nearly so confident in our conclusion were it not for the fact that, over the past three years, natural neuropharmacological experiments with psychiat-ric patients—that is, medical accidents—have exposed control levers on PG that can be manipulated by drugs. The drugs in question operate on exactly the part of the brain the neuroeconomic model would predict, and in the way it would predict. Science is ultimately about such delib-erate manipulation of real phenomena, its concepts, arguments, deduc-tions, generalizations, models, and theories all being devices to that end, and evaluated (by scientists, if often not by philosophers) in that light.

Because of the importance we attach to this kind of evidence, we devote chapter 7 to it. This is also where we again remind readers that the scientific problems involved cannot be detached from the underly ing clinical issues. Chapter 7 therefore considers nonpharmacological treatments of DG in addition to drug therapies. In the course of this, we begin to build our case for merely *local* reduction of *pathological* gambling to addictive gambling, in a wider nonreductive framework that continues to model *disordered* gambling in general as a behavioral (molar-scale) syndrome. This outcome, which philosophers who like their reductionism all-or-nothing might find inelegant, is, we suggest, typical of scientific progress in the conceptually messy world that is governed by chance and contingency, not logical order.

The concluding chapter 8 is devoted to several jobs of consolidation. First it takes seriously the clinical imperative, asking whether our proposed local reduction of PG to addiction threatens to inflate the concept of addiction in such a way as to encourage confused medical policies. As we point out, this is a worry to which we must be particularly alert if, as we argue, addiction will soon be most appropriately treated with powerful, and hence potentially dangerous, neurochemical agents. The most serious ground for such concern, we show, is the recent appearance of an industry built around "diagnosing" and "treating" a nonscientific idea of addiction to sex. Since this industry is mainly a part of an ideological campaign rather than a genuine medical one, its expropriation of a concept that is, according to us, neuroscientific in its basis should be resisted on both scientific and welfare grounds. We then argue that local reduction of addiction by the neuroeconomic model is likely to make such resistance more rather than less effective.

This returns us to more narrowly scientific challenges to our combination of local reductionism and global antireductionism regarding addiction. We conclude the chapter, and the book as a whole, by returning to these themes, which had been left partially argued at the end of chapter 3. Neuroeconomics and its investigative tools are so novel and liberating, the new paths to knowledge that they open so exciting, that it is only natural for scientists to want to push their application as far as it can possibly go. This should be encouraged, we believe; however, we reiterate and expand on our reasons for belief that PE, and therefore BE and standard microeconomics more generally, will continue to play essential roles in both generalizing our understanding and guiding clinical practice. Our overall model of DG, finally consolidated and summarized in chapter 8, is a hybrid picoeconomic–neuroeconomic model of the kind characterized by Ross (2005, 2007, forthcoming). Of course, we are in a position here to promote this hybrid only with respect to our particular subject of study—DG—but since we argue that DG is the basic form of addiction, and that addiction in turn is the form of reward system breakdown that best reveals the nature of the neuro-economic mechanism, we take our conclusion to have quite general significance.

2 Gambling in Scientific Focus

2.1 Knowledge for Policy

As reviewed by Gray (2004), in all historical and extant cultures except those that specifically enforce effective sanctions against gambling, the majority of human beings are disposed to regularly stake wagers against each other on the outcomes of natural and contrived processes. No one seriously doubts that one motivation of most people, most of the time they behave in this way, is enjoyment of the periods of uncertainty that fall between placing bets and seeing how they come out. On the occasions when people *win* bets they typically get a further shot of satisfaction over and above the enjoyment of suspense, since almost everyone enjoys becoming a bit richer. It is particularly pleasing when this results from something the person herself chose to do, as she can thus take credit for the outcome and congratulate herself. Much experimental evidence shows that nondepressed people systematically tend to inflate their own causal contribution to good outcomes and minimize it for bad ones. Perhaps this has a functional explanation, encouraging people to experiment with novel behavior and unpredictable consequences. The human conquest of the planet stemmed from our prodigious adaptability, both behavioral and cognitive. As every scientist knows, however, passive learning is extremely slow and unproductive; the world rarely yields up its surprising regularities unless carefully poked. Arranging novel manipulations of the environment to find out what will happen is as natural and central to humans as investigating scents is to dogs, and we are therefore hardwired in such a way as to be naturally rewarded for doing it. Gambling sets up opportunities for uncertainty resolution in which the natural, endogenous reward is supplemented by the prospect of an exogenous (monetary and/or social) one.

Saying that people gamble because they enjoy suspense is a truism, familiar to all gamblers. As with many obvious generalizations, stating it is a prompt for, rather than the foreclosure on, a series of further questions about underlying complexities. To judge from what they say, people gamble not only for excitement but also, at least often, in hopes of windfalls. Are some gamblers mainly motivated by this? Is there a correlation between attraction to gambling and some particular range in the relative motivational proportions of excitement and hopes of winning? Are there other rewards that significant numbers of people pursue by gambling, such as feelings of control or escape from unpleasant realities? One should not try to answer these questions by reflecting on one's own case or that of one's acquaintances, since these samples aren't likely to be representative. Furthermore, as psychologists have recognized for many years, people's reflective judgments about their own behavior more closely resemble story creation, for the sake of orienting their present and immediate future circumstances into a meaningful narrative arc, than objective reporting. Thus, subjective self-descriptions are inherently unreliable. A deeper understanding of gambling, including problematic gambling, requires that we make systematic efforts to collect and test samples of gambling behavior that are representative and objective—that is to say, we need to be scientific about it.

There are at least two main motivations for the scientific study of gambling. One is the fundamental engine of science: basic curiosity. Whenever we find a behavior common across most human cultures, we can be sure its deeper investigation will yield insights into our general ethological profile and its evolutionary origins—that is, into what sorts of creatures, at a relatively fundamental level, we are. After all, it wouldn't be obvious a priori that nature would have designed people to like to deliberately put their assets at risk, yet the majority of them clearly do. To the extent that we make progress in explaining why this is so, to a level of detail going beyond "because they enjoy suspense," we automatically make progress on answering further interesting questions, because the explanation of why people enjoy gambling is bound to imply explanations of other things they like and dislike doing.

The other main motivation for scientifically studying gambling is the hope of furnishing a basis for accurate guidance and self-regulation of behavior. There are benefits in improving our ability to forecast when people will gamble, and how much they'll gamble. These benefits are obvious for someone who's in, or considering entering, the business of supplying people with gambling opportunities by bringing prospective gamblers together with things to gamble on. In addition, people who enjoy gambling themselves have an interest in predicting the behavior of fellow gamblers. Next, governments have a direct interest, both as regards tax extraction and influence over social change and stability, in knowing who is likely to gamble, and how often and with what stakes, under different institutional structures. Finally, it is a common factor of both folk wisdom and scientific psychology that people usually need some knowledge of human behavior in general in order to best predict what they themselves will do in different kinds of circumstances. A very inefficient way of finding out what sort of things you'll do under different conditions is to actually put yourself under all conditions and find out directly; a more sensible approach, at least at a broad level, is to suppose that you're typical of some reference class (i.e., women in general, or South Africans in general, or South African women, or South African women in their forties, etc.) except where you have specific evidence to the contrary, and then find out by means of surveys what typical people in that reference class do.

Almost all human cultures not only include gambling as a recognized activity, but have in addition converged on institutionally established games with conventional rules for placing bets that require gathering and maintenance of some specific infrastructure (decks of cards, dice, fighting cocks, cowrie shells, specially shaped pieces of bark, etc.). This is important because, as noted above, *most* human activity involves gambling in a broad sense; over and above this, people establish institutions for what might be called "gambling per se" or "gambling for the sake of gambling." Provision of these institutional spaces can be a highly lucrative business where it is allowed (and, partly for that very reason, is often not allowed).

Gambling industries exist partly as solutions to coordination problems, providing geographical focal points where people who want to bet on things can find opportunities to bet and other people to bet against. Casual observation suggests that people value having preestablished, structured common focal points for gambling as social activity, with casinos catering to a distribution of preferences over how intensely social the activity should be; slot machines are on the low-intensity end of the distribution, whereas multi-person poker is on the high-intensity side. Casinos and other gambling brokers additionally supply the scenarios on which people gamble. What should these games be? At first glance this question might appear to be idle. After all, we know what sorts of games casinos and other commercial gaming businesses actually provide in modern industrial societies, and, in light of the profits available, we can assume that the industry has thoroughly done its research on the preferences of its current and prospective customers. Thus we might infer that people have natural preferences for slot machines, card and table games, and animal races. Are these preferences so strong as to explain why bookies and casinos are very handsomely compensated to facilitate betting? Almost every normal environment has naturally occurring elements of uncertainty we could exploit instead: people can (and sometimes do) bet on the weather, or on the color of the next car that will pass, or on whether a squirrel will run up a tree or down it, and no house need be paid to broker such wagers. People's willingness to pay for gambling industries indicates that they *do* like gambling on some kinds of uncertainties more than others, since casinos don't concentrate on finding games that cost as little as possible to set up, as they would if people were naturally indifferent and could be trained to prefer whatever was provided. As we've seen, the bald question "Why do people gamble?" admits of a truistic answer: for excitement. The absence of enlightenment from this answer indicates that a more interesting version of the question, one probing at what concerns psychologists, regulators, industry participants, and punters alike, is really: "Why are people especially attracted to certain distinctive sorts of gambling scenarios rather than others?" As we will see, this is also the crucial first question along the road to understanding why specific forms of gambling become, for some people, problems with the characteristics of addictions.

Internationally, the trend in public policy on commercial gambling over the past few decades has been in the direction of liberalization. As recently as the 1950s, legal gambling was limited to a few restricted jurisdictions (Las Vegas, Monaco, the Caribbean islands) where casinos were permitted, and to idiosyncratically tolerated special activities protected by local cultural traditions (e.g., dog racing in some southern states in America, or horse racing elsewhere, including the United Kingdom and Canada). Few jurisdictions had national lotteries, though several had smaller-scale lotteries and organized bingos for charitable fund-raising. Today, although some parts of the world—especially those with Muslim majorities—remain firmly closed to legal commercial gambling, the prevailing pattern is one of massively greater access. Many countries, provinces and municipalities get important revenue from supplying or licensing and taxing gambling opportunities such as lotteries and casinos. This in turn invites attention from economists, who try to predict the different levels of public revenue that should be expected from varying possible institutional arrangements.

Seeking public revenue from gambling proceeds implies some underlying normative assumptions behind policy. If legal gambling results in *extra* state revenue, this must be for one or both of two reasons: (1) legal gambling stimulates taxable economic activity in general, tending to raise formal-sector GDP; and/or (2) it is thought appropriate to tax gamblers in such a way that they will contribute more to public coffers than they would do from acceptable taxation on the activities they would substitute for gambling if access to the latter were more restricted. Specific liberalizing changes are typically promoted in political processes with greater emphasis on motivation (1) than on motivation (2). Evidence that expansion of gambling opportunities has a *generally* positive effect on GDP is far from compelling, however. As Collins (2003, p. 121) summarizes the research literature on this question,

From the point of view of promoting the economic interests of the general public, there are only two situations in which the legalization of gambling unambiguously provides such benefits. These are when an illegal industry is replaced by a legal one, and when legalization enables a jurisdiction to attract substantial gambling revenues from outside or retain substantial gambling revenues that would otherwise go "abroad."

When legal gambling was rare, areas could indeed recruit considerable tourist attention by joining the small club of gambling destinations; no one has any doubt what turned Las Vegas, for example, from a desert backwater into a major American city with soaring per capita income. However, diverting tax revenues from other jurisdictions is a zero-sum game unless the overall volume of taxable gambling is increased by legalization. This therefore brings us squarely to motivation (2). That in turn raises, for any specific liberalization policy, the question of who, demographically, are the people that the policy will lead to being taxed more highly. Are they richer than average, randomly distributed in wealth, or poorer than average? Are they older than average or younger than average? Are they more likely to be men or women? Better educated or less educated? In ethnically and culturally diverse societies, are they likely to be disproportionately drawn from one cultural community in comparison to another?

These questions are important partly for the same general reason that motivates any question about who is supplying what share of national income. The founder of modern welfare economics, A. C. Pigou, made a standing contribution to the taxation debate as it occurs in every modern democracy when he advocated using tax policy to modify people's behavior in socially desirable directions. It is now almost universally accepted that, for example, smokers, major environmental polluters, and people who park cars in crowded cities should be subject to special levels of taxation that claw back some of the negative externalities their dispositions impose on others. However, to the extent that Pigovian taxes on these activities are intended to disincentivize people from engaging in them, the tax, if carefully calibrated, should be revenue-neutral. If gambling legalization is defended on the grounds that it is revenue-positive, this must be either because people would otherwise gamble to the same extent but illegally—a proposition never supported by survey research in any jurisdiction—or because it is thought normatively appropriate that people who gamble pay higher taxes, to the extent that they gamble, than nongamblers, all else being equal. Perhaps underlying this belief is a vague assumption to the effect that gamblers, having shown themselves more willing, all things considered, to part with some of their disposable income than nongamblers, thereby signal that an efficient tax regime will take proportionately greater contributions toward public-good provision from their pockets.[1] Supposing this to be the real crux of the actual policy issue is surely too rationalistic, however. There is no doubt that many people are willing to impose extra taxation levels on gamblers in part to punish them for what is thought to be morally dubious, or at least morally second-rate, behavior.

Many people, for varying reasons, think that gambling is wrong. Others think that light gambling is morally harmless, but that heavy gambling—that is, gambling beyond some level of frequency or with stakes that exceed some approximate proportion of a person's resources—is morally improper. Still others think that gamblers themselves commit no moral offense, but that the state violates morality if it takes advantage of people's enjoyment of gambling to get extra taxes from them. This belief might in turn have one or both of two different bases: one might think that the state shouldn't exploit gamblers because gamblers are too likely to be economically vulnerable in other respects, or one might think that exploiting gamblers involves profiting from people's irrationality, and that this represents a form of preying on weakness, thereby resembling laying an extra tax burden on the physically or (in this case) mentally disabled.

Questions about whether certain kinds and patterns of gambling behavior, or certain public policies around gambling, are *in fact* morally bad, are philosophical questions. Questions about why people have the moral opinions they do, and about why and under what circumstances people do things they themselves think are immoral—thus opening themselves to immoral exploitation by their own standards—are anthropological and sociological questions. In this book, written from the perspective of scientists, we will set both of these kinds of questions aside, though we don't deny their importance. Readers who want to follow up on them in a careful way are referred to a recent discussion by Peter Collins (2003). At the same time, we do want to connect our discussion to policy debates—and many readers, especially philosophers, might then complain that policy issues must necessarily be distorted if their moral dimension is ignored. We agree that we cannot just ignore the normative dimension, even if we want to avoid explicit argumentation about it. We will therefore take one of Collins's main conclusions on moral attitudes to gambling as our undefended starting point, picking up, as it were, where he leaves off. This conclusion is based on first noting that, regardless of what one thinks is the right answer to the philosophical question, there is a clear majority opinion on the closely associated political/policy question that prevails at the moment in most democratic jurisdictions. This (several-part) opinion[2] is that

1. gambling at moderate frequency for moderate stakes (as referenced to people's own income levels) is something that people should be allowed to do if they wish;

2. the state should tax this activity at a rate comparable to the rate at which it taxes other forms of adult-focused entertainment that don't enhance health; but

3. the state should regulate and keep within normative bounds the visibility and extent of gambling, should not allow exploitation by either itself or by private parties of people who can't control their gambling, and should carefully monitor, with a view to managing, the extent to which gambling disproportionately draws resources from economically vulnerable people, especially children whose caregivers gamble.

Again, let us be clear that we neither endorse nor criticize this consensus that Collins identifies. Some (especially religious) people are inclined to doubt its moral soundness and therefore work to change it. One of the foremost scientific authorities on gambling behavior, Howard Rachlin (2000), has argued that, in light of the psychological factors that cause people to gamble, the current consensus doesn't lead to *stable* policy. That is, Rachlin thinks that commitment to norms (1) and (2) above almost inevitably leads governments to have problems maintaining coherent policies in line with norm (3), for two reasons. First, policies in keeping with norms (1) and (2) *cause* more people, according to Rachlin, to lose control of their gambling behavior, than policies that greatly restrict or ban commercial gambling. Let us call this the "pessimistic behavioral hypothesis." Second, Rachlin thinks that governments that depend on gambling for important revenues will be unable to avoid the temptation to exploit people who have trouble controlling their gambling because there is so *much* revenue to be had from doing so, and these people don't have a strong lobby working on their behalf. Let us call this the "pessimistic political hypothesis."

The scientific work we discuss in this book will not bear on the pessimistic political hypothesis; that is a subject for political economy. However, our discussion certainly will bear on the pessimistic behavioral hypothesis. We cannot claim to know whether liberal gambling policies contribute to the extent or severity of gambling problems except insofar as we have some idea why most people gamble, why some people gamble more than others, and why some people try to reduce or cease their gambling and find that they cannot (or, at least, that they cannot without special help).

It is the call for explanation of this last fact that confronts us with the supposed *irrationality* of some gambling behavior. We need to consider this idea carefully here, for two reasons. First, as we will see, the view that some or all gambling is irrational is crucial to the public policy issues around the legal status of gambling, the state's role in sponsoring it and profiting from its revenues, and the social obligations of the gambling industry. Second, it is because of the apparent irrationality of some gambling behavior, in a particular sense that we will define shortly, that economists can't study it using only the traditional analytical tools they bring to bear on other consumption behavior, but must resort to the microexplanatory synthesis described in chapter 1.

Let us begin with the role of irrationality in the public policy issues around gambling. Remember that we have put aside the philosophical question of whether gambling is *in fact* morally permissible, in favor of asking what kind of policy is best *given* a decision to abide by the approximate liberal-democratic consensus on this question identified by Collins. The third part of that consensus says that the state should act to soften the harm done by gambling to society in general, trading this off against our aim to specially tax more rational gamblers. This speaks to only a limited, negative degree of concern for problem gambling—don't encourage it for the sake of public revenues—because, as stated, it says nothing about whether or to what extent the public authority, if it tolerates and profits from gambling, should be obligated to help people who think that their gambling is a problem to themselves.

Modern democracies are, in general, deeply ambivalent and unsure about this sort of issue. On the one hand, most people shy away from too much paternalism—the view that some preferences people have are crazy in themselves and should be interfered with over and above the implications they have for the welfare of other people. For instance, most of us might think that handling cobras is mad, yet a few people enjoy doing it. The law of the home country of three of the present authors, South Africa, where there are wild cobras around, says not to transport cobras into circumstances where people don't expect them and where, if they escape from control, they are thus a menace to others. However, a few years ago a South African man made headlines by setting records for time spent living in rooms full of cobras and mambas, until his unsurprising demise at the fangs of one of his reptiles. The law did not try to interfere with him; and most South Africans probably think it was right not to have. If we say that this person was irrational, what we mean is that he wanted things out of life that we find strange, but which were dangerous only to himself. Many liberals think that intervention against that kind of irrationality is not the business of the state.

But now imagine that the snake enthusiast had told friends and the news media that, fearing for his life, he was desperate to stop consorting with cobras, but found himself unable to follow through on his resolutions to do so. No matter how sincerely and fervently he swore off snakes, he reported, when the moment to leave them safely on the other side of some glass screen arose, he could not resist the impulse to place himself on the dangerous side of the partition. Many or most people of liberal-democratic views might in these circumstances think they had an obligation, or at least a legitimate reason, to help the unfortunate "cobraholic" achieve *his own* stated goal in life by making it more difficult for him to come within range of his siren's call.

The different judgments in these two cases—the real one and the hypothetical one—stem from recognition of the fact that our cobraholic is irrational in a more profound way than was the late real-life individual. The latter, as we saw, just had peculiar preferences. In the case of the imaginary cobraholic, it is hard to say that he even *has* clear preferences. If he merely *said* he wanted nothing more to do with snakes, but never took any actions consistent with this declaration, we might think he was just being disingenuous to keep his audience on edge. But suppose he took time and trouble and spent money to keep snakes out of his life, and then spent yet more time and trouble and money getting around these very barriers he'd set up for himself. We might then judge either that "he doesn't know what he wants" or that "he really wants to stay away from snakes but can't pull this off on his own." In either case, we might think we could, and/or should, help him to achieve the less eccentric of his two conflicting goals.

The case of the imaginary cobraholic is fanciful; the real snake man did his thing while observers shook their heads in bemusement, before meeting his predictable end. But it is easy for anyone to understand the made-up case because it has close parallels in the situations of the many people who take actions to try to stop drinking, taking drugs, or gambling, but fail in their attempts.

Economists use the ideas of rationality and irrationality in a narrower sense than most people. To economists, only the more profound kind of irrationality exhibited by the cobraholic really *counts* as true irrationality. This isn't because economists don't recognize strange preferences, like the real snake man's, as being strange. Instead, it is because they begin by taking note of the distinction made just above— between cases of strange but clear preferences and cases where people don't seem to even *have* straightforward or consistent preferences—and then, for the sake of avoiding confusion in their professional discourse, agree to *call* only the second kind of phenomenon "irrationality." This reflects more than just an arbitrary taste in the use of words. It stems from deep facts about the relationship between the subject matters of economics and psychology as neighboring sciences of behavior. Economics is concerned with the consequences on behavior, both individual and aggregate, of changes in incentives (costs and benefits). To address this, it must assign potential costs and benefits to stable units of accounts—that is, to points at which the costs and benefits are compared. As a first approximation, we can think of people as such units. However, psychology, taking biological organisms as *its* basic units, tell us that people don't evaluate costs and benefits from consistent baselines, because they change their tastes over time and with the adoption of new evaluative *frames*. Some economists have tried to resist this (rather obvious) psychological observation, but for reasons discussed in Ross 2005 (pp. 148–166), we don't think such resistance is an ultimately promising way of defending the value of distinctive economic generalizations. Instead, what economists should recognize is that their direct objects of study aren't whole people but abstract entities that strive for efficiency against stable sets of preferences in certain situations or for certain periods of time. People sometimes approximate such entities, especially when social pressures strongly encourage them to do so; thus, economists can explain behavior in financial markets with only limited recourse to psychology. But even where people most manifestly *fail* to demonstrate stable valuations in the ways in which they invest their resources, economics can play a contributing role in helping to understand their behavior by modeling it as if it were the consequence of conflicts and bargains among simpler subpersonal agents with different goals of their own. This is similar to the way in which social scientists study the policy lurches of countries as consequences of coalitional competition involving broadly rational individual citizens. From the economist's point of view, an "irrational" person is "irrational" in the same sense as a national legislature that votes for expensive new social programs one year and then struggles the next year to shake off the obligations incurred by those programs so as to balance the budget. In both cases, recognizing "irrationality," in the sense of inconsistency, does not require throwing economics aside in favor of psychology. Economists must pay attention to psychologists' data showing that people *are* "irrational" in that sense; but then they can contribute to explaining such irrationality by showing the ways in which it too is a response to incentives by fleeting or standing interests within people that prevent them from maintaining steady control over the direction of behavior as a whole.

Let us illustrate this by drawing attention to another aspect of the imaginary case of the cobraholic that the reader will likely have noted. Irrationality as economists understand it corresponds to a core *part* of what we mean in everyday contexts by the concept of "addiction." The historical origins of this concept are closely related to the concept of "enslavement," which at one time was called by the same word. Gradually, "addiction" came to mean "enslavement to an object or to a kind of behavior" (to what some psychologists generalize as "a reinforcer"), as opposed to enslavement to a person. Modern democracies have outlawed literal enslavement to persons.[3] But there is plenty of "addiction" around, and modern societies are less sure about how they should handle it. There may be no actual cobraholics (or maybe the real snake man actually *was* a cobraholic—we'll come back to this question later, in chapter 8). But there are certainly people who try to drink less or nothing but end up drinking a lot and severely harming themselves. There are also significant numbers of people who try to gamble less, or with smaller stakes, or not at all, but end up gambling themselves to ruin. These people invest resources in both gambling *and* in efforts not to gamble or to gamble less, and that is exactly and precisely equivalent to irrationality as economists understand it. We think it is obvious that, according to large majorities in contemporary democracies, such people (and, at least as importantly, their families) are appropriate, indeed obligatory, potential beneficiaries of public health interventions. We will show over the course of this book how economic theory, conjoined *in the right way* with applications of cognitive and behavioral science, can directly contribute to figuring out *how* to help those whose inconsistencies imperil their social networks, sanity, and lives.

2.2   Classifying the Phenomena

We will come back, at various points over the next three chapters, to the question of how helpful (or unhelpful) it is to lump people who are irrational (in the economist's sense) about gambling in with people who are irrational about alcohol and drugs. For the moment, we put this aside in order to stipulate a more precise way to talk specifically about different sorts of gambling behavior. We'll need a finer set of distinctions than just the bare one between people who have an unusually strong but not irrational (in the economist's sense) taste for gambling and people who would like to change their gambling behavior but have trouble doing so. Psychiatrists have developed some conventions for separating kinds of cases here, and we need to follow these conventions, both to avoid confusions and so that we can measure the extent of different social phenomena with consistency from one survey or experiment to the next.

One of the most crucial steps in setting up a problem for scientific study is the definition of fundamental concepts. Carelessness here can, all by itself, predetermine or overwhelmingly influence the later interpretation of results and so make whole investigations useless. At the same time, we do not want to follow a vice that often carries philosophers away, that of becoming slaves to our initial conceptual distinctions; ultimately we want empirical inquiry to guide our ways of distinguishing phenomena. The correct approach is to begin with clear, pragmatically justified, stipulations on what we will mean by what, and then, if scientific discovery motivates reform of these stipulations, to be fully explicit about this when we make the change.

Let us now begin to apply this policy to the case of different grades of problematic patterns of gambling behavior. Suppose on the one hand that one adopted a very liberal definition, according to which anyone who had ever regretted any particular participation in a game or any particular bet was said to have a "problem" caused by gambling. In that case, everyone who has ever gambled more than two or three times would be declared to have a gambling problem, since almost everyone who has bet that often has lost at least once, and everyone who has lost a bet regrets *that* bet in at least the mild sense that if they were given the option of taking the bet again, knowing the outcome, they'd decline it. In that case "problem gambling" would be made almost synonymous with "gambling," and whatever facts we later said we'd found about problem gambling would really just be facts about gambling in general. On the other hand, suppose we adopted a very stringent definition. For example, we might say that someone only has a clear, serious gambling problem if it leads them to bankruptcy. We know that if we use that definition, we're very likely to "discover" that only a tiny proportion of gamblers have problems, so the costs of problem gambling aren't likely to come out as large in comparison to the benefits derived from less regulated gambling. In the cases of both the overly liberal and the overly stringent definitions, we make it more difficult for subsequent empirical study to come to grips with measurements that bear on interesting questions, from either the purely scientific or purely clinical point of view.

This potential problem caused by careless definition is obvious enough, but the solution to it is far from simple. What definition of problem gambling *is* the right one? Scientists don't and won't find it written on a rock somewhere. It looks, therefore, as if *any* definition we try will be arbitrary, a pure *decision* made prior to doing any investigative work but which then, at least to some extent, shapes and restricts those very findings.

Scientists such as psychologists and psychiatrists, whose disciplines (unlike, for example, physics and economics) lack an underlying, fully specified mathematical theory, partly overcome this problem by distinguishing between theoretical definitions—or, speaking more properly, *analyses*—and *operationalizations*. When you operationalize an idea, you don't think of yourself as trying to state the truth about its deep nature. Rather, you just take yourself to be stipulating what you'll mean by it for the duration of some enterprise in which you'll use it. Analysis is then something to be done after the data, for the gathering of which the operationalization was among the tools, have come in. The only test of a good operationalization is usefulness: does it divide the phenomena being studied into two or more piles that are *both* interesting? Notice that if we used either the overly liberal or overly stringent definitions of problem gambling as operationalizations, they'd fail this test: the overly liberal operationalization would put almost all gambling in one pile and leave in the other pile only gambling by people who have hardly ever gambled, and the second pile here isn't interesting; the overly stringent operationalization would leave in one pile only gambling by people who have gone bankrupt as a result. That pile isn't completely uninteresting, but it's not nearly as interesting as the pile we really want, which is the one containing all and only the gambling by people who, if asked "Is your life made significantly worse by your unsuccessful struggles to stop or cut down on gambling?" would answer "Yes."

One way to increase the probability of useful operationalizations is to deploy more of them than analysis might ultimately find necessary. For practical (as opposed to theoretical) purposes, having too many distinctions is harmless (since ones that turn out to be redundant can just be ignored), but having too few distinctions invites failure to make some potentially informative measurements. In the case of patterns in gambling behavior, this is what scientists and clinicians have done. The psychiatric and psychological research community has attempted to operationalize three categories of gambling behavior:

Pathological gambling
A chronic inability to refrain from gambling to an extent that causes serious disruption to core life aspects such as career, health and family. The diagnostic criterion established by *DSM-IV* (American Psychiatric

Association 2000) is that a person is a pathological gambler if they agree with five or more of the following statements:

1. You have often gambled longer than you had planned.

2. You have often gambled until your last dollar was gone.

3. Thoughts of gambling have caused you to lose sleep.

4. You have used your income or savings to gamble while letting bills go unpaid.

5. You have made repeated, unsuccessful attempts to stop gambling.

6. You have broken the law or considered breaking the law to finance your gambling.

7. You have borrowed money to finance your gambling.

8. You have felt depressed or suicidal because of your gambling losses.

9. You have been remorseful after gambling.

10. You have gambled to get money to meet your financial obligations.

Problem gambling (PG)
This idea is intended to capture people whose gambling behavior is at least a *nuisance* to them, and is so along the same dimensions as are used to operationalize PG. Ideally these operationalizations should line up in this way so that we can use the concept of problem gambling to clinically pick out people who might be thought to be at risk of becoming pathological gamblers. President Clinton's Committee on the Social and Economic Impact of Pathological Gambling[4] operationalized problem gambling as "gambling behavior that results in any harmful effects to the gambler, his or her family, significant others, friends, coworkers etc." In this the committee members simply reflected what they found in the research and treatment literature. But this operationalization is too liberal for our purposes here; losing $5 on a football bet or being late for lunch with a coworker because of a queue at the betting window constitute "harmful effects," however trivial. It would be natural, and maximally helpful, to operationalize problem gambling as "PG lite" (which might indicate incipient PG) by describing the problem gambler as someone who agrees with some number of the statements in the operationalization of PG less than five. However, this confronts us with the problem that the statements don't all seem to be

equally diagnostic. Anyone who agrees with (5), (6), or (10) probably
has or has previously had a relatively serious problem associated with
gambling, and likewise for (8), if "depressed" is interpreted clinically.
But this cannot be said of the other statements unless their interpretations are specially restricted. It cannot be said of (1) under *any* plausible
restriction.

Disordered gambling (DG)
This denotes the inclusive disjunction of the two ideas above, i.e., gambling that is either PG or problem gambling.

We said that researchers "have attempted to" operationalize these
three terms, and it will now be evident why we used this cautious formulation. "PG" is indeed operationalized by *DSM-IV*. But "problem
gambling" is not; nor can it readily be operationalized by reference to
the operationalization of "PG." And then, "DG" automatically inherits
all the problems attaching to the lack of clarity around "problem
gambling."

The lack of a settled operationalization for any term other than "PG"
raises a problem for the writing of a synthesis of knowledge about DG.
A synthesis must consolidate and compare many studies. This is precisely the activity in which one most depends on confidence that
different groups of researchers mean at least approximately the same
thing by every term they use to describe the phenomena they take
themselves to be measuring.

We could get around this problem, in principle, by strictly confining
our discussion to PG and remaining absolutely silent on everything
else. This would be deeply unsatisfactory procedure, however. Suppose,
as seems clearly the case, that there are substantially more problem
gamblers, on some reasonable but necessarily (at this point) vague
understanding of that concept, than there are pathological gamblers.
In that case, the lion's share of the social costs associated with a given
gambling policy might be accounted for by the problem gamblers, and
no major policy recommendations could be based on studies that
ignored them. That would be a situation we'd just have to live with for
now if it could honestly be said that the study of problem gambling
hasn't yet progressed far enough to license any policy recommendations. But we don't think this can honestly or sensibly be said.

Fortunately, we believe that the union of disciplinary perspectives
from which this book is written—the microexplanatory union of neoclassical microeconomics, BE, and NE described in chapter 1—affords

a way around the difficulty. In chapter 4 we will introduce George Ainslie's (1992, 2001) BE-oriented concept of a "personal rule." We'll eventually operationalize "problem gambling" in terms of this idea. (That is, we will identify problem gamblers as people who both struggle to maintain and regularly break personal rules, but who lack a distinctive variety of neurochemical pathology described in chapters 5 and 6.) We will use "PG" as per the *DSM-IV* operationalization. Since we'll thus have operationalizations of both "problem gambling" and "PG," we'll be able to clearly use "DG" in the way indicated above.

We have explained that an operationalization is not yet an analysis. This is important: whereas an operationalization is a tool for doing scientific study and therefore must precede it, analysis is one of the things one wants to get *from* scientific study. That is, scientific investigation aims at telling us, among other things, what problem gambling and PG "really are." This is not a matter of idle metaphysics, but is directly relevant to public health policy. Policy makers and industry participants need to know whether there's a qualitative "jump" between problem gamblers, as just typical consumers of gambling services who sometimes have bad days at the casino—in the same way that people have bad days in all their activities—and pathological gamblers, as people for whom special policies and practices need to be adopted. (Most carefully regulated and administered casinos *do*, at present, implement an assumption like this as a prudential matter and aim to identify and then exclude pathological gamblers. They don't, obviously, exclude or have special policies for those who merely occasionally gamble a bit more than they intended to.) If there is not such a qualitative jump and all people who gamble are on a smooth continuum without "bright lines," then policy problems are going to be relatively more challenging. Louise Sharpe (2002) points out that we get divergent interpretations of some research data depending on which of these hypotheses we consider most probable. Addressing this question about continuity is one of the basic underlying aims of our book.

The perspective we'll defend with respect to problem, but not pathological, gamblers is that there are probably no systematic biological differences between them and people who like to gamble from time to time but haven't experienced problems. (Some people who don't like to or for some other reason never gamble might also have distinctive biological properties, and this is a topic we'll touch upon briefly in the final chapter.) We'll maintain, that is, that problem gambling isn't a property of an organism considered in isolation, but of a typical person in a kind of situation. Where pathological gamblers are concerned, we'll maintain, matters are different. Surveys from a number of countries and regions of countries tell us that between 1 percent and 3 percent of the population of any country or province-sized jurisdiction will tend to be incapable of gambling nearly as moderately as they themselves wish to unless they're assisted with clinical intervention. In chapter 6 we'll present reasons for thinking that all or almost all of this population should be categorized as *addictive* gamblers because they have brains that physically malfunction in the same way that drug addicts' brains do. We'll show why we think it will very soon be possible to reliably diagnose people in the addictive group by (non-invasively) examining their brains (or perhaps even their genes), and why there are also grounds for optimism that the day isn't far off when they'll be able to control their problem with medication.

There is a good deal of careful ground to cover before we'll be able to get to this. As we've stressed, in advance of arriving at a basis for categorization that is supported by a marriage of theory, systematic observation, and experiment, behavioral researchers must gather subjects for study and sort them according to some operationalization or other. For this they use "screens," questionnaires that are administered to people in order to classify them for data-gathering and experimental purposes. Here we encounter another problem related to definitions of phenomena. With respect to conditions that cause serious harm, such as DG, the clinical imperative—the need to help suffering people—has higher social priority than scientific research.[5] In screening people to determine which are pathological or problem gamblers for clinical purposes, the treatment community rightly prefers to err on the side of avoiding false negatives. That is, there is a preference for diagnosing risk in some people who aren't really in trouble over missing people who need help. Clinical screens build in this bias, and are criticized if they don't. But then we face a dilemma in choosing a screen for research purposes. If we use the clinical screen, we will find in most populations we survey a higher prevalence of the target condition than is really there. If we instead develop a research screen that differs from clinical screens, we'll get mismatches between clinical and research samples. This is problematic for two reasons. First, subject recruitment for studies of conditions that affect only small proportions of the population, such as PG, is difficult and expensive. Practical purposes require that we usually rely on samples already assembled (often by self-selection) for treatment purposes (so-called "convenience samples"). This is especially true, for obvious reasons, when an aspect of a research project is evaluation of a therapeutic approach. Second, there are serious ethical problems in sorting clinical populations into those we scientifically classify as "really" manifesting the condition for which they are being treated and those we admit we have merely diagnosed for cautionary reasons. Since scientific research on subjects cannot be concealed from those subjects, doing this would send signals to the subjects as patients and thereby undermine the point of having designed our clinical screens to minimize false negatives in the first place.

These objections carry the day in practice. In the study of DG, research subjects are generally recruited and pooled using clinical screens. This has several implications, which we now consider.

First, we should be cautious about estimating prevalence. One can do so only by application of a "double filter." That is, if one has run statistical tests to determine the *extent* to which a screen gathers false positives, one can then use this to systematically down-weight prevalence estimates in a population obtained using that screen.[6] Notice that this requires that we have already made some progress in the direction of analysis; if you have nothing beyond a bare operationalization of your phenomenon with which to work, then you have no distinction on which you can base the statistical testing. To a considerable extent, this is where we still stand with respect to research on DG. This is why, for example, we had to report prevalence for PG as "between 1 percent and 3 percent"—not a very exact figure, since the upper bound is three times the size of the lower bound. The problem isn't lack of data; it's ineliminable error when all one has to work with are operationalizations instead of analyses.

Second, when considering any research report, especially of research into the efficacy of a therapy or policy, one needs to know where the screen used to recruit and pool subjects stands comparatively on the question of the average *severity* of pathology found in these subjects. Consider two hypothetical screens *a* and *b*. Suppose that screen *a* consistently produces samples in which the median subject agrees with eight statements in the *DSM-IV* operationalization of PG, while the median subject recruited by screen *b* agrees with six of them. If one knows that, then one also has reason to suspect that research using screen *b* is more likely to find that a given policy or therapy is effective than is research on that same policy or therapy that recruits and pools subjects by means of screen *a*, because the *a*-screened samples will contain higher proportions of "hard cases." (One can't be quite sure of this, however, because of the fact that, as noted above, not all the *DSM-IV* criteria seem to be of equal diagnostic weight. Suppose, for example, that more of the *b*-screened subjects agree with statements (5) and (6).[7])

Third, one of the "big" questions about DG we identified above as central at the moment is whether there is a qualitative "jump" (which should be indicated by some quantitative discontinuity) between subgroups of disordered gamblers. As we have also explained, if there is such a discontinuity then it is highly unlikely that our current operationalizations will exactly line up with it; bringing our operationalizations closer into line with it, so that they approach analyses, is precisely one of our goals here. This means that we can't fully trust results derived from work using just one screen, because each screen will have its own bias with respect to the population proportions it selects on either side of the discontinuity[8]—but we can't know in advance where these biases are, at least until we've clearly identified the basis of the discontinuity. To complicate matters further, Blaszczynski and Nower (2002) argue that there is more than one kind of pathological gambler, thus suggesting the possibility of two scales with discontinuities at different measurement points and of different magnitudes.[9] We should therefore ideally run every study we think is important on several groups of subjects recruited using different screens; but this practice is expensive and logistically tedious.

This set of circumstances confronts us with a trade-off. On the one hand, it is very helpful for cross-comparability of studies that one particular screen has so far dominated DG research. On the other hand, this also limits our ability to bootstrap our way around the inadequacies of our initial operationalizations. In an ideal world we'd have a matrix: we would use all available screens on subsample populations in all studies, thus having cross-comparability *and* controlling for screen biases.

Unfortunately, we don't live in an ideal world. Here in the actual one, the dominant instrument mentioned above is the South Oaks Gambling Screen (SOGS) introduced in 1987 (Lesieur and Blume 1987). The SOGS is closely based on the *DSM-III-R*[10] criteria for PG. (It has not been updated to reflect changes subsequently introduced with *DSM-IV*.) As of a 2000 survey by Dickerson and Baron, these diagnostic criteria had been used in over 90 percent of published research on DG.

The SOGS can be self-administered by prospective subjects, which is convenient and cost-efficient. Petry (2005, pp. 39–41) recommends that for research purposes SOGS be used as an initial screen, with a more discriminating instrument then employed as a further filter. She reviews four such existing instruments, among which the comparatively new Diagnostic Interview for Gambling Severity (DIGS) developed by Winters, Specker, and Stinchfield (2002) has been suggested by validation studies to be especially promising. Another recently developed, more intensive instrument is the Canadian Problem Gambling Index (CGI) (Ferris and Wynne 2001a), which facilitates distinguishing between pathological and problem gamblers. Its psychometric properties as measured to date are also encouraging (Ferris and Wynne 2001b).[11]

It must be made clear, however, that such double-filtering hasn't thus far been the norm in DG research, and that establishing it as the norm would add significantly to the average cost of studies. Instruments like the DIGS and the CGI are time-consuming to administer. Their use thus multiplies research staff time, laboratory usage time, and the amount of subjects' time that must be requested. It thus also multiplies all of the main items in the cost budget of a typical behavioral study.

In many cases, even double-filtering of the sort just discussed is inadequate. A number of studies have aimed at identifying the extent to which pathological gamblers tend to have additional psychological–behavioral problems ("comorbidities"), such as substance dependence (Crockford and el-Guebaly 1998a; Feigelman et al. 1995), depression (Cunningham-Williams et al. 1998; Dannon et al. 2004), schizophrenia (ibid.), and antisocial personality disorder (Lesieur 1987). Determination of comorbidity rates that are stable across populations of pathological gamblers, if there are any such rates, would be helpful for a number of reasons. First, it would assist in predicting the likelihood that a given person is at risk of becoming a pathological gambler, since establishing the comorbidity factors in question would carry at least some information about this. Second, it would be highly relevant to design of treatments and interventions, possibly helping to explain patterns of success and failure. Interventions that work for pathological gamblers who lack certain specific comorbidities might fail for others who do. For example, Ladd and Petry (2003) report that PG is more persistent in subjects who have been treated for substance abuse than in otherwise comparable subjects who have not been so treated. Third, efforts to explain such stable comorbidity patterns as we find might lead us to the explanation of PG itself, to the extent that PG and comorbidities are sometimes or often consequences of a common causal factor. Comorbidity data are what mainly lead Blaszczynski and Nower (2002) to the view that there are three different kinds of pathological gamblers. They report that across studies with larger numbers of subjects, stable proportions of pathological gamblers show comorbidity with, respectively (1) nothing, (2) depression and other mood disorders, and (3) antisocial personality disorder. Unsurprisingly perhaps, subjects in these groups respond differentially to therapy. Blaszczynski and Nower then argue, more controversially, that the different comorbid factors causally contribute to PG in different ways (hence explaining the varying susceptibility of these groups to different interventions).

Obviously, the more we discover about the significance of comorbidity for predicting, explaining, and treating PG, the more importance we will attach to screening research subjects for the identified correlated conditions. This does not imply anything especially onerous for research methodology where substance abuse is the possible factor in question, since substance abuse can be effectively screened for by comparatively basic instruments. However, reliable screening for psychiatric disorders requires use of sophisticated instruments and qualified expert administration and analysis. This can drive up the cost and complexity of research.

Note that an approach that focuses on searching for comorbidity factors is almost inevitable to the extent that PG is conceptualized as a kind of disease—that is, as a specific breakdown in the functional constitution of the person. Thus, the reason Blaszczynski and Nower conclude from three comorbidity patterns that there are three different kinds of PG is that they implicitly identify any case of PG with its *etiological* pathway. This assumption sets researchers off in search of the site of damage. They often suppose it to be unlikely that something could go wrong with a person's mind or brain that would produce *only* PG, in which case such searches are bound to be, at least in part, searches for comorbidity factors. This has tended to be the perspective of much recent psychiatry, and its promised implications for policy and intervention are straightforward. If we could identify the site of damage in the pathological gambler, then we could either seek to repair the damage in question or, if that is not possible, use diagnosis of the damage as a basis for knowing whose access to legal gambling opportunities should be restricted or blocked. And perhaps we could set up mechanisms to identify those people who are at risk of becoming pathological gamblers and effectively intervene to stop the onset of the condition. In chapter 6 we'll present evidence that this approach looks likely to bear fruit because pathological gamblers appear mainly to be addicts, in a specific sense captured by neuroeconomic models of the reward pathways in their brains. Furthermore, this seems to be a common element to PG that is independent of differences in comorbidities or etiologies.

Where policy is concerned, however, what about disordered gamblers who *aren't* addicted? Or suppose we found a reliable diagnostic but not a cure for addictive gamblers? We could probably prevent many of them from going to casinos or racetracks. Preventing them from buying lottery tickets or playing Internet poker would be more difficult. But would it even be appropriate to try to prevent such people from "playing" the stock market? If so, what about real estate markets? Should pathological or addictive gamblers be prevented from reselling houses or other assets? These are issues with which the organizers of Gamblers Anonymous and other treatment groups wrestle; there is no consensus on them in the clinical and helping communities.

Such questions help to remind us that gambling per se is a normal, not a deviant, kind of human behavior. By this we don't just mean that it is widespread; we mean to reiterate a point made earlier, that a disposition to gamble is adaptive and a disposition *never* to gamble is severely *mal*adaptive, because the urge to gamble is in part just the urge to explore and take risks. Few people aspire to have the kind of personality that tries to avoid all risks. More to the point, few people aspire not to *enjoy* taking some risks. Aversion to risk, or mere inability to appreciate the pleasure of moderate risks, amounts to aversion to novelty and absence of both curiosity and ambition. This suggests that, except where addictive gamblers are concerned, it may be mistaken to take for granted that our main question must be: What, specifically, is wrong with disordered gamblers? Is it possible that gambling problems arise, at least in the first place, when people fail to learn to effectively manage some natural dispositions shared by almost everyone?

Behavioral economics, inheriting from the history of economic thought an ambition to establish universal generalizations and then model special cases by adjusting specified theoretical parameters, incorporates this perspective. In our opinion, the BE perspective generally, and the picoeconomic (PE) perspective more specifically, currently promise to be the most fecund source of insights and productive

research procedures for studying the broad class of behavioral dispositions popularly associated as "compulsions" and "bad habits" specifically including (at least) non-addictive DG. PE has been thought by
some of its founders to be in tension with neuroscience, a matter to
which we return—in application to pathological–addictive gambling—
in chapters 5 and 8. Our view is that this tension, however natural,
must be overcome, since both PE and neuroscience offer crucial insights
into the phenomena of interest to us here, and many others. How can
we maximally exploit their complementarities? To this we turn over
the next three chapters.

Picoeconomics, Impulsive
Consumption, and
Disordered Gambling

3.1   Behavioral Economics and Picoeconomics

DG (in general) has sometimes been grouped with stereotypical substance dependencies (e.g., alcoholism) by reference to "mental" symptoms, including sensed loss of control and preoccupation in consciousness. But DG and substance abuse have also been associated by appeal to the way in which these behavioral patterns both supposedly manifest *impulsivity*. The report of President Clinton's Committee on the Social and Economic Impact of Pathological Gambling (1999) said that "there is considerable consensus that gambling involves impulsiveness" (p. 37). The report was ambiguous with respect to its interpretation of impulsivity, however, which provides a useful way of introducing the distinction between the frameworks of traditional psychology and BE.

According to *DSM-IV* (American Psychiatric Association 2000), a person manifests an impulse control disorder when he or she shows recurrent and significant "failure to resist an impulse, drive or temptation to perform an act that is harmful to the person or to others" (p. 609). On this interpretation, impulsivity is an "inner-referenced" pathology, a tendency of some sort of behavioral "organ" to misfire. This is the perspective that the great psychologist Richard Herrnstein and others dubbed "molecular." It presupposes some notion of "normally non-impulsive molecular behavioral causation," and it is by implicit reference to that notion that we are to understand the idea of the subject's doing harm to herself. Traditional psychology often asks us to contrast "healthy" with "unhealthy" behavior in this way. The definition just given more or less *identifies* impulsivity with unhealthy behavior.[1]

This way of thinking is in tension with the fact noted previously that virtually everyone gambles in one way or another, and that a person who absolutely refused to gamble would not likely be regarded as "healthy." This implies that "health" must be compatible with harm caused by gambles, since the idea of a gamble that is guaranteed not to produce harmful consequences makes little sense. Reflecting the different usages found in the literature (Evenden 1999; see chapter 8, section 2 below), the committee's report *also* understands impulsivity in a different sense: as a tendency to choose smaller, sooner rewards (SSRs) over larger, later rewards (LLRs). The alcoholic could have sobriety, accomplishment, and social respect today and tomorrow, with all the possible streams of subsequent reward these can produce; but she chooses instead the vivid but transient pleasure of a high now, from which she must subtract the costs of hangover and social disapprobrium tomorrow. Likewise, the disordered gambler *could* have money to pay his bills and so secure his welfare for the month, but instead chooses to experience the satisfaction of a brief thrill, from which he must subtract the value of his expected loss.

Describing these scenarios in terms of choices immediately raises the possible relevance of economic analysis. Economics is, in its broadest sense, the study of the way in which people (and other organisms and groups) try to promote their welfare in the face of scarcity. "Scarcity" has two complementary connotations. First, an economic agent's wants exceed what the environment provides, especially given other agents with wants who share that environment. Second, capturing one stream of benefits typically precludes capturing another possible stream. The value of what is forgone as a result of choice is referred to as the "opportunity cost" of that choice. Conceiving of impulsivity in this framework amounts to seeing the impulsive person as choosing to forgo LLRs as the opportunity cost of SSRs. As soon as we frame things this way, we can introduce all of the technical apparatus of economic analysis. If indulging in a drink or taking a bet is a trade-off between benefits and costs, then we can ask questions about how much change would have to be made to the goods on either side of the ledger to produce the opposite decision.

In fact, there is now a very large scientific literature on such economic analyses of the consumption of abused substances (e.g., Bickel, Madden, and Petry 1998; Carroll 1996; Chaloupka 1991; Chaloupka, Grossman, and Tauras 1999; DeGrandpre et al. 1992; Higgins, Heil, and Lussier 2004; Leung and Phelps 1993). That literature has been concerned primarily with how consumption of abused substances varies with (1) the price (broadly conceived) of the substance and (2) the availability of alternative rewards. This research has consistently found an inverse relation between consumption and price: consumption decreases as price increases (and vice versa). It has also consistently found an inverse relation between consumption and the availability of alternative rewards: consumption decreases as alternative rewards are more readily available (and vice versa). The generality of these relations is impressive, having been found in different species (including humans), for different abused substances, in normal and clinical ("addicted") populations, and in laboratory and natural environments. It is particularly important to note that both these relations hold for individuals clinically regarded as "addicted" to the substances in question. Such findings indicate that the consumption of abused substances can be usefully described with the same analytic tools that apply to all commodities. We will shortly return to and explain the significance of this literature for how we conceptualize the family of disorders in which DG has usually been included by psychologists, the clinical community, and policy makers.

Before that, however, we must say more to introduce and explain the nature of BE itself. Confusion can readily arise here because the term is widely used with two sharply opposed connotations in different circles of opinion. Indeed, so much dust has lately been stirred up here by rhetorical controversies that we will have to indulge upon the reader's patience for a few paragraphs while we try to clear the issue out of our way.

Most economists, most of the time, study phenomena in which individual agents' preferences and behaviors are aggregated in consequence of interaction and cannot be systematically disaggregated. Underlying this in principle, though usually not in practice, is a body of inquiry, both empirical and theoretical, that aims to model individual preference structures and dispositions in a way that is consistent with, and might to some extent explain, the kinds of assumptions used to model aggregated situations. More specifically, this literature begins from one or another abstract conception of an individual with wants, and with certain restrictions on how these wants are related to one another, and models ways in which such an individual's behavioral dispositions respond to shifts in external incentive structures, particularly in the schedules and relative prices of scarce commodities that service their wants (e.g., Camerer, Loewenstein, and Rabin 2003; Kagel and Roth 1995). Because this modeling has often aimed at very high degrees of generality, it has frequently taken as its question what an "ideally rational" agent *would* do in a kind of incentive situation or parameter shift, given a particular quantified profile of preferences (a "utility function") and a budget constraint. We will say more about the meaning of "ideally rational" in this context shortly. In addition, those concerned with the *foundations* (as opposed to applications) of economic theory, in modeling both individuals and their aggregates, have searched for generalizations that hold in any set of institutional conditions. Against this background contrast, BE refers to any approach that aims at theories and models of what *actual* people do in *particular* institutional settings. This question needs separate study because actual people are not ideally rational agents, and because real institutions cannot be maintained for free; they impose so-called "transaction costs," and will survive only to the extent that some agents deem themselves to be best off if they pay these costs. Furthermore, institutions are often based on, and perpetuated through feedback mechanisms by, asymmetries of information among agents that interfere with the generalizing reach of foundational theory. That is to say, institutions affect the properties of the individual agents in the first place, and this is why, in practice, most aggregates as modeled in economics do not rigorously decompose into relations among the kinds of individuals featured in the abstract models of ideal consumers. (They nevertheless often so decompose *approximately*, and for many practical purposes that is good enough.)

Upon first encountering this contrast, many people think that BE should *supplant* traditional idealized modeling in economics. Shouldn't we always care more about what actual people do in concrete conditions than about what ideal but non-existent agents could do in completely abstract situations? Although the question seems reasonable, it is profoundly misleading. The concepts we use to represent—to, as it were, stand in for—actual people (or actual firms, or actual governments, or actual agents of other kinds) are given their exact meanings in models by their definitions in the general theory of ideal rational agency. Without this theory, we wouldn't be able to state clear economic hypotheses about actual people in actual circumstances in the first place. Such hypotheses *begin from* the idealized definitions and then modify and amend them in various particular ways for particular purposes of application. Despite a good deal of recent "revolutionary" rhetoric from BE practitioners interested in strongly contrasting their work with that of supposedly unworldly, old-fashioned economic theorists, we are unaware of any important economist who has argued that economics should not study actual behavior or the impacts of actual institutions. Indeed, most of the difference between an excellent and a mediocre economist lies in the art of modeling—that is, in the extent to which the economist can see how to capture the features of a particular situation using theoretical concepts that were not developed with that situation in mind. This is as we should expect: if every theoretical model was built de novo as a customized application, there would be no possibility of *general* economic knowledge. The point of economics, as with any science, is to show how particular phenomena are explained and predicted by reference to more general ones. Even where the particular phenomena themselves are concerned, the aim should never be to try to capture *every* detail of a situation, since that makes theory redundant and bars any hope of applying or extending generalizations (which is the entire point of theory). At the same time, *relevant* details whose exclusion would distort analysis and render it a misleading basis for prediction must be carefully shoehorned into the exact terms that are well defined in theoretical representation. Skillful trade-offs between generality and accuracy rely crucially on the modeler's insight, judgment and experience—in a word, on her pragmatic professional know-how—not on applications of a priori methodological rules (as some philosophers imagine).

In this context, all that "BE" sensibly ought to connote is a body of research that explicitly measures and models more psychological and institutional detail than does economics that begins from the points of maximum abstraction. The number of economists with preferences for this sort of work has greatly increased of late, which we regard as a good thing. However, as noted above, this has been accompanied in some such economists with self-consciousness about constituting a methodologically radical "movement." This should mainly be understood in the context of competitions for authority, prestige, and funding within the professional community of economists.

So, in this book, we will use "BE" without connotations of opposition to "old-fashioned" economics. The term will refer to the economic study of people with psychological properties as identified by current cognitive and behavioral sciences, as opposed to abstract agents stripped of all properties other than utility functions.

For the most part, our focus *within* this ideologically neutral conception of BE will be on a specific family of models, one developed mainly by psychologists rather than economists. This family has been dubbed "picoeconomics" by the theorist who has done most to elaborate it,

George Ainslie. The basis for this label will be made clear shortly. PE models aim to explain and predict the consumption behavior of actual people and other animals who manifest a particular kind of pattern in their consumption behavior discovered and initially modeled by the late Richard Herrnstein. That is, they choose consumption bundles, at least when they don't pay costs in effort to do otherwise, according to what Herrnstein called "the matching law."

We will explain the matching law by contrast with the standing model of choice that the law was proposed (in some contexts) to supplant. In the economic theory of the ideally rational consumer, the agent is modeled as *maximizing* a consistent utility function over the agent's whole life. As we will discuss later in this chapter, Ross (2005) argues at length that the empirical interpretation of "the agent's whole life" here is left open by economic theory, and the modeling discretion that results from this freedom is importantly useful. For the moment, however, we will defer this point and think of agents in the way they are uncritically interpreted in most of the BE and related literature, as being more or less equivalent to individual people.

The utility maximizing agent of microeconomic theory is held to be "rational" in the sense of having *consistent* preferences. Consistency comprises three main properties: (1) if the agent prefers choice bundle a to choice bundle b and bundle b to bundle c, then in otherwise identical circumstances she will not choose bundle c over bundle a; (2) there are no bundles over which the agent has no preferences; and (3) the agent will not reverse a preference for some bundle a over b merely because a bundle c becomes available, unless c includes some elements that complement an element in b (i.e., increase its value to her). These very abstract consistency properties, which characterize "rational choice theory," are typically extended to more specific restrictions in microeconomic modeling. The agent will choose a greater quantity of b the lower its price and will vary her choice patterns between any given stream of benefits b and all possible alternatives to b only on the basis of changes in: (1) her stock of b in proportion to other goods, (2) her expectations about any exogenous fluctuations in the flow of b she'll face, and (3) her expectations concerning the future price of b relative to prices of other goods. Add finally that the maximizing agent will accept higher opportunity costs for b the less of it she has, and we have the standard generic model of the rational consumer. This agent, to the extent that she knows what consumption opportunities her environment will provide, will allocate her resources over time in such a way that she'll get the highest possible welfare over the course of her life as an agent. This means that she'll forgo possible temporary welfare increases at a given time for the sake of this general maximization. Uncertainty about future consumption opportunities complicates matters technically, but as long as she calculates her probabilities rationally, the agent will choose in such a way that her overall welfare will be maximized except insofar as she suffers from bad luck. An uncertain agent who allocates resources as wisely as possible and then encounters bad luck will be *disappointed* but has nothing to *regret*, unlike the agent who contributes to her own misfortune by suboptimal allocations or failure to use information that was available to her.

In this framework, the economic analyst must interpret chronic impulsivity and addiction not as marks of irrationality, but simply as signs of preferences that, given the distribution of opportunity costs in the world, happen to make the agent's life hard. If we see a person waste away from alcoholism, application of the model directs us to infer that this person considers drunkenness to be worth very high opportunity costs. Like any other utility maximizer, she gets as much welfare overall as is possible for her given this preference. That she becomes less and less well off (against some arbitrary reference point of her own) over time is because alcohol consumption causes tolerance to increase, so the opportunity cost of the same high, for which her preference must persist lest she exhibit inconsistency, rises steadily during the history of drinking. In this frame, so far as the alcoholic's harm to herself is concerned, the only policy response by others that isn't cruel and oppressive is to try to avoid unnecessary increases in the price of drinks, and to help her minimize her opportunity costs by helping her to avoid situations that are potentially dangerous or embarrassing. It would make no moral sense in this framework for others to help the agent avoid alcohol, since (once potential harm to second and third parties is minimized) this would just amount to lowering her welfare. This way of applying the traditional economic model of utility maximization to addiction was originally worked out in technical form by the Nobel Prize–winning economist Gary Becker and his students (Becker 1976; Becker and Murphy 1988), and continues to be refined and extended.

Critics of the standard microeconomic model often think it suffices for them to point out that real people don't have psychological profiles analogous to economic consistency, and then regard the case against use of the model as closed on that account. This will not do.

Expected-utility maximization is a mathematical modeling technology, not a psychological hypothesis, and we should evaluate it as we would any other practical tool: can it do the job of systematizing behavior for purposes of prediction and explanation with no more sweat and strain than we'd face if we used an available alternative tool? Addiction is one of the leading behavioral patterns—perhaps *the* leading behavioral pattern—for which it has seemed to many critics that the answer to this question is "no." A principal objection is that most addicts don't just consume their substance of abuse until they've run out of all resources (due to their high preference for the substance, which persists as their budget runs down), as the straightforward application of standard economic theory with expected-utility maximization predicts they should. Instead, most of them spend resources trying to *stop* consuming their substance of abuse. It isn't *impossible* for models like Becker's to accommodate this. One might conjecture, for example, that some or most addicts periodically stop consumption so they can recalibrate their tolerance levels and then temporarily enjoy their highs less expensively. But a more serious problem for expected-utility maximizing accounts of addiction that identify whole biographical people with single agents is that most addicts eventually successfully quit. Becker-style theories *must* infer from this that addicts did not initially know that addiction was going to be bad, and only learned this through experiencing lower welfare levels than they expected. Again, this is possible—but then it is difficult to reconcile with the strong tendency of addicts to *relapse*. We must suppose on the one hand that each time an alcoholic stops drinking but then relapses, she's aiming to get drunk more cheaply for a while. But then, on the other hand, we must hypothesize that when she at last stops once and for all, this was because she *finally* realized that she was doing herself more harm than good. If she never stops once and for all, we have to suppose that she was *not* doing herself more harm than good, in her own terms. Thus, by traditional economic accounts, we can characterize the most common course of addiction, consisting of starting, deepening, repeated relapse, and eventual successful abstinence, as involving a radical psychological discontinuity between unsuccessful and successful attempts at quitting: the former are for the sake of enhanced enjoyment of the addiction, and the latter result from a decision to abandon this enjoyment. Unfortunately for ease of modeling, this psychological hypothesis is entirely ad hoc and has no empirical evidence in its favor.

In the face of this, most commentators with close experience of addicts and addiction reject the model of the consistent expected-utility maximizing addict as empirically inadequate. The appeal of Herrnstein's alternative generic model, based on empirical measurement of animal behavior (including human behavior) under experimental manipulations, must be understood in this light.[2] His original work (Herrnstein 1961) shows that animals allocate responses to two choice alternatives proportionally to the relative frequencies of reinforcement received from them. The empirical relation $B_1/B_2 = R_1/R_2$, where the Bs and Rs refer to responses allocated to and reinforcements received from the two alternatives respectively, became known as the "matching law" because relative behavioral allocation matches relative reinforcement received. Herrnstein later showed (1982) that a choice rule that directly compares the local rates of reinforcement on the two alternatives and selects the alternative with the higher local rate describes the process that produces matching, which he termed "melioration."[3] Subsequent work building on these basic relations showed that we get accurate predictions of human and animal choice behavior if we model organisms as maximizing *local* rather than *overall expected* utility. The family of models that technically represent melioration specify that a person or animal will distribute their resources to a range of activities during a time interval in exact proportion to the value of the rewards they experience for each activity *in that time interval*. Importantly, the time interval over which local rates of reinforcement are computed and compared is not set in stone and so may vary. Obviously, if variation in the temporal interval over which rates are computed changes the estimate of those rates, this changes the valuation of the choice options and leads to a change in behavioral allocation. Thus the standard microeconomic assumption of choice that reveals consistent preferences may be violated. What Ainslie later called PE begins as the family of models at the intersection of economics and psychology that represent choice behavior by applications of the matching law.

Herrnstein did not merely show that this way of modeling *addicts'* behavior captures the data; he demonstrated that it applies to people and other animals *in general*. People popularly thought of as addicts are merely ideally vivid cases for illustration. All agents who match and meliorate will tend to behave, from the traditional economist's point of view, short-sightedly, failing to take full account of their long-run welfare. We must say "tend to" rather than the more straightforward "will" for two reasons. First, both the matching law and expected-utility maximization predict the same behavior when an agent chooses between two streams of benefits *a* and *b* in which *a* is more rewarding than *b* over *all* intervals. For example, an alcoholic will display consistent choice between good whiskey and bad whiskey. Second, many human institutions are set up so as to incentivize people who meliorate to act as if they were maximizers; financial institutions are the outstanding examples here, finding devices like compound interest and derivatives to ensure that all failures to respect the logic of maximization can be efficiently exploited for someone else's profit. (This simultaneously ensures that resources don't go to waste and that investors have incentives to adjust their accounting of time intervals until they're acting like maximizers.) But for the phenomena of concern to us here—first, addiction-like behavior patterns in general, and then DG specifically—PE makes distinctive predictions and offers distinctive explanations. As we will see, these predictions and explanations have been strongly supported by empirical behavioral research.

Most importantly, PE (like all BE, but unlike the NE described in chapter 5) explains behavioral patterns in a *molar*, rather than a *molecular*, way. That is, it doesn't aim to trace out causal sequences whereby some particular event in a person's life, or in their brain, or in their consciousness, leads to this particular drink or to that particular refusal of a drink, to this specific ante at the blackjack table, or that specific decision to go to a movie tonight instead of to the casino. What PE explanations aim to account for are *patterns* of behavior, the relative opportunity costs that people pay over a given stretch of time for different rewards. Pathological gamblers are, in the first instance, people who pay what seem to the rest of us to be—and what they themselves eventually agree to be—extravagant opportunity costs for whatever it is they find rewarding about gambling. They don't offer this payment on every single possible occasion, but that isn't what PE aims to explain. What is of interest in PE is that they offer the payment significantly more often than problem gamblers, who in turn offer it significantly more often than nondisordered gamblers. Note that on this perspective it makes no sense to think of the returns to gambling—either the excitement or the winnings, whichever turn out to matter more motivationally—as *bad* things for the gambler. They are, after all, what the gambler *likes*—what she gambles *for*. Indeed, almost everyone gambles for these rewards to *some* extent, regardless of whether they ever play structured games of chance and pay third parties to set them up. What is bad, for the gamblers, about DG is that they pay more for these rewards, over time, than they themselves want to.

PE is a *general* framework for thinking about behavior. As will be discussed in the next few sections, melioration and matching are compatible with several specific models of the phenomena traditionally grouped together as "addictions," including PG. PE also implies a particular set of experimental *methods* for trying to choose among these different models. We describe these experimental approaches and what has been learned about DG from their application in chapter 4.

3.2   Intertemporal Choice and Impulsivity

The scientific community has not reached a consensus regarding whether or not DG and substance abuse are fundamentally the same or different types of behavioral disorders (Petry 2006; Potenza 2006). We will argue in chapters 6 and 7 that the basis for a particular such consensus is now upon us, but in advance of that argument we must treat the question as still open. To the extent that the phenomena are similar, knowledge gained regarding substance abuse would also apply to DG. To date, PE has been much more extensively applied to substance abuse than to gambling, so we will summarize some of the PE work on substance abuse as an illustration of what can be gained from the PE perspective.

3.2.1   *The Matching Law*

As noted earlier, studying choices between SSRs and LLRs provides a framework for understanding impulsivity. The valuation of delayed outcomes presumably is a critical issue for understanding substance abuse, and also gambling, because substance users and gamblers repeatedly choose between immediately available but relatively small rewards (substance consumption or the fun of betting) and engaging in alternative activities that could produce delayed but more valuable rewards in the future (e.g., positive intimate, family, or social relations; vocational or academic success; purchase of something for which savings have been set aside). In such choices, gaining access to the more valuable but delayed rewards depends on, or at least is facilitated by, forgoing the less valuable but more immediate reward. Conversely, repeatedly enjoying the SSRs risks reduced future access to the LLR. When someone's choices in these life areas go awry (e.g., excessive drinking or gambling at the expense of marriage and family), it is natural for us to introduce "irrationality" into the analysis. As argued above, most such individuals, if modeled as single economic agents over time, are in fact irrational in the economist's sense. Like the fanciful cobraholic, their preferences are inconsistent over time: at time t_1 they (truthfully) report a strong desire to drink less or not at all in order to maintain a happy marriage and family life, but at time t_2 they drink to excess and thereby further threaten the very things they desired at time t_1. Research derived from the matching law has produced large strides in our understanding of such choices and their disorders. We will now describe the theoretical and empirical basis of this progress.[4]

Experiments on the matching law typically give subjects opportunities to respond on two options, manipulate some dimension of reward (e.g., frequency, amount, or delay) derived from option 1 and option 2 choices, then relate the pattern of choices to the pattern of rewards received. In these experiments, both animals and humans make a very large number of choices across multiple sessions, and the individual rewards typically are small amounts of food for animals and small amounts of money for people.[5] The first dimension of reward studied was frequency (Herrnstein 1961), with the same size of reward occurring more or less frequently from option 1 and option 2 choices. Herrnstein found, for example, that if reward occurred twice as frequently from option 1 as from option 2, then option 1 was chosen twice as often as option 2. Later studies investigated varying the amount (Catania 1963) and varying the delay (Chung and Herrnstein 1967) dimensions of reward, and produced results similar to those that studied frequency of reward. For amount variation, if rewards occurred equally often from option 1 and option 2, but the option 1 rewards were, for example, twice as big, then option 1 was chosen twice as often as option 2. For delay variation, when the same size rewards occurred equally often on option 1 and option 2, but receipt of the option 2 rewards was, for example, delayed twice as long as receipt of the option 1 rewards, option 1 was chosen twice as often.

The leap forward in our understanding of impulsivity and self-control occurred when scientists began studying choice between rewards that varied in both amount and delay, with one reward being smaller but sooner and the other reward being larger but later. Equation 3.1, below, is a version of the matching law concerning choice between rewards that vary in both amount and delay (Rachlin and

Green 1972). In equation 3.1, B_1 and B_2 represent the number of choices of option 1 and option 2 respectively, A_1 and A_2 represent the amount (size) of each reward received from option 1 and option 2 respectively, and D_1 and D_2 represent the delay between the choice and receipt of the reward from option 1 and option 2 respectively. The equation shows that relative choice of the two options is directly proportional to the relative amount of reward and inversely proportional to the relative delay of reward:

$$\frac{B_1}{B_2} = \frac{A_1}{A_2} \times \frac{D_2}{D_1} \tag{3.1}$$

This relation shows an unsurprising tendency in both animals and people to prefer larger rewards to smaller rewards, and to prefer sooner rewards to later rewards. But these two tendencies are put in conflict when the smaller reward is sooner and the larger reward is later. Choice of the SSR is understood as impulsive, and choice of the LLR is understood as self-controlled. The critical importance of this form of the matching law for understanding impulsivity and self-control is the manner in which the value of rewards is predicted to vary with their delay. This prediction is that preference between the two rewards will depend on the temporal distance from those rewards at which the choice occurs. At some choice points the individual will be impulsive (choosing the SSR) and at other choice points the individual will be self-controlled (choosing the LLR), even though nothing differs between the choice points except the temporal distance from reward. Moreover, this predicted preference reversal is in sharp contrast to more traditional views of changes in reward value over time, as we discuss shortly.

These choice dynamics are best described with a hypothetical but concrete example, as shown in figure 3.1. Suppose choice of option 1 (the LLR) leads to a six-unit reward ($A_1 = 6$) and choice of option 2 (the SSR) leads to a two-unit reward ($A_2 = 2$), and that the LLR is available eight time units after the SSR. (The reward units are measures of value—we can think of them in terms of how much a subject would pay for the reward. The time units can be any regular unit of time—hours, days, seconds, etc.) In figure 3.1, time is along the horizontal axis, reward value lies along the vertical axis, and the rewards are represented as vertical boxes at the times they are available; the two-unit reward (A_2) is available at time 14, and the six-unit reward (A_1) is available at time 22. As derived from equation 3.1, the value of any delayed

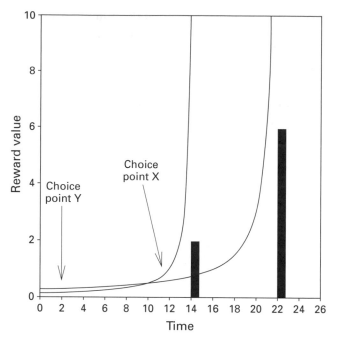

Figure 3.1
Choice between SSR and LLR

reward at any point in time along the horizontal axis is given by dividing the reward amount by the reward delay at that point (A/D), as shown in equation 3.2:

$$v_i = \frac{A_i}{D_i} \tag{3.2}$$

In equation 3.2, v_i is the present value of a reward of amount A_i that is available after a delay of D_i. In figure 3.1, the curves to the left of the rewards were drawn using equation 3.2; they trace the respective A/D fractions for the SSR and LLR as delay changes. Thus, these curves represent the value of the rewards during the times before they are available. Importantly, the reward with the highest value curve at the time the choice is made will be preferred. This change in reward value with delay is termed "temporal discounting," because the present value of a delayed reward is discounted below what its value will be at the time it is received in the future. Equation 3.2 is one form of a temporal discounting function, because it describes how reward value changes with delay.

In equation 3.1, the B_1/B_2 ratio measures whether the subject prefers option 1 or option 2: a behavior ratio greater than 1.0 indicates a preference for A_1, while a behavior ratio less than 1.0 indicates a preference for A_2. At choice point X at time 12 in figure 3.1, the LLR is delayed by ten time units ($A_1 = 6$, $D_1 = 10$), and the SSR is delayed by two time units ($A_2 = 2$, $D_2 = 2$). Inserting these amount and delay values into equation 3.1 yields a B_1/B_2 ratio of .60, indicating a preference for option 2, the SSR (impulsivity). At choice point X, the absolute values (from equation 3.2) of option 1 and option 2 are .600 and 1.000 respectively. But preference is predicted to change if we further delay both rewards by ten time units so that choice occurs at a greater temporal distance from both rewards. This is shown as choice point Y at time 2 in figure 3.1. Now option 1 is six units of reward delayed by 20 time units ($A_1 = 6$, $D_1 = 20$), and option 2 is two units of reward delayed by 12 time units ($A_2 = 2$, $D_2 = 12$). Inserting these modified amount and delay values into equation 3.1 yields a B_1/B_2 ratio of 1.80, indicating a preference for option 1, the LLR (self-control). At choice point Y, the absolute values of alternative 1 and alternative 2 (from equation 3.2) would be .300 and .167 respectively. Thus, the values of both rewards are less at choice point Y than at choice point X, because of temporal discounting, and the shape of the discount function inherent in the matching law predicts that preference between the rewards will reverse simply with the passage of time. For example, someone offered a choice between one pizza at 1pm seven days from now and two pizzas at 1pm eight days from now would probably prefer the two pizzas delayed by eight days. At 12.55pm on the seventh day, however, if the same person were offered a choice between one pizza in five minutes and two pizzas in 24 hours and five minutes, their preference may have reversed, leading them to choose the more immediate single pizza.

This research derived from the matching law has revealed that irrationality, in the technical sense of the economist, is in fact normal. This is critically important and worth repeating: matching law research reveals that both people and other animals are naturally disposed to have inconsistent preferences for future rewards as time passes toward the availability of those rewards. At time t_1 they prefer a larger but temporally more distant reward, but at time t_2, when a smaller but sooner reward is available, their preference reverses and they choose the smaller reward. In the hypothetical example in figure 3.1, our subject preferred the LLR at choice point Y but later this preference reversed and our subject preferred the SSR at choice point X. This is just like the problem drinker or disordered gambler who says she wants to indulge less so as to have a happy marriage, but then later changes her mind and drinks or gambles. According to the prevailing interpretation of this work, having inconsistent preferences over time is the normal state of affairs. Thus, the question of why we sometimes behave irrationally is replaced with the question of how we ever can resist imminent temptations and behave in ways that are consistent with our long-term interests, a question we'll address shortly.

Subsequent research (e.g., Mazur 1987) revealed inadequacies with the simple A/D fraction in equation 3.2 as a generally useful temporal discounting function, and led to the slightly modified version in equation 3.3:

$$v_i = \frac{A_i}{1 + kD_i} \tag{3.3}$$

In equation 3.3, v_i, A_i, and D_i represent the present value of a delayed reward, the amount of a delayed reward, and the delay of the reward respectively. The 1 in the denominator of equation 3.3 prevents the infinite rise in reward value when delay is zero, as in figure 3.1. The k parameter is a constant that is proportional to the degree of temporal discounting, with higher and lower k values describing greater and lesser degrees of discounting respectively. Thus, an individual with a higher k value would discount delayed rewards more than an individual with a lower k value, and the former individual would therefore be more impulsive than the latter individual.[6] As discussed below, such individual differences in temporal discounting are critical to understanding substance abuse and DG.

The discovery that hyperbolic temporal discounting is natural implies a significant departure from earlier models of intertemporal changes in the value of outcomes over delays. In the standard formulation of Samuelson's 1937 discounted utility model, both economists and psychologists model discounting using an exponential function, as in equation 3.4:[7]

$$v_i = A_i e^{-kD_i} \tag{3.4}$$

Here, v_i, A_i, k, and D_i are the same as in equation 3.3, and e is the base of the natural logarithms. The key difference between exponential and hyperbolic temporal discounting is that the rate of discounting is constant at all delays in the former but varies with delay in the latter. That is, with an exponential discounting function, equal increments in delay

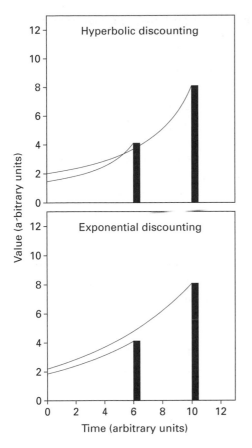

Figure 3.2
Hyperbolic and exponential discounting

produce constant proportional decrements in reward value. With a hyperbolic discounting function, in contrast, equal increments in delay produce larger decrements in reward value at short delays than at long delays. This critical difference is illustrated in figure 3.2. Again, time is along the horizontal axis, reward value is along the vertical axis, and the vertical bars represent the rewards at the times they are available. The top and bottom panels show hyperbolic discounting and exponential discounting respectively. The curves to the left of the rewards represent their values during times before they are available. The hyperbolic and exponential curves were drawn using equations 3.3 and 3.4 respectively. The key difference is in the shape of the curves; the exponential curves show a constant change in slope, but the hyperbolic curves are relatively flat at the left of the figure and then rapidly rise as the rewards become closer in time.

3.2.2 Temporal Discounting and Substance Abuse

The choice dynamics described in the previous two sections obviously are important for our understanding of impulsivity, substance abuse, and DG. The SSRs and LLRs described in section 3.2.1 are analogous to an alcohol or drug consumption episode and a more valuable but delayed nondrinking or nondrug activity respectively. The choice dynamics that result from hyperbolic discounting are consistent with the ambivalence that is a critical feature of impulsive behavior patterns. That is, even when reward availability does not change, individuals will show ambivalence over time, and their preference for substance use will vary depending on the temporal distance to the availability of the substance and the alternative activity. The LLRs will be preferred before the point at which the reward value curves cross, and substance use will be preferred after that point. But once the person exits the situation involving imminent substance use, preference will revert back to the LLRs and the individual may regret the substance use episode. Such ambivalence is a key feature of impulsive behavioral phenomena.

PE makes a straightforward prediction regarding differences in temporal discounting between problem substance users and normal populations. This prediction is displayed in figure 3.3, which again shows an SSR that is available at time 6 and an LLR that is available at time 10. The reward value curves in both panels of figure 3.3 were drawn using the hyperbolic function in equation 3.3, with the top and bottom panels showing the curves for relatively high and relatively low values of k respectively. The higher k used in the top panel produces steeper value curves than the lower k used in the bottom panel. Preference between the SSR and LLR reverses with the passage of time in both panels, with higher and lower discounting producing sooner and later preference shifts respectively. As suggested by figure 3.3, an individual with a high degree of temporal discounting (top panel) would spend more time preferring the SSR (i.e., substance use) than an individual with a low degree of discounting (bottom panel). This leads to the prediction that k values would be larger among substance abusers than among normal individuals. This prediction has been supported in numerous studies of temporal discounting that compared normal indi-

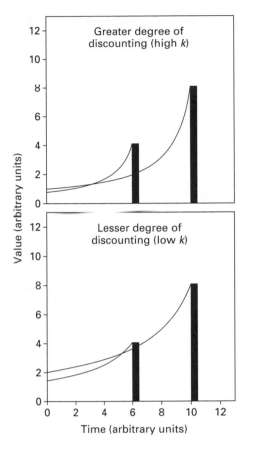

Figure 3.3
Greater and lesser discounting

viduals with problem drinkers, heroin addicts, smokers, cocaine addicts, and disordered gamblers (reviewed in Bickel and Johnson 2003; Bickel and Marsch 2001).

To summarize the discussion so far: BE research on substance abuse and related phenomena has produced significant advances in our knowledge about the nature of these disorders. We now know that demand for addictive substances can be analyzed with the same economic concepts and methods as other commodities. From matching law research we now know that maximizing local rather than global rates of reinforcement, and inconsistent preferences over time between an SSR and an LLR, is the normal state of affairs for humans and other animals. And we now know that one aspect of individuals with substance abuse and other impulsive behavior problems is that they discount the value of future rewards much more so than do individuals without those problems. These basic empirical facts have provided a solid foundation for the development of PE accounts of chronic impulsivity, which are described over the next few sections.

3.3   The Picoeconomics of Impulsivity

To those who suppose that whole adult people maximize a single consistent utility function over the course of their lives, it is surprising and often disconcerting to learn that normal human choice is better modeled by hyperbolic discounting with a systematic tendency for intertemporal preference reversal. As argued by Ross (2005), it does not follow from this, as many suppose, that there is anything wrong with economic theory as the theory of how agents minimize payment of opportunity costs: treating people as meliorators over time is simply equivalent to modeling their behavior as equilibria in bargaining games among shorter-lived agents, following Ainslie (1992, 2001). We will now explain.

In the economic theory of the ideally rational consumer, the agent is modeled as *maximizing* a consistent utility function over the agent's whole life. Ross (2005), following the lead of Schelling (1978, 1980, 1984), emphasizes that the "whole life of the agent" need not mean the "whole life of a person," since there is no reason why biological and psychological persons cannot be modeled as *sequences* of agents that succeed each other over time when their tastes change in ways that, if modeled as changes in the preferences over which a single agent's utility function is defined, would make that function inconsistent. The axioms of microeconomic theory (revealed preference theory, plus Houthakker's axiom) say nothing whatsoever about which entities in the world implement consistent economic agency. Nor is there any metaphysical fact of the matter about which general kinds of things must count as instances of agency a priori. If standard economic theory turns out to be useful in describing the choice behavior of any entities, then let us regard the entities in question as economic agents. Note also that "choice" here carries no necessary connotations of consciousness (although conscious choice is one kind of choice). "Choice" simply denotes implementation of a behavior when alternative behaviors are practically possible and economically assessable, in model-relative senses of "alternative" and "possible" that must be specified in any application. (The point here is simply that we have a meaningful instance of economic choice wherever we can motivate assignment of opportunity costs.) Ross argues that two interesting classes of agents that show the kind of consistency described by conventional micro-economic theory are cephalic animals without a cortex, such as insects, and individual neurons and functionally fused neuronal groups. The agency of the second of these classes, also emphasized by Glimcher (2003), is important for the interpretation of the new research program of NE that we will introduce in chapter 5 and elaborate upon in chapter 8.

For immediate purposes, another class of consistent agents is more important. We will shortly describe Ainslie's (1992, 2001) account of the way in which most people prevent their natural inclination to hyper-bolic discounting from leaving them vulnerable to exploitation and, in general, to lowering their welfare by undoing investments. This account involves modeling the behavior of a whole person as a product of bargaining (in the sense captured by game theory) among *interests* in different possible, alternative consumption schedules. For reasons extensively reviewed by Ross (2005, 2007, forthcoming), and to which we will return in chapter 8, Ainslie's "interests" should not be identi-fied with physical parts of a person's brain. These interests are cases of what philosophers of science call "theoretical entities" (van Fraassen 1980; Ladyman and Ross 2007)—that is, posited kinds of things con-structed as elements of theories that predict empirical phenomena. In this instance, as we will soon see, we can predict and systematize molar-scale behavioral dispositions in people by modeling them as patterns in the bargaining dynamics among conventional economic agents with rival preferences over short-range and long-range con-sumption. Because these subpersonal agents are biologically and socially yoked together, they are forced into strategic interaction that involves both competitive and cooperative aspects; that is, they play non-zero-sum games together.

More details of this picture, with demonstration of its utility as applied to understanding impulsivity and addiction, will be given shortly. For now we want simply to state its implications for the rela-tionship between economic theory and related behavioral sciences as theorized by Ross. A person is a biological, sociological, and psycho-logical entity, not, in the first place, an economic one. Ainslie's subper-sonal interests are, fundamentally, economic entities. (Insects and neurons are biological entities that turn out to map unusually neatly onto economic entities.) Because game theory allows us to model stable patterns—dynamic Nash equilibria—that emerge from the bargaining among these entities, people behave with *enough* consistency that we can model them for periods of time, regulated by institutional and other social constraints, as approximate economic agents. They are analogous to countries in this respect. Countries pursue goals over time, choosing means that promote these goals and paying or refusing to pay opportunity costs for them against limited budgets, with highly imperfect but far from zero consistency. They can and usefully should thus be modeled as utility maximizers in carefully restricted senses. Because of their chronic susceptibility to inconsistency, their economic agency breaks down—across drawn-out time periods, or if their strategic contexts are significantly reframed, or often simply because of unpredictable (from the molar scale) internal disruption. This is just how matters stand, logically, with people. However, their stability as economic agents is in general far more reliable than that of countries because (1) subpersonal interests live in more intimate and repetitive strategic relationships than do compatriot citizens and (2) people are under intense social and cultural pressure from others to be predictable and stable for purposes of interpersonal project coordination. Factor (2) induces people to use their learned public languages to narrate distinctive "characters" for themselves, a process that induces extra consistency through recursive feedback. The relative importance of factors (1) and (2) in explaining the details of personal economic agency vary across people and societies and are regulated by both biological and cultural evolutionary dynamics.

In summary, Ross thus understands the relationship between economic theory and the behavioral and cognitive sciences as follows. Economics is made distinct as a science by its commitment to modeling consistent agency. People are not, in the first instance, economic agents because they are too complex, in both their constitution and their embedding in social and cultural environments, for such agency. However, economics is usefully applied to them in two complementary ways. First, their behavior can be theoretically synthesized as equilibrium patterns in bargaining among subpersonal economic agents, both neuronal and (separately) virtual. Second—and thanks to the first point—economics can be applied to temporal slices of whole people within socially and institutionally constrained contexts. The extent to which a given whole person approximates an economic agent within a frame is variable and requires situational judgment on the part of the modeler—but only the usual kind of situational judgment in using models as filters on reality that all good economists must master as the basic skill of their profession.

In this framework, we can understand the general policy and clinical challenge raised by substance abuse and DG in two complementary ways, so far as economic theory is concerned: (1) Given that individual human beings, not their short time slices, are the units of social accountability, how can we help them better approximate consistent economic agency? (2) How can we help teams of subpersonal agents whose bargaining equilibria have broken down get back onto, and remain on, equilibrium paths?

In the framework of Ross's interpretation, we now outline complementary PE accounts of chronic impulsivity,[8] derived principally from Ainslie (1992), Herrnstein and Prelec (1992), and Rachlin (1997). PE models are grouped into a class as those that take matching, melioration, and hyperbolic temporal discounting as their starting points. They may differ in details regarding which choice dynamic is of primary interest, the breadth of the temporal intervals over which matching occurs, how the alternative objects of choice are organized, and whether there is anything special and distinctive to be said about DG by comparison with the classic pattern of substance dependence as recognized in *DSM*.

Far more than any other author, the behavioral economist and psychiatrist George Ainslie (e.g., 1975, 1992, 2001) has vigorously and extensively pursued the implications of the preference reversals caused by hyperbolic temporal discounting for understanding impulsivity and impulse control in substance abuse, as well as in obsessive-compulsive disorders, dissociative disorders, bulimia, itches, physical pain, and flaws of character.

Hyperbolic discounting can explain impulsive choices that are later regretted, and thus can explain a chronically impulsive person's repeated surrender to temptation, despite earlier resolutions to quit or curtail substance use. That immediately leads to a new puzzle about how such impulsivity can ever be avoided. How do most people, most of the time, resist temptation and exercise self-control? More precisely, why is the LLR ever preferred to the SSR, especially when the SSR is immediately available? Ainslie describes four processes that can be used to subvert preference reversals and thus can lead to choices that are more consistent with long-term interests. All are to be understood as devices whereby interests in long-range welfare improve their strategic bargaining power vis-à-vis shorter-range interests in the sub-personal marketplace.

External commitment

The most obvious self-control tactic is precommitment, meaning the deliberate engineering of the physical or social environment so that the impulsive choice becomes impossible or much more difficult to make. Consider, for example, figure 3.1, in which the LLR is preferred at time 2 but the SSR is preferred at time 12. A long-range interest might induce an individual with this preference pattern to do something at time 2, when the shorter-range interests are weak because their temptations are not at hand, that makes it impossible or very difficult to reverse course and choose the SSR when short-range interests are ascendant at time 12. This device is exemplified by the myth of Ulysses and the Sirens, in which Ulysses chained himself to the mast of his boat before sailing past the deadly temptation of the sirens, whose charms he knew he'd be unable to resist if he left himself free to succumb. Notice that Ulysses thereby showed awareness of his own disposition for intertemporal preference reversal, and used this foreknowledge to block its dangers. According to Ainslie's interpretation, Ulysses' long-range interests stole a march on short-range runs by organizing the world so as to block their efficacy. An obvious example from the substance abuse field is voluntary ingestion of the drug disulfiram, which a problem drinker knows will make her feel very ill if she consumes alcohol. Even pigeons will make precommitments of this sort under carefully set-up conditions (Rachlin and Green 1972); there is bargaining among subpigeonal interests.

Control of attention

Long-range interests sometimes act to restrict in advance the processing of information about the availability of an SSR. This is somewhat similar to the Freudian concept of repression, although it originates from a very different theoretical base. From Ainslie's viewpoint, the avoidance of information, unlike in repression, can be conscious as well as unconscious. For example, a recovering alcoholic may avoid walking past her usual pub. Since interfering with access to information, or with information processing, is a manipulation of the external environment in which subpersonal bargaining takes places, it is possible to see control of attention as a subspecies of external commitment.

Preparation of emotion

This describes attempts by long-range interests to inhibit emotional responses that boost the power of interests in an SSR, or to augment emotions that are incompatible with the individual's appetite for it. In the case of substance abuse, it mainly applies to the cognitive control of so-called "craving" responses. For example, people trying to quit smoking may absorb themselves in pictures of diseased lungs, or put the money they had been spending on cigarettes in a kitty used to reward themselves with periodic indulgences, so as to make vivid to themselves the financial costs of smoking in addition to its health costs.

Personal rules

This process is by far the most important category of methods of self-control described by Ainslie, and the one that is used to create a major extension to Herrnstein's theory as Ainslie found it. This part of Ainslie's work provides a PE account of willpower, the vaguely conceptualized force that is widely believed to be responsible for human resistance to temptations. We will explain personal rules at greater length than the other devices, both because this idea will feature most prominently in later chapters, and because it involves more complexities. It is attention to the dynamics of personal rules that mainly brings out the value of modeling the person's global dispositions as equilibria in bargaining games among subpersonal interests.

The basic case of temporary reversals of preference due to hyperbolic discounting involves a single SSR-LLR pair, as in several of the previous figures. But, of course, in life outside the laboratory many identical or very similar SSR-LLR choices occur repeatedly over time. Personal rules apply to whether and when an individual will perceive a given SSR-LLR pair as a separate choice, or whether she will perceive the choice as being between a whole series of SSRs and a whole series of LLRs. If she perceives the choice in the latter way, she is engaging in the potentially powerful self-control process of reward bundling. Reward bundling is illustrated in figure 3.4, in which time is plotted along the x-axis and reward value is placed along the y-axis. Figure 3.4 shows four SSR-LLR reward pairs spread out at the times they will be available. The solid curves to the left of the rewards were drawn from equation 3.3 and represent the value of the rewards during the times before they are available.

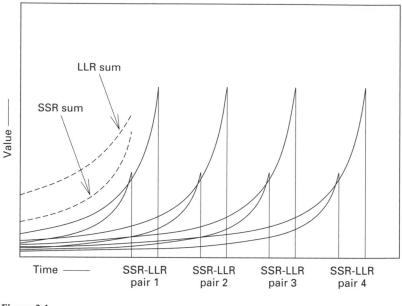

Figure 3.4
Reward bundling

If the person facing this series of choices takes the SSR-LLR pairs one at a time, we would see repeated preference reversals. At the far left of the figure she prefers the pair 1 LLR, but when the pair 1 SSR is imminent, its value rises above that of the pair 1 LLR, so her preference reverses and she chooses the SSR. After pair 1 is past, she faces pair 2. Initially the pair 2 LLR is preferred, but again as the pair 2 SSR becomes imminent, its value rises above that of the LLR and her preference once again reverses. The same thing would then happen for SSR-LLR pairs 3 and 4. This is a common pattern for individuals with chronic impulse control problems. Many people wake up each morning preferring not to do what they did yesterday—not to drink or smoke or gamble or indulge in whatever other self-control problem they have—but then later in the day as the object becomes available they succumb to temptation and indulge.

On the other hand, if the person facing this series of choices did not take them one at a time, but instead viewed her objects of choice as the whole series of SSRs and the whole series of LLRs, we could see more self-control. In figure 3.4, the reward value curves for all four SSRs and all four LLRs are summed during the times before the pair 1 SSR is available. These summed value curves are the dotted lines at the left.

The key point is that the LLR sum is greater than both the SSR sum and the value of the pair 1 SSR at the time the pair 1 SSR is available. So, an individual who viewed this as one choice between series of rewards would prefer the LLR series even when the SSRs are immediately available. This is also a common pattern for individuals without (major) self-control problems. Many people wake up each morning not even thinking about drinking, smoking, or gambling, because they didn't do it yesterday, or the day before yesterday, or the day before that; some time ago they made the choice not to engage in the SSRs and so now are reaping the greater benefits of the LLRs. Research with both animals (Ainslie and Monterosso 2003) and people (Kirby and Guastello 2001) shows that bundling rewards in this fashion produces choices more consistent with long-term interests than with short-term interests.

To avoid a reversal of preference, a person can bundle a whole series of choices together in anticipation of the higher aggregate reward that would be obtained from preferring the LLRs. She does this by adopting personal rules that dictate the choice to be made in a whole class of conflict situations involving the need to delay gratification. These personal rules correspond to the idea of "principles" or "universal rules" of behavior that have been recommended as a means of achieving willpower by philosophers down the ages. The person is seen as committing themselves to a course of action by making private side-bets, a form of personal rule making in which the current choice serves as the best predictor of what future choices will be. If the current SSR is successfully resisted, the bet is won, the expectation of future reward is proportionately strengthened, and the ability to overcome similar temptations in the future is enhanced. On the other hand, if the SSR is not resisted, the bet is lost, and also lost is whatever elements of the person's view of herself had been staked, with a decreased expectation of being able to resist SSRs of the same kind in the future.

Personal rules and private side-bets can be illustrated with figure 3.4. Say the individual has a strict rule mandating her to "only go to the bar for a few drinks on Fridays and legal holidays." If followed, this rule would allow enjoyment of drinking on the designated days but would also produce choices of the LLR over the SSR (drinking) the rest of the time. But when the pair 1 SSR is immediately available on a regular weekday, there is nothing in the physical or social environment that prevents the individual from choosing the SSR or that even makes choosing the SSR much more difficult. What is at stake in the private side-bet is the difference between the summed LLR and SSR value curves at the time the pair 1 SSR is available, because the reward that is chosen from pair 1 strongly predicts the reward that will be chosen from subsequent pairs. If the first SSR is resisted, the individual gets the first LLR plus the enhanced expectation of also getting subsequent LLRs reflected in the LLR sum. On the other hand, if the first SSR is not resisted, she gets that SSR but also gets a reduced expectation of getting any of the subsequent LLRs. Because of the predictive value of current choices for later choices, which is a reward the chooser gets right now as she makes the choice, personal rules can bring into the present the value of rewards in the future and thus allow people to overcome the effects of their natural hyperbolic discounting.

Take, for example, an overweight person who wants to lose weight primarily for health reasons. If he thinks truly seriously about his situation, he can notice that when he chooses to fix or not to fix himself another sandwich, he isn't just choosing between satiation now and sticking with his diet today. If he prefers to be trim in the distant future, his choosing a sandwich now provides him with evidence that he won't choose his diet then either; for hyperbolic discounters, present choices predict future choices. In light of this, perhaps he can frame his present choice to reflect the fact that it isn't just between immediate streams of benefits and costs, but has implications all the way along the flatter part of his discount curve into the future. If all those preferred states of fitness in the future are at stake now, then their value, added together, might be enough to trump the present value of the sandwich. It won't typically be enough for the person just to tell himself this; if it were, self-control would be easy and impulsivity would be mysterious. The would-be dieter needs to arrange his patterns of action so as to make it impossible for him to avoid keeping the future implications of his action in mind while he makes his present choice. Suppose he therefore frames a personal rule to the effect that an extra sandwich is allowed only on a day after he visits the gym. Then, if today isn't a day after a gym session, his choice is between a sandwich *now* and *now* facing the long-term ruin of his personal rule. The key thing to see here is that because present choices predict future choices the personal rule is a presently valuable asset. It bundles a whole series of future benefits and puts them at stake in the present moment. If the individual in our example throws his rule away by breaking it, he will suffer from his knowledge of the loss of it *here*, where discounting is at a minimum.

As explained earlier, Ainslie models personal rules as analogous to laws in a community, which are negotiated by conflicting subpersonal interests in different and competing rewards that, because of hyperbolic discounting, achieve dominance over each other at different points in time. Each appetite for and motivation to acquire each type of reward is described as an interest in that reward, and the interaction between these competing interests is portrayed as an internal economic marketplace. In particular, according to this model, the interests of a present self compete strategically with those of an anticipated future self that may attempt to subvert them. This battle may be complicated by the existence of mid-range interests against which short- and long-range interests may combine forces. This strategic interaction of interests can be illustrated by further complicating the above example of the overweight person. In this example, the short- and long-range interests are vested respectively in the extra sandwich now and being slim and healthy in the future. But there are other interests at intermediate ranges between short and long that may interact with the short- and long-range interests and impact the critical choice to have or not to have that extra sandwich. Say, for example, the man has a mid-range interest in following his favorite football team, and another mid-range interest in getting dates with attractive women. Suppose that on a day he didn't go to the gym, his team happens to be playing a televized game. In this situation, his extra sandwich interest may recruit his sports interest; together the pair will then overcome his future-slim-self interest, and he will choose to watch the game and eat the extra sandwich. Alternatively, imagine that on a day he didn't go to the gym, he meets an attractive woman but makes no overtures because he is overweight. Later, when he gets home, he will be tempted to make the extra sandwich, but the future-slim-and-healthy-self interest could recruit the attractive-date interest, and both together may overcome the extra-sandwich interest; in this case the individual will resist the extra-sandwich temptation, moving him closer to his intermediate and long-range goals of dating attractive women and being slim and healthy.

How are relatively stable choices ever made in this intrapsychic free-for-all of successive motivational states attached to short-range, mid-range, and long-range interests? Here Ainslie borrows concepts used to analyze interpersonal and international conflict and applies them to the intrapersonal bargaining situation. In particular, he models the typical strategic interaction between short-range and long-range

	Defect	Cooperate
Defect	2, 2	0, 4
Cooperate	4, 0	3, 3

Figure 3.5
The prisoner's dilemma

interests using that most famous of all games, the two-person prisoner's dilemma. Its standard strategic form is shown in figure 3.5.

"Cooperate" here denotes strategies by which short-range and long-range interests support one another. "Defect" denotes strategies by which they undermine one another. As is well known, the only Nash equilibrium of the one-shot version of the game is (defect, defect). Since short-range interests are called into being by consumption opportunities and then perish, the partial conflict is not, at least in general, a *repeated* prisoner's dilemma in which every strategy pair is a possible Nash equilibrium. Thus the only way to achieve outcomes not equivalent to war between short-range and long-range interests—which will be manifest as chronic subversion by the person of her own best plans—is for the players to take strategic actions that change the form of the game. We have reviewed Ainslie's list of common examples of such actions, with establishment of personal rules being the most important and ubiquitous. The intricate and subtle arena of competing personal rules and complex intrapersonal bargaining strategies leaves plenty of room for the evasions, distortions, and other forms of self-deception well recognized in the behavior of anyone with chronic impulsivity problems, as well as in ordinary human conduct, and these are carefully deduced by Ainslie from his model.

Ainslie's model might appear to some readers to be too strange and unexpected to be a plausible molar-scale account of such phenomenologically familiar processes as choosing in circumstances that involve temptations. (Note that this objection would not arise if Ainslie's were intended as a molecular-scale account, since people should expect not to have direct perceptual access to mechanisms at that scale.) However, Howard Rachlin (1995) has produced a more intuitive redescription of reward bundling in language consistent with his (and our) version of behaviorism, according to which intentional terms (e.g., beliefs, desires) refer to temporally extended patterns of behavior rather than to internal states.

Rachlin first reminds us that naturally occurring LLRs (e.g., vocational success, marital happiness, health) are typically not discrete, tangible, and temporally circumscribed events. Rather, they are abstractions comprising many smaller rewards that occur over extended temporal intervals in complex but coherent patterns. An individual's behavior is allocated over time to activities that produce a series of relatively small but immediate gratifications (e.g., SSRs associated with alcohol consumption) or that may produce a more temporally extended but more valuable pattern (e.g., the constituent events in the LLR associated with vocational success). But even if an individual were to let every discrete drinking opportunity (SSR) pass by, vocational success would not suddenly arrive fully formed at a specific future time. Rather, as more actions are chosen that are consistent with the molar pattern of vocational success, and as less behavior is devoted to activities that may undermine it, more of the constituent parts of the overall LLR pattern accrue over an extended interval. Rachlin thus proposes a shift away from the discrete SSR versus LLR view of intertemporal choice in order to accommodate those considerations. Hyperbolic discounting indeed produces temporal inconsistencies between short-range and long-range preferences, but rather than focusing on the changing value of a discrete SSR and a discrete LLR over time, perhaps we should consider the idea that the key distinction is between the value of discrete acts and the value of patterns of acts. Rachlin argues that the temporal inconsistencies often found between individuals' preferences at different points in time are better characterized as differences between the value of discrete acts that determine short-term preferences and the value of temporally extended patterns of acts that determine long-term preferences. In this view, behavior in accordance with the higher-valued, long-term preferences entails temporally extended patterns, but the development and maintenance of such patterns may be undermined because their component acts are often relatively less valuable than alternative particular acts that are inconsistent with the patterns in question. Thus, a key issue becomes whether objects of choice are perceived as discrete acts or as parts of patterns.

For example, assume that act x and act y are, respectively, a mildly enjoyable evening at home with the family and a boisterous evening out drinking with friends. Further, assume that pattern a is comprised of a long series of act xs (solid family life) and that pattern b is a long series of act ys (alcohol abuse). When considered as discrete outcomes, act y may have greater value than act x. On the other hand, when considered as single components of wider behavior patterns, pattern a (which includes act x) has greater value than pattern b (which includes act y). When the choice is perceived as being between particular acts in the present, act y is more valuable (in the short term) than act x, so act y tends to be preferred. When the choice is between patterns of acts that extend into the future, pattern a (comprised of a series of act xs) is more valuable (in the long term) than pattern b (comprised of a series of act ys), so pattern a tends to be preferred. Thus, patterns of behavior that are more valuable over long temporal intervals may be comprised of single component acts that individually are less valuable than alternative particular acts. Conversely, patterns of behavior that are less valuable over long temporal intervals may consist in single component acts that alone are more valuable than alternative particular acts.

Viewing the primary units of analysis as patterns of acts, rather than as discrete and atomic acts, is a recent development in the behavioral literature and has not yet inspired much research designed in its light.[9] There is, however, some empirical evidence relevant to the value of behavior patterns. In laboratory experiments, Rachlin and colleagues have shown with both humans (Kudadjie-Gyamfi and Rachlin 1996) and animals (Siegel and Rachlin 1995) that if contingencies are established that generate cohesive patterns in subjects' behavior, then behavioral allocation is more consistent with long-term preferences. There is also some empirical evidence relevant to the relative valuation of patterns of events versus discrete events. Several studies have shown that if future events are part of a temporally extended sequence or pattern, they are assigned greater value than if they are independent events in separate, discrete choices (Chapman 1996a; Frank 1992; Loewenstein and Prelec 1993).

These findings regarding the value of patterns of acts as opposed to atomic acts are inconsistent with a simple model of behavior valuation, according to which values of patterns are computed as the sum of the discounted values of their individual components. For example, assume that four rewards assigned values of 5, 10, 15, and 20 (arbitrary) units will occur in either increasing or decreasing sequence at delays of 2, 4,

6, and 8 (arbitrary) temporal units respectively. Using equation 3.3 with $k = 1.00$, the discounted values of the components of the increasing sequence (5, 10, 15, and 20) would be 1.67, 2.00, 2.14, and 2.22 units respectively, which sums to 8.03 units. The discounted values of the individual rewards in the decreasing sequence (20, 15, 10, and 5) would be 6.67, 3.00, 1.43, and .56 units respectively, which sums to 11.66 units. Even though the decreasing pattern yields a greater sum of the discounted values of the individual components, the studies cited above find that increasing patterns are preferred when the objects of choice are temporally extended sequences of outcomes. Thus, preferences tend to be more future-oriented when the objects of choice are perceived as multicomponent sequences, the value of which accrues over extended time frames. In choices between discrete outcomes, preferences tend to be more present-oriented or impulsive.

Rachlin's account is not an alternative to Ainslie's but a redescription of the framing underlying self-control. We think it is a good deal more intuitive to most people than positing internal prisoner's dilemmas. However, the problem of how to perceptually group discrete acts into extended patterns for purposes of behavioral motivation is simply equivalent to Ainslie's question of how to put the value of future rewards at stake in the present by associating them with personal rules. Then Ainslie's model has the advantage of being amenable to modeling using the well-developed formal resources of game theory. Questions about whether there are "really" subpersonal interests that bargain with one another introduce inappropriate metaphysics into science. These interests are "virtual" entities constructed by models that are empirically adequate to the phenomena. Being virtual—like a user interface programmed by some software—is not a way of being fictitious but a way of being real (Ladyman and Ross 2007, chapter 4).

Ainslie's distinctive contribution to PE (aside from its name) is the account of intrapersonal bargaining around personal rules. The core predictions concerning impulsivity, however, all arise directly from the discovery of hyperbolic discounting and its implication of melioration as the dynamic of intertemporal choice. It follows from this that an individual's choices will tend to be relatively insensitive to global utility and more sensitive to the comparison of local utilities. Obviously, this should make the existence of patterns of chronic substance abuse and other impulsivity less surprising than it would be if people were straightforward implementations of economic agents who discounted exponentially.

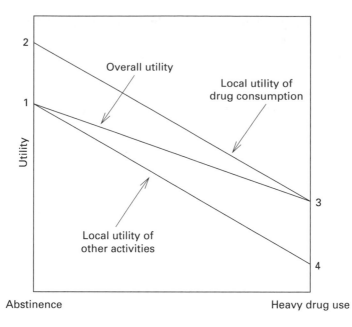

Relative behavioral allocation to drug consumption
(drug consumption/[drug consumption + other activities])

Figure 3.6
Melioration chronic impulsivity

As noted above, a key aspect of the standard pattern of substance dependence according to all BE models, both Becker-style and PE, is that repetitive use lowers the marginal utility derived from each successive episode of consumption while also lowering the marginal utility derived from non-substance use activities. This process is shown in figure 3.6, in which utility is plotted along the vertical axis, and the relative behavioral allocations to substance use and to non-substance use activities are placed along the horizontal axis. The farther to the right along the horizontal axis, the more the individual is choosing substance use and not choosing other activities—the pattern of chronic impulsivity—and conversely for movement to the left. So, at the far right the individual is consuming the substance and doing little else, and at the far left, she is doing a lot of other things and not consuming the substance at all. The local utility of substance use, the local utility of other activities, and global utility are signified by lines 2–3, 1–4, and 1–3 respectively, at the various distributions of choices along the x-axis. Choice according to melioration occurs when the selected options are those yielding the highest local utility at the time. As seen in figure 3.6, increasing levels of substance consumption—movement to the right along the horizontal axis—reduces both local and global utility, but the melioration process continues to drive impulsive consumption because the local marginal utility of that consumption remains higher than the local marginal utility of not consuming.

This model assumes that only events during substance use episodes are included in the computation of local marginal utility derived from substance use. So, the marginal utility derived from an evening of heavy drinking is kept separate from the next morning's hangover. As noted earlier, however, the time intervals over which local marginal utilities are estimated can vary, which can alter the utility calculations. If the temporal boundary of what counts as a source of local marginal utility is expanded, this may alter the computation of local marginal utility so that the value of a substance use episode is changed. In the case of a hungover individual described above, if the time interval over which local marginal utility is calculated is expanded to include the time spent drinking plus the hangover, and not just the drinking, this would reduce the local marginal utility derived from drinking and therefore lower its value. Thus, in principle, the process of altering a chronically impulsive behavior pattern may involve a restructuring of how the choice alternatives are perceived. This is, of course, just another redescription of reward bundling; so once again we are led to Ainslie's methodology for the relevant application of economic analysis.

Rachlin (2000) adds a distinctive element to the general PE model of consumption impulsivity in arguing that targets of such consumption are substitute goods for social interaction. When economists refer to two commodities as substitutes, this amounts to claiming that their consumption varies inversely. Then, according to Rachlin's model, the marginal utility derived from substance consumption and that derived from social interaction changes in opposite ways as these activities are indulged. We noted earlier that, because of tolerance, the marginal utility derived from a given level of substance consumption decreases with increased consumption. On the other hand, the marginal utility derived from a given amount of social interaction increases with total consumption. So, if you have two drinks tonight, those two drinks would provide higher marginal utility (all else being equal) if you haven't had any alcohol for several weeks than if you've been having two drinks every night for several weeks. Conversely, if you encounter a stranger at a bus stop and converse for five minutes, that brief interaction would provide higher marginal utility if you'd recently been socially interacting regularly than if you'd recently been socially isolated. (The assumption here, which we think highly reasonable, is that comfortable socialization requires a standing sense of immersion in society; re-entry from solitude is to some extent awkward.)

Rachlin refers to these changes in utility as the price habituation of substance consumption (because consumption and utility are inversely related) and the price sensitization of social interaction (because consumption and utility are directly related). He frames this in terms of price changes because a given increment of marginal utility costs more or less over time. The more a substance is consumed, the higher the price for a given increment of marginal utility (and vice versa). Conversely, the more one interacts socially, the lower the price for a given increment of marginal utility (and vice versa).

How the price habituation of abused substances and the price sensitization of social interaction can lead to chronic impulsivity is illustrated in figure 3.7. As in figure 3.6, movement to the left along the horizontal axis signifies less substance use and more social interaction, and movement to the right along the horizontal axis signifies more substance use and less social interaction. The utility derived from a given choice of substance use and social interaction is signified by lines 1–3 and 2–4 respectively, at the various distributions of choices along the horizontal axis. The price habituation and price sensitization of substance use and social interaction, respectively, are shown with (linear) curves sloping down to the right. Movement to the right raises the price of both substance consumption and social interaction. (A given increment of marginal utility from either consumption alternative costs more because substance use has been increasing and social interaction has been decreasing.) Conversely, movement to the left lowers the price of both substance consumption and social interaction. (A given increment of marginal utility from either consumption alternative costs less because substance use has been decreasing and social interaction has been increasing.) Given the melioration process, the person will choose the option that provides the highest marginal utility at the time the choice is made.

As an example, assume that over a period of time an individual's choices are stable with a pattern of drinking and social interaction at the point of intersection of lines 1–3 and 2–4 in figure 3.7. This choice pattern involves relatively more social interaction and less substance use. However, suppose an event (e.g., marital separation) then occurs

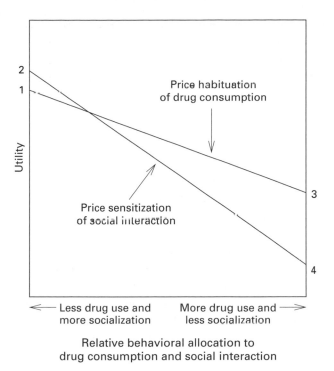

Figure 3.7
Relative chronic impulsivity

that makes social interaction more expensive in the sense that it is now
more difficult to obtain, which would reduce the rate of choice of social
interaction. Because drinking and social interaction are mutually substitutable, the individual begins after the event to drink more in order
to make up for less social interaction (movement to the right along the
horizontal axis in figure 3.7). Because of the price habituation and price
sensitization of drinking and social interaction respectively, drinking
more and socializing less will reduce the marginal utility derived from
both drinking and socializing. But even though both rates of marginal
utility are decreasing as the individual moves to the right, the choice
dynamic of relative addiction theory continues to drive impulsive
choices because the marginal utility from drinking exceeds the marginal utility from social interaction.

Given its focus on the relative benefits and costs of substance consumption and social interaction, Rachlin's model directs our attention
to these variables in trying to predict or alter a chronic impulsivity

behavior pattern. Interventions or other changes that produced a large enough increase in the price of substance consumption and/or a large enough decrease in the price of social interaction could tip the balance of the cost/benefit ratios so that an impulsive individual could successfully implement a personal rule to reduce or eliminate impulsive consumption.

3.4   Extensions of PE Research to Gambling

From the perspective of PE, what is problematic about substance abuse and DG is the same: the person systematically and recurrently invests in both the substance or in gambling, and in measures to curtail substance use or gambling. Economists regard such manifestation of cycling preferences as problematic to a typical person for one basic reason: it allows her to be exploited by consistent agents and/or by institutional structures in such a way as to extract her assets without compensation. In the standard phrase among economists, she can be used as a money pump. Economists have often used this consideration to justify the idea that rationality requires intertemporal preference consistency. The classical money-pump argument works as follows: suppose that an agent prefers (in the sense of behaviorally choosing) some commodity bundle a to bundle b, b to c, and c to a. Then another agent with acyclical preferences could offer her a sequence of trades in which she first surrenders her stock of c for some marginal gain in her stock of b, then surrenders her stock of b for some marginal gain in her stock of a, then finally surrenders her stock of a for some marginal gain in her stock of c. If the agent's utility function in fact conforms to the preference ordering $c > a > b > c$, then there must exist a quantity of c she could be offered in the final trade such that the total value of her final endowment is smaller than that of the stock she started with. Thus, by a series of such sequences, the agent could be drained of all but an infinitesimal proportion of her initial asset stock. Therefore, if agents with acyclical (and otherwise consistent) preferences can exist or evolve, market selection will favor them over agents with cyclical preferences and the latter will go extinct. This could mean either that they perish as entities, if they cannot adjust their behavior, or that the underlying biological or psychological entities are induced to become different economic agents by changing their preferences.

As pointed out by Ross (2005), economists sometimes try to get more work from this argument than it can perform. First, it should not be wheeled out as an ultimate normative *justification* for intertemporal consistency. Such a prescriptive-normative view of the money pump requires an assumption that maximization of the long-run stock of tradable assets must trump all other values as a matter of rationality, a premise that is ludicrous. More subtly, money-pump arguments have been used to justify descriptive claims that actual agents in markets at equilibrium will behave in ways that respect acyclicity because the cyclical entities will have been driven out. The relevance of this claim is doubtful for everyday behaviors that occur in dynamic out-of-equilibrium contexts. A basic limitation on the relevance of money-pump arguments is given by Cubitt and Sugden (2001): serious consequences of vulnerability to money pumps require exploitation by near-omniscient pump operators, and it is far from obvious that such exploiters arise in normal human environments.

This all being admitted, Ross (2005, pp. 346–351) points out that people who exhibit *recurrent* attempts at and breakdowns in establishing personal rules truly are at a socioeconomic disadvantage. It hardly requires omniscience to predict that the person with a history of alcoholism who swears to drink only when she has a reason to celebrate is likely to gradually lower the bar on what is worth celebrating. People usually make their personal rules known to others, because this partially recruits the others in question into the enforcement of those rules: if the personal rule collapses, witnesses are likely to be at least disappointed and perhaps contemptuous. But this is a two-edged sword. People whose personal-rule maintenance behavior has the pattern of which addiction is the stereotype have low social status in most communities (except in outcast communities consisting entirely of other addicts). Ross (2005) suggests that this is especially and increasingly the case in information-intensive societies in which management of risk becomes a preoccupation. There is a sound reason why those regarded as addicts tend to be stigmatized: they make unreliable partners in coordination games, the basic recurring strategic interactions in societies, because their preferences are visibly and chronically unstable. To cite the most obvious manifestation of this, disordered gamblers with even short histories at casinos are likely to be known as such by credit ratings bureaus, and this is likely to harm their prospects. The most serious penalties attached to those who are bad at maintaining personal rules, however, are more subtle: regular demotion to the backs of queues when network favors are allocated in small sets of acquaintances. In these most pervasive clusters of exchange, those regarded as addicts are often allowed or forced to drop out.

We therefore think there is justification, from the perspective of PE, in regarding anyone who exhibits recurrent attempts to erect personal rules against overconsumption of one or more commodities that they also recurrently consume because their personal rules collapse as sharing a problem—that is, as falling into a class for some clinical and policy purposes. This class includes far more people than just substance abusers: it also takes in overeaters, extreme procrastinators, and even, as Ainslie argues, those who have difficulty sleeping because they can't stop thinking while lying in bed about itches they could scratch. Obviously, the class includes all those to whom *DSM-IV* intends to refer in its definition of PG, along with many other people who do not meet enough of the criteria to fit the diagnosis, but who repeatedly try to reduce their gambling frequency or amounts gambled or both, and who repeatedly find these variables creeping back up again. This wider class is the class of disordered gamblers, in the usage we have adopted.

Evidently, the class of disordered gamblers (like any class of agents individuated using elements of economic theory) is constructed on the basis of *behavioral* criteria. It is thus open to someone to wonder whether the members of this class have any interesting *non*behavioral properties in common that are also distinctive to those with their shared problem, and not simply common consequences of it. In the case of disordered gamblers (as for cocaine abusers, heavy smokers, etc.), an obvious question to ask is whether they also exhibit distinctive neural properties. People with strong prior reductionist hunches might suppose that they must. It is true, of course, that everyone who gambles more than they like to has to have this behavioral disposition coded somewhere in their brain. However, it is very far indeed from obvious that all people who share the behavioral profile of DG share *similar* relevant neural correlates, especially of clinically marked subtypes; compare, imaginatively, the disordered gambler whose problem is an excess of machismo with the disordered gambler from a poor community who finds the glamour of the casino irresistibly alluring. Are they likely, a priori, to have a common clinical neural signature?

In chapter 6 we will present evidence for thinking that almost all *pathological* gamblers—that is, the class to which *DSM-IV* tries to refer—in fact *do* share a common clinical neurochemical profile, and that this licenses our regarding them as true addicts. This will make the new subdiscipline of NE relevant to modeling them. However, since the class of disordered gamblers is larger than the class of pathological gamblers, and since it is highly doubtful that the disordered gamblers who are not pathological gamblers share any one distinctive clinically marked neural condition, we think that the "top-down" modeling principles of PE need to be integrated with the "bottom-up" modeling principles of NE in developing the overall science and policy of DG. Thus we think that the domain of DG exemplifies the relevance of the hybrid PE/NE account of the frontier between economic theory and cognitive science promoted by Ross (2005).

In the remainder of this chapter and throughout the following one, we will focus on PE models of, and PE-inspired studies of, DG. We will turn to PG more specifically, and to NE, in chapter 5.

As applied to DG, the LLRs would appear to be the same as those contrasted with substance abuse: adaptive functioning in key life-health areas such as intimate, family, and social relations, and vocational success. The SSRs are different, however, because the gambler does not take anything into her body as the substance abuser does. Neuroscience is now telling us about this difference in detail, and we will describe these advances in chapter 5. In any case, the apparent irrationality of the disordered gambler and of the substance abuser or addict are the same: at time t_1 they truthfully report that they want to gamble less or not at all so as to improve their lives in more important ways, but at time t_2 that stated preference reverses and they gamble. Later, at time t_3, when regret sets in, they are confronted again with their inconsistent preferences for a better life and excess gambling.

In the remainder of this section we will discuss Ainslie's and Rachlin's specific perspectives as applied to DG. Both models are entirely consistent with each other, but they focus on different aspects of impulsivity and self-control. Because Rachlin's model of impulsivity in general is consistent with Ainslie's, and then adds to it a particular account of DG, all policy and intervention implications of Ainslie's model will carry over to Rachlin's and then be supplemented by it. We should make clear that all that is being attempted at this point is logical extrapolation from theoretical perspectives. We will turn to the implications of direct empirical studies in the succeeding chapters of this book. Also note that at this point we will only briefly mention practical implications, as they will be spelled out in considerably more detail in chapter 6.

We will first discuss how Ainslie's model can be used to conceptualize the choices faced by the disordered gambler. As noted earlier, in this case the SSRs are opportunities to gamble and the LLRs are quality of life concerns in other areas. As in figure 3.4, the gambler faces a long series of such choices. Any of Ainslie's self-control tactics discussed earlier (external commitment, control of attention, preparation of emotion, and personal rules) could be brought to bear to make current choices more consistent with long-term interests. We will focus, however, on personal rules (reward bundling), because this is by far the most important self-control tactic and the one with the most extensive implications.

An individual could develop personal rules that are in force before she even enters the casino. As with the earlier discussion of rules regarding drinking, a gambler could, for example, generate a rule according to which she can only go to the casino on Fridays and holidays. If followed, this rule would allow her to enjoy gambling (the SSR) on a relatively small number of designated days, and also enjoy the greater benefits of the LLRs on days she is not gambling. The more times the rule is followed, the stronger it will become as she develops heightened expectations of continuing to be governed by it in the future and in reaping the benefits of the LLRs. As with all personal rules, however, it will always be vulnerable to being broken if a strong enough coalition of interests assembles to subvert it. If given an opportunity, the short-range interest in gambling could recruit a mid-range interest to its side of the conflict and subvert the rule. Suppose, for example, that on a Friday in the casino the gambler meets an attractive man who asks her if she will be back on Saturday night. Rigid adherence to the rule would require her to say "no," which she may well do. But as Saturday night approaches, her mid-range interest in dating attractive men could combine with the short-term interest in gambling again on Saturday, which may be enough to overwhelm the long-range interest, and the rule. If she gambles on Saturday she has broken the rule, and in so doing has now reduced her present expectation of rule following in the future and of receiving future LLRs.

Gamblers can (and do) also develop personal rules that are in force while they are in the casino. As an example, suppose there are two gamblers, a and b, and that a has no personal rules regarding the extent of his gambling while in the casino. For a, with no rule, there is nothing at the moment that can bring possible future LLRs to bear on his current decisions. With nothing to connect his present self, which strongly prefers the SSRs of gambling, to his future self, which will prefer the LLRs, the SSRs will have their way with his decisions and he will gamble until he runs out of money or the casino closes. On the other hand, suppose b has a rule that states: "I'll count my money every hour. If I'm losing money at the count I'll leave the casino. If I'm winning money at the count I'll stay another hour, but under no conditions will I stay longer than three hours." At each count b faces the choice of doing what the rule dictates, or continuing to gamble. If he follows the rule, then it becomes stronger and he has increased his present expectation of continuing to reap LLRs in the future; if he breaks it he will bring on the reverse present expectation. If the rule collapses and he fails to generate another, effective one, he will be in the same situation as gambler a. Of course, like rules in force outside the casino, rules for choices inside the casino can be subverted by a coalition of interests. Suppose that b is losing money at the hour-two count, and the rule enjoins him to leave the casino. But it happens that 15 minutes ago a valued business contact arrived at the table and had been looking at him expectantly. His short-term interest in continuing to gamble could coalesce with the mid-range interest in networking, and together they may subvert the rule.

Rachlin's relative account of impulsivity supplements Ainslie's emphasis on intrapersonal bargaining with additional, specific implications for gambling behavior. Rachlin assumes that gambling behaves like the consumption of addictive substances in two ways. First, the more one gambles, the less utility one derives from a given amount of gambling. In other words, gambling is price-habituated like drugs and alcohol, so there is an inverse relation between the extent of gambling and the utility derived from gambling. Second, gambling is mutually substitutable with social interaction, so the less one gambles, the more one interacts socially (and vice versa). We note that although the second hypothesis is plausible where young or middle-aged people are concerned, it is probably backwards in the case of many older people. To the extent that we find elderly people who simultaneously experience gambling problems and enjoy a large share of their social contacts in casinos or other betting venues, humane policy would not simply consist in an aggressive campaign against DG.

Rachlin (1990) is the only PE theorist to date who has an explicit and specific model of DG. According to this model, a person at risk for PG is prey to an insidious perceptual process or accounting scheme. We will introduce the idea by referring the reader back to our earlier discussion of Herrnstein's point that the size of the behavioral unit over which utility is calculated is not carved in stone. With drinking, for example, is the utility calculated by adding up each individual sip, each drink, or each drinking episode, or each drinking episode plus the hangover? In that same discussion, we also noted that recovery from chronic impulsivity may involve a process of restructuring the alternatives so that the behavioral unit over which utility is calculated is made larger. An individual whose drinking behavioral unit also included the next day's hangover would be more likely to reduce their drinking than an individual whose behavioral unit included only the night of drinking itself.

In the case of gambling, the question of the behavioral unit over which utility is calculated concerns how bets are aggregated into larger units. At one extreme end of a continuum, each bet could be seen as a single, independent event. Alternatively, at the other end of the continuum, each visit to the casino could be seen as a single, independent event (where an "event" just names the unit used for cost-benefit analysis by the person). Rachlin (1990) argues that the disordered gambler sorts her gambles into strings in which each string terminates with a win. That is, she thinks of each win as redeeming the sequence of losses that preceded it, regardless of how long that sequence was in any given case. Her losses redeemed, the disordered gambler is ready to start a new sequence, with a clean record (to her internal regulator) following every nod from lady luck. This perceptual or bookkeeping scheme interacts with hyperbolic discounting in an insidious way. Each string the gambler perceives will have the form of a win preceded by n losses where $n \geq 0$. It is the sequences in which n is largest that account for most of the financial distress—this is what makes problem gambling a problem. But now: the overall outcomes of long sequences will have their values hyperbolically discounted relative to the elements of short sequences. Long sequences, as noted, are where the losses are disproportionately concentrated. Thus, the gambler weights wins after short strings at closer to their full value than wins after long strings, with the average discrepancy being greater the worse the ratio of wins to losses.

Let us show an example. Ls and Ws below represent sequences of losses and wins, respectively, in a simple game of tossing a coin:

WLWLLWWLLLWLLLWWWWLLWW

	W	LW	LLW	W	LLLW	LLLW	W	W	W	LLW	W
Undiscounted	+1	0	−1	+1	−2	−2	+1	+1	+1	−1	+1
Discounted	+1	0	−.33	+1	−.67	−.67	+1	+1	+1	−.33	+1

Figure 3.8
Gambling accounting schemes

There are 11 wins and 11 losses in the string, so as a whole it is neither positive nor negative in value. In the same W–L sequence somewhat modified above in figure 3.8, the outcomes are organized as in Rachlin's model, with each substring terminating with a win. The numbers in the top row of figure 3.8 represent the overall outcome for each substring. Summing the outcomes of the substrings again results in zero, so the overall outcome is neither positive nor negative. Importantly, however, because the W that terminates each substring is some distance into the future when the string begins, the present value of the overall outcome of the substring will be discounted. Using the hyperbolic discount function in equation 3.3, with k equal to 1 and delay arbitrarily indexed as unit-equivalent to the number of coin tosses in the substring, the discounted overall value of each substring is shown in the bottom row of figure 3.8. Summing the discounted values of each substring yields a value of 4, a decidedly positive overall outcome. Because of this perceptual organization of behavioral units into strings terminating in a win, the disordered gambler perceives positive value when in reality, in this example, the overall outcome is neutral. As a result of perceptual organization and hyperbolic discounting, the disordered gambler fools himself into perceiving positive value where in fact there is none.

This looks like a disastrous way to think, so it is initially surprising that, as Rachlin documents, animal behavior suggests it to be common in nature. Why would natural selection have built so perverse a perceptual quirk? The answer, presumably, is that in normal environments rewards are distributed in a patchy way. Thus, when an animal finds any reward in an area, it should persist through some disappointments in searching the region further. But modern gambling environments, unlike any in nature, are built to exploit the bias for following up reward. Lucky rolls of the dice are *not* distributed in patches. Thus a disposition that was helpful to our ancestors is harmful to many contemporary people.

3.5   Temporal Discounting Revisited

Our earlier discussion of temporal discounting mentioned only Samuelson's standard exponentially discounted utility model and the PE alternative to it. We thereby passed over most of the huge literature on the topic, which has been comprehensively reviewed by Frederick, Loewenstein, and O'Donoghue (2003). Their historical summary shows that pre-Samuelson economists had speculated about a number of psychological factors, based on introspection and casual observation, that may influence intertemporal choice, and that all these factors were collapsed together into Samuelson's exponential discount rate. Frederick, Loewenstein, and O'Donoghue (p. 15) assert that the warm embrace by economists of the discounted utility model was "due largely to its simplicity and its resemblance to the familiar compound interest formula, and not as a result of empirical research demonstrating its validity." They therefore regard it as unsurprising that the exponential discount function has fared poorly in empirical studies of the issue. Frederick, Loewenstein, and O'Donoghue conclude their review by arguing that the post-Samuelson unitary concept of time preference should be "unpacked" to better reflect the pre-Samuelson acknowledgement of diversity of psychological motives in intertemporal choice, but this time with a vigorous empirical agenda.

We agree that understanding intertemporal choice in people and other animals requires empirical (including experimental) research rather than a priori speculation or formal modeling by itself. However, for reasons mustered by Ross (2005) and Gul and Pesendorfer (forthcoming), we do not favor the collapse of economics into psychology. In PE models, subpersonal interests are conventional economic agents. As we will see in chapter 5, the same is true of neurons and groups of neurons in NE. It is of course true that Samuelsonian microeconomics generally empirically fails if applied to people over inappropriately long timescales, across significant shifts in institutional context, or without regard to the vulnerability of personal rules against preference reversal to collapse. However, it is perfectly possible to apply standard microeconomics with careful attention to all of these considerations. We will return to these issues at greater length in chapter 8.

Where problematically impulsive consumers are concerned, we have the paradigm class of instances in which people do not behave like economic agents. A main burden of argument in this book is to show that even with respect to this phenomenon, the best recourse is not to simply abandon economics in favor of psychology. PE uses standard microeconomics to model subpersonal interests, and classical economic game theory to model their interactions, equilibria of which constitute patterns in personal behavior. NE, as we will see in chapter 5, indispensably deploys economic theories of value to deliver understanding of the brain dysfunctions that constitute true addiction. Finally, we will argue in chapter 8, PE and NE are both required for comprehensive explanation of impulsive consumption in general. Of course, we do not deny that psychology and other behavioral sciences have essential roles to play. Our point here is just that their contributions can be distinguished from those of economics.

The BE literature on time preference massively exceeds what we could attempt to cover in a book for which this is only an indirect, although crucially important, topic. In this chapter devoted to PE theory, we will introduce a subset of the critical literature relevant to two purposes: (1) defending our selection of equation 3.3 as currently the best expression of the relation between delay and reward value, and (2) preparing the groundwork for our later efforts, in chapter 8, to defend the combined use of PE and NE in modeling DG against alternative approaches that would collapse PE entirely into NE.

Daniel Read (2001, 2003) and George Loewenstein (1996) challenge the current dominance of the hyperbolic discounting model of intertemporal choice, preference reversals, and impulsivity. We will describe these challenges here, along with some critical commentary, and then return to a more extensive discussion of these issues in chapter 8. The later discussion will benefit from availability of the extensive body of knowledge about DG that will have been laid out in the intervening chapters. However, the present outline of PE would be grievously incomplete if we did not mention its important critics. The reader should know that our review of theory and evidence about DG in the following chapters comes filtered through a conceptual model that is not entirely uncontroversial.

Read (2001, 2003) argues that discounting is subadditive rather than hyperbolic. Subadditivity refers to assignment of different values or different estimates of probability to reward bundles when they are judged as wholes and when they are judged on the basis of decomposition into their component parts. The summed judgments of the values of the decomposed parts do not always equal the judgments of the values of whole bundles, according to Read. As applied to temporal discounting, if a whole interval, say 24 months, is divided into three eight-month intervals, subadditivity implies that the aggregated rate of discounting over the three eight-month intervals might not equal the discounting that would be applied over the 24 months as a whole, with discounting being proportionally greater over the shorter intervals. Read's (2001) experimental data are consistent with this prediction.

Read distinguishes between *interval* and *delay*, where interval is the time between the SSR and the LLR, and delay is the time between the present (the moment of choice) and the LLR. Based on this distinction, he advances a critical methodological point against the main discounting literature in noting that the vast majority of studies have had subjects choose between an immediate reward and a delayed reward at various delays. The typical finding from those studies, consistent with hyperbolic discounting, has been decreasing impatience—i.e, lower degrees of discounting at longer delays. But, as Read points out, because the SSR is usually immediately available in this paradigm, the paradigm confounds interval and delay, raising the possibility that observations interpreted as decreasing discounting at longer delays may actually be due to decreasing discounting over longer intervals, and may have nothing to do with delay per se. This point is important and needs to be incorporated into future research on hyperbolic discounting, but it does not undermine the entire literature. Both animal (Chung and Herrnstein 1967; Mazur 1987) and human (Green, Myerson, and Macaux 2005; Kirby and Herrnstein 1995) studies that do not confound interval and delay nevertheless find hyperbolic discounting to be a function of delay.

Read (2001, 2003) attributes some "predictions" to hyperbolic discounting models that these models in fact do not make. For example, after computing some hypothetical hyperbolic discount rates of magnitudes similar to those suggested by Ainslie, Herrnstein, and others for food rewards, Reid complains that "Someone who discounts the future in this way would choose $27,000 today over $1 million in one year, $14,000 over $1 million in two years, $8,000 over $1 million in three years, and so on" (2003, pp. 316–317), which he says is "absurd" (p. 317). A theory that made such predictions would indeed be absurd, but the main hyperbolic discounting literature does not do so. Ainslie (1992, pp. 228–234) discusses at length the several reasons (e.g., cash pricing over myriad goods, interpersonal competition) why financial transactions are especially amenable to reward bundling, which makes choices in this realm strongly resemble those of an exponential discounter. As we noted, the fact that people are imperfect examples of economic agency does not imply that they never approximate such agency. This is why economic theory works especially well in application to institutional domains governed by exchanges of money.

Loewenstein (1996) and Read (2001) also criticize PE for not dealing adequately with "visceral" factors that influence intertemporal choice. Loewenstein's main point in this connection is that impulsivity, behaving now in a way contrary to one's long-term interests, mainly occurs when "under the influence of visceral factors such as hunger, thirst, or sexual desire" (p. 279), and that "the hyperbolic discounting perspective has difficulty accounting for such situation- and reward-specific variations in impulsivity" (p. 279). We regard this criticism of PE as deeply misplaced. Loewenstein (1996, p. 289) explains that "[t]he decision theory paradigm . . . is the product of a marriage between cognitive psychology and economics. . . . Decision theory is thus the brilliant child of equally brilliant parents. With all its cleverness, however, decision theory is somewhat crippled emotionally, and thus detached from the emotional and visceral side of life." This ignores the fact that economics has had more than one lover, and the union of economics with the behavioral analysis of choice (e.g., Rachlin and Laibson 1997) is what begat PE as a specific branch of BE more generally. Unlike the emotionally stunted decision theory, PE is well adjusted and fully appreciates the power of motivational states over choice. In fact, it would be fair to say that "visceral factors" are at the very foundation of PE. After all, the initial data that revealed hyperbolic discounting (Chung and Herrnstein 1967) were from animals responding for food while they were very hungry—that is, while they were under the influence of raging visceral states, as is true of the vast subsequent animal literature on the topic. Ainslie (1992) extensively discusses the role of drive and appetite in the bargaining between subpersonal interests, and convincingly shows how hyperbolic discounting could have evolved via natural selection operating in periods of intense scarcity and deprivation (pp. 85–88). More empirically, Logue and colleagues (Kirk and Logue 1997; Logue and Peña-Correal 1985) showed that humans' choices for food and liquid rewards under varying levels of deprivation (i.e., visceral states) were well accounted for by the matching law, including hyperbolic discounting. Clearly, then, PE has neither conceptual nor empirical difficulties with visceral factors in the situations so far studied. It is *because* of a reward's visceral properties that it constitutes an SSR in the first place, and conjures into being a short-range interest in its consumption.

Nevertheless, several of Loewenstein's arguments are important and deserve comment in connection with our perspective. First, Loewenstein (1999) emphasizes conditioned craving as an important determinant of relapse among substance abusers. Such classical conditioning effects do not in any way contradict the PE account. Instead, they merely indicate that no single perspective can explain every aspect of these complex phenomena. For example, Vuchinich and Tucker (1996) found that alcoholic relapse episodes due to the imminent availability of alcohol were less severe than episodes due to reduced access to rewards in important life-health areas. This difference may correspond to the difference between Loewenstein's visceral factors and more molar changes in the economic context that promote substance use. Similar distinctions between biological (e.g., exposure to food or to cues correlated with different rates of reward) and economic (contingencies of reward) influences are routinely made in the animal literature (e.g., Green and Holt 2003; Green and Rachlin 1975), and these influences complement rather than contradict one another.

Second, Loewenstein (1996, 1999) emphasizes that people routinely underestimate the effect that past and future visceral states will have on future behavior, thus neglecting to incorporate the influence of these states in making present choices. For example, an abstinent substance abuser may reinitiate consumption in part because he fails to remember the effect of past craving on drug use, and thus underestimates the extent to which future craving will make it difficult to quit. We are unaware of any direct empirical evidence for this suggestion, but in any case it is quite consistent with a general notion of discounting in which temporally distant events have diminished effects in the present.

Third, Loewenstein, comparing dessert and petrol (Hoch and Loewenstein 1991), and Read (2001), comparing hamburgers and computer paper, make the useful point that issues regarding impulsivity and self-control arise much more often around the former than the latter types of rewards. This must surely be admitted. However, we think that Loewenstein and Read both exaggerate the significance of the point when they cite it as evidence that instances of impulsivity are completely explained by imminent visceral factors and that temporal discounting of reward value is unrelated. In Read's words (2001, p. 28), "Dynamic inconsistency of this sort does not require hyperbolic discounting, but only an *immediacy effect*. . . . This means that we put a lot more decision weight on immediate relative to delayed pleasure or pain. An immediacy effect is *not* declining impatience, but rather a one-time-only charge for delaying consumption." This is obviously incompatible with the PE account, but our full response to this issue must wait until chapter 8, when we will have more elements of our thesis in place. Here we will simply note and emphasize that time-based preference reversals, which are predicted by hyperbolic discounting, do occur with purely instrumental goods and with money (e.g., Kirby and Herrnstein 1995) under conditions in which Read's distinction between delay and interval is not confounded.

We'll now begin to lay the groundwork for our later efforts to relate the concepts of PE to those of NE. As noted repeatedly, hyperbolic discounting predicts preference reversals in intertemporal choice. Laibson (1997), studying savings-related financial transactions, shows that this *qualitative* property of hyperbolic discounting can be captured by a discount function of the form $v_i = A_i \beta \delta^D$, with v_i representing the present value of a delayed reward, A_i the amount of that reward, β a constant discount factor for all delayed rewards, δ the per-period exponential discount factor, and D the delay of the reward. This discount function was originally employed by Phelps and Pollack (1968) to study intergenerational wealth transfers. In such so-called "β-δ" (beta-delta) discounting, value drops precipitously from no delay to a one-period delay, but then declines more gradually (and exponentially) over all periods thereafter. Laibson's (1997) initial motivation for employing β-δ discounting was apparently primarily pragmatic, as he noted that "When $0 < \beta < 1$, the discount structure . . . mimics the qualitative property of the hyperbolic discount function, while maintaining most of the analytical tractability of the exponential discount function" (p. 450). β-δ discounting has in fact proven to be a powerful analytic tool in the analysis of a number of intertemporal choice phenomena in economics (e.g., Laibson 1998; Laibson, Repetto, and Tobacman 1998; O'Donoghue and Rabin 1999).

Although β-δ discounting may initially have been viewed primarily as a pragmatic analytic tool, more recently it has acquired deeper theoretical significance through being merged with Loewenstein's (1996) ideas regarding the centrality of visceral factors in explaining intertemporal choice pathologies (e.g., McClure et al. 2004). In this merger, the δ discount factor refers to a more deliberative cognitive process mainly concerned with long-range interests, while the β discount factor refers to a more impetuous discounting process concerned with visceral factors. Thus, a reward at any delay is judged *in the absence of visceral factors* (the presence of β discounting), but visceral factors can then overwhelm the more deliberative δ process when the reward is immediately present (and β discounting is absent). As summarized by Rachlin (1996, p. 297), in this model "behavior is the outcome of a fight taking place somewhere in the brain between an internal cognitive decision process and visceral factors." In an fMRI study, McClure et al. (2004) attempted to locate these opposing discount factors in different brain regions—the δ factor in cortical areas, and the β factor in areas associated with the midbrain reward system. Their results showed increased (attributed) β system activation only when one of the choice options was immediately available, and increased (attributed) δ system activation across all choices regardless of delay, which they took to support their hypothesis.

On this account, which we might appropriately call "neural realist complex discounting," β-δ discounting is a challenge to hyperbolic discounting rather than an approximation to it made for analytical purposes. The implications are much more general, however. PE is a molar account of intertemporal choice that makes no pretense to describing any molecular mechanisms. In identifying molar-scale behavioral patterns with molecular-scale discounting by parts of the brain, McClure, Laibson, and colleagues implicitly promote the elimination of PE by NE. This meets with favor from economists Gul and Pesendorfer (2001, 2005, forthcoming) because, among other considerations, it allows economics to remain strictly partitioned from psychology: the former can study discounting by itself, while the latter studies impulsivity as a response to visceral influences. As noted, our contrary perspective is that while (micro)economics should indeed not be collapsed into psychology, it offers a valuable, indeed essential, contribution to our understanding of substance dependence and DG. These contributions arise both on the molar scale of explanation, through PE, and on the molecular scale, through NE. We turn now to making this case.

4

Behavioral and Psychological Investigations of Disordered Gambling

4.1 Models and Experiments

This chapter reviews empirical findings regarding substance abuse and DG from behavioral fields, and assesses their implications with respect to the PE theoretical model. The later part of the chapter looks forward to issues around the methodological and modeling interface between behavioral and neuroscientific studies, which will occupy the subsequent chapters of the book. The concepts around which the review of research is organized are consumption impulsivity as defined by BE, PE, and personality psychology. We will also consider data bearing on our behavioral thesis emerging from cognitive neuroscience. Behavioral and cognitive approaches to choice and decision-making have been pursued in relative independence for decades (but see Rachlin 1987 for an interesting integrative effort). We will not dwell here on the various causes of this bifurcation or on what has kept it alive. Rather, we mention the (happily disintegrating) split because our hybrid model of DG, to be defended in chapter 8, aims among other things to repair it where our target phenomenon is concerned.

Though scientists are and should be opportunistic in assimilating empirical data, clear progress requires that experiments be designed around the predictions and conceptual regimentation afforded by a clear underlying model of the phenomena under investigation. Among the social and behavioral sciences, the glory of economics is its tradition of rigorous and exact models. PE offers a platform for exploiting this tradition in the psychology of intertemporal choice. A preliminary way of making this point is negative: some leading research paradigms in the area, while useful up to a point, yield at best equivocal insight because they are not model-driven.

A popular tool for investigating the interanimation of choice behavior and cognition has been the so-called Iowa Gambling Task (IGT) (e.g., Bechara, Tranel, and Damasio 2000). In this experimental paradigm, subjects choose cards from four decks. The cards are face down, so subjects are uncertain about the consequences of each choice. Each subject can choose a card from any deck at any time, and is told to try to maximize her earnings over the course of the task. Each card leads to some combination of winnings and penalties—for example, winning $250 and paying $50. Unknown to the subjects, two of the four decks are "bad" decks in which large wins are on average more than cancelled out by regular penalties, so that consistently choosing from those decks is guaranteed to result in net loss. The two other decks are "good" decks in which the balance of rewards and penalties favors the subject who persists with those decks, even though the rewards associated with individual cards are generally smaller. A standard implementation of the test involves turning 100 cards, although subjects aren't told this. The performance measure is determined by counting the changing proportion of choices from good and bad decks made as the subject is exposed to more and more cases of the effects of choosing from each deck. Most subjects start allocating their choices roughly equally, and a "normal" or "healthy" subject should learn to make increasingly fewer selections from the bad decks as they proceed through the task.

Some researchers have found that subjects with substance dependence (including for alcohol, cocaine, and methamphetamine) perform poorly at the IGT compared to normal controls (Bechara and Martin 2004[1]). The same has been found for patients on a methadone maintenance program attempting to recover from heroin addiction (Mintzer and Stitzer 2002); furthermore, the effect is worse for subjects who are also smokers (Rotheram-Fuller et al. 2004). Long-term heavy users of marijuana are also poor at the IGT (Whitlow et al. 2004). This suggests that, at least some of the time, the IGT sorts relatively impulsive people into one pile and the others into another pile in the same way, roughly, as measures of discounting.

From the perspective of PE, the IGT is a rather peculiar instrument. Apparently there is no good reason to have four decks rather than two. Indeed, a variation of the task developed for use with children dispenses with half of the decks for the very reason that the extra two aren't required, or even distinguished in scoring the performance of subjects (Kerr and Zelazo 2004). There is also enough that the subjects don't know to confound interpretation of some of their behavior. They don't know for sure what the gains from any deck will be, even though those are fixed for each deck. This means that, unlike options in a PE discounting task, choices don't directly convey information about the individual subject's response to risk, even though the risk of gains and punishment is important in the procedure. As subjects perform the task they do get exposed to information about the frequency and magnitude of penalties in each deck, but don't ever know those contingencies in advance of their choices. Again, interpretation of the results cannot clearly say whether the behavior of subjects is telling us something about their preferences, for example that they favor the bad decks just as they favor all risky options, or their ignorance, in cases where they fail to come to understand that these decks are bad at all. (There is a variation on the Iowa task that makes the likelihoods known up front for this reason [Brand et al. 2005].) No matter what subjects know, their choices involve a confusing mixture of delayed and probabilistic rewards and penalties. That is, if they assume (tacitly) that the remainder of each deck is roughly similar to what they have so far experienced the rest of the deck to be, their view of that deck will include a mixture of frequencies and probabilities of gains and losses of various sizes in a way that leaves it quite unclear without additional measurement how their choices relate to their individual discount curves for delay and probability.

More recent work has suggested that some of what the IGT has purportedly measured may not be what it was intended to measure. A team of Taiwanese researchers has developed a variant of the task, called the Soochow Gambling Task, in which the "good" and "bad" decks have the same average net earnings as in the IGT, but where the frequency of rewards is different. This research has found that normal subjects (that is, subjects who were not brain-damaged in areas known to correlate with bad IGT performance) who did "well" at the IGT made mostly bad choices in the Soochow Task when the frequency of reward from the bad decks was high. On the basis of this work some of the early research on the IGT has been reinterpreted, suggesting that frequency of reward is a much more important determinant of how normal subjects behave (Chiu et al. 2005). It also appears as though nearly half of normal subjects perform poorly at the IGT (Glicksohn, Naor-Ziv, and Leshem 2007).

Given this, some dissociations between IGT measurements and discounting ones are not surprising. In contrast to some results we consider shortly, showing that cigarette smoking is associated with steeper delay discounting, it seems as though worsened IGT performance is *not* associated with smoking (Harmsen et al. 2005). This result tentatively suggests that IGT performance is to some extent independent of discounting. Nonetheless, in a population of methadone-maintenance subjects, smoking *was* associated with further worsened performance at the IGT than was the case for nonsmoking patients (Rotheram-Fuller et al. 2004). This result has been tentatively taken to suggest that IGT performance, like discount rates, is cumulatively associated with multiple consumption problems.

A further complication is that the association between education and IGT performance seems to be the opposite of what is found in the case of delay discounting. That is, more years of education is associated with less steep discounting for delay (Jaroni et al. 2004), but with worse performance at the IGT (Evans, Kemish, and Turnbull 2004).[2] This is despite the fact that in general IGT performance improves with age (Hooper et al. 2004[3]), even if some older subjects undergo a decline (Denburg, Tranel, and Bechara 2005). We also know that administration of testosterone leads to worsened performance on the IGT in young women (Van Honk et al. 2004).

Because no stable underlying model motivated the demonstrations of these various and conflicting correlations, they don't seem to take us far in the direction of enlightenment about relationships between gambling and the wider cognitive and behavioral economy in which it is integrated. Let us hasten to add that data are data and should never be resented. But steady forward progress requires an experimental agenda driven by a model. PE furnishes us with a candidate.

4.2　Distinguishing Delay and Probability Discounting

Having stressed the importance of modeling, let us remind ourselves that useful models are not based on mere hunches about mechanisms. Establishment of carefully isolated and accumulated correlations is an essential part of the input. A body of work has been directed at testing the simple idea that substance abusers and disordered gamblers are more impulsive, in one or another more general sense (but see chapter 8), than appropriate control subjects. Of course, such correlations do not by themselves tell us anything about causation. That is, they don't indicate whether the individuals in question became abusers because of an earlier predisposition to be more impulsive, or whether use (or abuse) of a substance made them more impulsive. Both these paths of influence could hold: some people may be more prone to immoderate substance use because of being less patient, and consumption might then make them still more impulsive, so that they become addicts with time.

One obvious way to shed clearer light on causal issues is through collection of longitudinal data. For this we would need to measure discounting in cohorts over a number of years, ideally beginning when they were young, so that follow-up study could establish the extent to which the degree of impulsivity in youth, and in the absence of disordered consumption, was a *predictor* of self-destructive patterns of behavior, including DG, later in life. At this point in time there are some suggestive studies with a longitudinal component, indicating that larger-scale efforts are worth making. Vitaro et al. (1999) find that impulsivity at age 12–14 is a significant predictor of involvement in problem gambling at age 17.[4] In their study, younger boys who more strongly preferred SSRs to LLRs were more likely than their peers to be disordered gamblers a few years later. Related findings are that low behavioral impulsivity is a good predictor of academic success (Kirby, Winston, and Santiesteban 2005) and high impulsivity is a good predictor of self-reported alcohol consumption and poor academic performance (Hair and Hampson 2006).[5] In the laboratory, early behavioral impulsivity is a predictor of the extent of later cocaine self-administration in rats (Perry et al. 2005). Such results suggest that behavioral problems later are at least partly the result of an earlier predisposition to be impulsive, or share a common cause with early impulsivity.

Other work, however, suggests the opposite (not, as noted, necessarily contradictory) causal direction between substance abuse and discounting. For example, Bickel, Odum, and Madden (1999) compared the discount rates of matched current, former, and never smokers and found that ex-smokers and never smokers both discounted less steeply than current smokers, suggesting either that smokers with low discount rates are more likely to quit smoking or that stopping smoking leads to reduced delay discounting. Our view is that the most likely outcome of future research on this question will be causal arrows pointing in both directions.

Even though the studies just reviewed shed only ambiguous light on causation, they help to establish that the behavioral notion of impulsivity, as measured by relative discount rates, is a good tool for sorting disordered consumers from normal ones, and a good basis for trying to work out what it is that makes the difference.

Most empirical work aimed at testing models of discounting has focused on delay discounting. Being removed in time, however, is not the only way in which a reward can be separated from consumption. Nor, for anyone interested in gambling, is it the most interesting form of separation. The other main way in which the value of a reward can be manipulated is by varying the probability that it will be delivered.[6] Just as the present value of $100 after a delay of one month is, for most people, lower than that of $100 right now, so the value of a 50/50 chance of getting $100 is (again for most) less than that of a guaranteed $100. Since gambling essentially involves risk and uncertainty, it is plausible to suppose that gamblers, and especially disordered gamblers, might be distinguished specifically by different responses to risk compared to control subjects.

Delay and probability discounting are measured in similar ways, and both are empirically best characterized by the hyperbolic discount function of PE (Green and Myerson 2004). A common theme in the literature has been to view delay and probability discounting as arising from similar if not identical choice processes. Some theorists (e.g., Rachlin et al. 1986; Rachlin, Raineri, and Cross 1991) have supposed that probability discounting is a derivative form of delay discounting, while others (e.g., Myerson and Green 1995) have suggested the reverse. Another logical possibility is obviously that they are independent. Both clearly are involved in most choice situations, in that a series of probabilistic outcomes necessarily involves delays to receipt of any reward, and any delayed reward involves some risk that it won't be received— that the hopeful recipient won't still be there to collect it, or that some misadventure including the efforts of a competitor will take it away between now and its scheduled delivery. Thus, delay and uncertainty are connected in everyday contexts relevant both to phylogenetic evolution and individual learning. In the ethological literature, delay is standardly studied and modeled in environments with competitors who can help themselves to a subject's unexercised options (see, e.g., Houston, Kacelnik, and McNamara 1982; Stephens and Anderson 2001; Stephens, Kerr, and Fernandez-Juricic 2004). Data related to this point are provided by a recent study that found that subjects rated delayed rewards as increasingly uncertain the more they were delayed, even though the original delayed rewards were offered in the form of a standard instrument intended to measure sensitivity to delay only

(Patak and Reynolds 2007).[7] There is also some evidence that rates of delay and probability discounting are correlated (Richards et al. 1999). Given the importance of risk to gambling, considerably more study of probability discounting (in populations with mixed gambling severity) is in order.

Against the suggestion that the two kinds of discounting might be manifestations of a single process, there are ways in which they clearly dissociate. Green, Myerson, and Ostaszewski (1999) found that reward amount is inversely related to the degree of delay discounting but directly related to the degree of probability discounting in human subjects. Another study (Ostaszewski, Green, and Myerson 1998) asked subjects about the relative preferability of pairs of immediate and delayed rewards in each of two different currencies. One (the Polish zloty) was undergoing rapid inflation at the time, while the other (the American dollar) was not. The experimenters found that subjects treated the chances of immediate rewards of the same magnitude equivalently irrespective of currency. That is, their discounting for reduced likelihood was the same for both. However, when considering guaranteed delayed rewards, subjects discounted the rapidly inflating currency more steeply. In a complementary study it was found that subjects' cultural background could make a selective difference to one or the other kind of discounting independently (Du, Green, and Myerson 2002); Chinese subjects discounted delayed rewards more steeply than Japanese subjects and vice versa, whereas American subjects discounted relatively steeply in both areas. Other work found that while smokers discounted more steeply for delayed rewards than nonsmokers, and were less sensitive to reduced probabilities, the difference between smokers and nonsmokers was more pronounced in the case of delay discounting (Reynolds et al. 2004). A further study (Mitchell 1999) found that smokers were more impulsive behaviorally and on most scales in five different personality measures, but that they were not different in their responses to uncertainty or to a procedure that measured discounting for effort independent of delay or uncertainty.[8]

Not only are delay and probability dissociable, then, but most real choices, fairly obviously, involve elements of both kinds of separation, as well as variations in effort required and so forth. That is, most real choices concern rewards that won't arrive immediately, and which are also not absolutely guaranteed to arrive. In particular, when people gamble, they explicitly make such choices.

4.3   Studies of Discounting in Substance Abusers

As explained in chapter 3, PE models substance abuse and DG as similarly structured consequences of failure to successfully bundle hyperbolically discounted rewards. As substance abuse has received far more empirical study in light of this model than DG, we review work that focuses on the former before considering studies of the latter.

In one of the first studies of discounting and substance abuse, the discount rates of a mixed population of inpatient substance abusers was compared to the discount rates of hospital employees, and it was found that the substance abusers discounted delayed rewards more steeply (Ainslie and Haendel 1983). More recently, Mitchell (1999) compared regular smokers with nonsmokers on a variety of clinical and personality measures of impulsivity, as well as three distinct behavioral tasks assessing impulsivity as a function of delay, reduced probability, and effort required to obtain a reward. Smokers had higher impulsivity scores than controls on the personality questionnaires, and were more impulsive on delay discounting, but not on the other behavioral tasks.[9] A more recent study has found that lower behavioral impulsivity predicts greater success in a smoking cessation program for adolescents (Krishnan-Sarin et al. 2007). A complementary study of current smokers, ex-smokers, and never smokers found that current smokers discounted the value of delayed money more steeply than both never smokers and ex-smokers (Bickel, Odum, and Madden 1999). Smokers also discounted the value of delayed cigarettes more steeply than they did money. Never smokers and ex-smokers were not significantly different from each other. This work suggests, but does not show, that smoking is associated with a temporary and reversible change in discounting. The result that current smokers discount more steeply than nonsmokers has been confirmed in other research (Reynolds et al. 2004[10]).

In the case of alcohol, Vuchinich and Simpson (1998) found that heavy and problem drinking college students discounted delayed rewards more steeply than light drinkers. Petry (2001c), comparing currently drinking alcoholics, abstaining alcoholics, and non-alcoholic controls, found that drinking alcoholics discounted more steeply than abstaining alcoholics, who in turn discounted more steeply than nonalcoholics. Alcoholic subjects also discounted delayed alcohol more steeply than delayed money. Finally, Kollins (2003) found that discount rates among college students were associated with a number of substance consumption variables, including age of first use of alcohol, tobacco, and marijuana, number of times incapacitated by alcohol, and total number of illegal drugs used.

Turning to drugs other than alcohol or nicotine, a pair of careful studies (Madden et al. 1997; Madden, Bickel, and Jacobs 1999) compared the discount rates of opioid-dependent subjects recruited from a treatment program to those of control subjects matched for age, education, gender, IQ, and income, and drawn from the same community. Opioid-dependent subjects discounted the value of delayed hypothetical money substantially more steeply than did controls. In addition, they discounted the value of delayed hypothetical heroin still more steeply than they did money. These studies, and the second of the investigations of discounting and alcohol described above, jointly show that there are subject-specific variations in the rate at which different sorts of reward are discounted, and that discount rates can be significantly higher for rewards that are commonly abused.

A further study using real (i.e., nonhypothetical) money also found that heroin-using subjects discounted dramatically more steeply than non-heroin-using controls, who had again been matched carefully in other respects (Kirby, Petry, and Bickel 1999). The same relation held in a different study of cocaine abusers (Kirby and Petry 2004). A complementary study found that among a population of heroin users, all of whom discounted very steeply, those who discounted most steeply were also those most likely (on the basis of self-report) to share a needle in a case where sufficient sterile ones were not available (Odum et al. 2000). It has also been found that mild deprivation from opioid drugs leads to steeper discounting of delayed rewards in already dependent (according to *DSM-IV* criteria) subjects (Giordano et al. 2002).

This collection of results encourages the view that steepness of delay discounting is an important factor distinguishing a variety of substance abusers from non-abusing subjects. At the same time, it suggests that the PE framework for the study of decisions is appropriate for designing cumulatively informative research into the decisions of addicts, or at least substance addicts. We now turn to similar work with disordered gamblers.

4.4 Studies of Gambling

We begin with Holt, Green, and Myerson (2003), who found that gambling subjects (some of whom scored in the "probably PG" range on the SOGS) were less sensitive to reduced probability than nongamblers, but did *not* discount delayed rewards more steeply than nongamblers.[11] This result is in conflict with other studies (Petry 2001a; Dixon, Marley, and Jacobs 2003[12]) finding that pathological gamblers *do* discount more steeply for delay than nonproblem controls. The preliminary data from an ongoing empirical project of our own also suggests that greater gambling severity is correlated with greater sensitivity to delay (Murrell et al. 2006).[13] Petry (2001a) also found, consonant with prior work on abusers of more than one substance, that pathological gamblers with substance abuse problems discounted yet more steeply for delay. This suggests that PG is behaviorally similar in a key way to substance abuse in that having more than one consumption problem, even if only one is related to a substance, seems to be associated with more severely impulsive discounting than having only one such problem.

Direct comparison of the Petry and Holt, Green, and Myerson studies is difficult given that the gamblers in the Petry study (finding an effect in the case of delay) had much more severe gambling problems (with SOGS scores of around 12–13, compared to 6–7) than those in the study by Holt and colleagues (finding an effect for probability but not delay). Subjects in the Petry study were also older (with a mean age of 44, compared to 19.6) and with an average of eight years of gambling problems each. The subjects in the Dixon, Marley, and Jacobs (2003) study were also older (mean age 38) but the gamblers had lower SOGS scores (around 6). Holt, Green, and Myerson's outlying result might be explained by the possibility that their subjects were not addicted gamblers, in the sense we will describe in chapter 6. Other results support the more common finding that disordered gamblers are more impulsive in response to delay. Alessi and Petry (2003) found that steepness of delay discounting was well predicted by SOGS scores, *and* that SOGS scores were a significantly better predictor of discounting than scores on the Eysenck Impulsivity Scale.[14] (This foreshadows our discussion of the relevance of the general impulsivity construct to consumption pathology and addiction in the next section and in chapter 8, section 8.2.) A more recent and very thorough study assessing the divergent validity of a selection of discounting, impulsivity, and cognitive measures with respect to a population of nonpathological gamblers, potential pathological gamblers and pathological gamblers (sorted by SOGS scores), and also using young subjects, found that increased gambling severity was clearly associated with greater sensitivity to delay (MacKillop et al. 2006).

Yet further support for the idea that gamblers are more impulsive can be found in the following results. First, a measure of a person's attitude to risk, or alternatively to the value of the future, and hence a proxy measure for delay discounting, is willingness to engage in risky sexual activity. Petry (2000) finds that substance abusers with gambling problems are more likely to engage in risky sexual behaviors than abusers without gambling problems. Second, disordered gamblers who smoke cigarettes have been discovered to have more severe gambling problems than nonsmoking disordered gamblers, further confirming the association between smoking and disordered decision making (Petry and Oncken 2002). Finally, DG substance abusers have directly shown dramatically higher discount rates than nonproblem gambling substance abusers (Petry and Casarella 1999). In connection with this, it is worth noting that the prevalence of DG has been shown by several studies over the years (e.g., Shaffer, Hall, and Vander Bilt 1999; Petry and Pietrzak 2004) to be much higher among substance abusers than in the population at large.

There is little doubt, then, that disordered gamblers are, like others with widely studied consumption pathologies such as smokers, alcoholics, and other substance abusers, more impulsive in the behavioral sense and may also differ in their responses to risk. There is much more we could aim to find out in order to more precisely characterize the impulsivity of disordered gamblers. It would be especially useful to know how gamblers of differing problem severity differ with respect to discounting. Perhaps, for example, moderately disordered gamblers are more like substance abusers in being relatively more sensitive to delay but don't differ much from suitable control subjects in their probability discounting, whereas severely disordered gamblers are both impatient and insensitive to risk or to their own losses. If there are indeed subjects (and severely disordered gamblers are a likely example of this) who are impulsive and risk-insensitive, then we need to conduct research on how particular situations, and particular series of choices and results of choices, might be especially dangerous for such people. Casinos, for example, may turn out to be exquisitely tailored traps for those with dispositions to impulsive consumption. And perhaps sufficiently extreme discounting makes the whole world a trap.

The variously reported finding that people with substance abuse problems are more behaviorally impulsive for the target of abuse suggests additional work in the case of gambling. While most discounting procedures concern money (real or hypothetical), it isn't money itself that is the target of DG. To our knowledge nobody has yet attempted to measure the impulsivity of anyone, disordered gambler or not, for the activity of gambling itself (asking questions like "Would you rather play the machines for two minutes now, or for ten minutes after a delay of one hour?") or for increases or decreases in money in the context of gambling. What we have in mind here would most obviously start with wins and losses—gamblers may, for example, be more impulsive for money (described as) won than they are for "mere" money. This work would not be difficult, and some neuroeconomic research to be considered in chapter 6 has taken steps in this direction already.

4.5 Other Impulsivity Constructs

Behavioral economists are not the only scientists who model and study impulsivity. Personality and clinical psychologists use frameworks for classifying humans that analyze personality into varying sets of dimensions ("sociability," "neuroticism," etc.). Most theories of personality employ a concept labeled "impulsivity," but there is considerable variation among theories regarding whether impulsivity as modeled is a dimension itself or treated as a complex construct from subjects' scores on two or more other dimensions.

The typical measurement instrument in this field is the self-report questionnaire, which solicits answers on a so-called Likert scale, and assigns scores on one or more dimensions. There are many instruments of this sort. One example, widely used in addiction research, is the Barratt Impulsivity Scale (BIS). The BIS is intended to measure patterns of behavior by asking subjects to report levels of agreement with statements concerning how they act and think (e.g., "I do things without thinking"). The current version, the BIS-11, has three subscales, measuring the following constructs: cognitive or attentional impulsivity (tendency to make decisions in the moment), motor impulsivity (tendency to act without thinking), and nonplanning impulsivity (see Patton, Stanford, and Barratt 1995). The UPPS Impulsive Behavior Scale (Whiteside and Lynam 2001; Whiteside et al. 2005), on the other hand, identifies four distinct components: urgency, lack of premeditation, lack of perseverance, and sensation seeking.

Behaviorists are apt to worry that the questions asked in these instruments call for more self-interpretation than do the reports on preferences required by a discounting procedure, and offer less clear incentives for honesty than discounting procedures, which can use real money. Also, whereas humans and nonhuman animals alike can express preferences in ways suitable for measuring discounting, questionnaires cannot be administered to nonhuman animals, isolating results gained with them from the wealth of work in the field and the laboratory on the preferences of such animals. Much behavioral work, and a great deal of NE, depends on cross-species comparisons. Fortunately, protocols have recently been developed and applied for assessing personality variables on the basis of field observations and experimental manipulations of nonhuman animals (Gosling and Vazire 2002). As these instruments are applied to humans, comparative personality results can be accumulated.

Reservations about the current state of this knowledge duly noted, some comparative research suggests that disordered consumers known to be behaviorally impulsive are also impulsive by one or more personality measures. Billieux, Van der Linden, and Ceschi (2007), for example, recently showed that urgency on the UPPS scale was a significant predictor of strength of tobacco cravings. Furthermore, disordered gamblers are sometimes classified correctly with psychiatric impulsivity measures, but with less effective discrimination than by behavioral ones (Alessi and Petry 2003, mentioned above[15]). Given this, it is not surprising that various studies report that disordered gamblers are more impulsive than controls on personality measures of impulsivity (Steel and Blaszczynski 1998; Blaszczynski, Steel, and Mcconaghy 1997; Blaszczynski and Nower 2002; Petry 2001b), or that high scores on these measures at one age is a predictor of DG later in life (Vitaro et al. 1999). A recent useful study by MacKillop et al. (2006) found that the Gamblers' Beliefs Questionnaire (Steenbergh et al. 2002), the Gambling Passion Scale (Rousseau et al. 2002), the impulsivity subscale of the Eysenck Impulsivity Questionnaire (Eysenck and Eysenck 1978), and a delay discounting task all discriminated effectively between nonpathological gamblers, pathological gamblers, and potential pathological gamblers in a sample divided by SOGS scores.

Various attempts to work out whether discounting procedures measure the same thing as this or that impulsivity instrument have turned up a mixture of results that, considered collectively, show partial overlap between some components of common impulsivity measures with discounting, but also considerable dissociation and conflict. The following reviews some of the recent results in this area. Krishnan-Sarin et al. (2007) found that delay discounting, but not impulsivity according to the BIS-II, predicted treatment outcome in a smoking cessation program, with the additional complication that only one of two delay discounting measures was a predictor. Dom et al. (2007) found only weak correlations between impulsivity measured with the BIS and scores at a delay discounting task (DDT), and similarly between DDT and the Iowa Gambling Task. Monterosso et al. (2001) did find a significant DDT—IGT correlation in a population of cocaine-dependent subjects. De Wit et al. (2007) found that steeper delay discounting was significantly but weakly correlated with the nonplanning scale of the BIS-11, and that it was significantly but *negatively* correlated with the cognitive scale of the BIS-11, and with IQ. Reynolds et al. (2006) found that scores on various self-report measures (including the BIS-11, the Multidimensional Personality Questionnaire [Patrick, Curtin, and Tellegen 2002]) were highly correlated with each other but *not* with various behavioral tasks including a DDT, and concluded that "self-report measures and behavioral measures assess different forms of impulsivity" (Reynolds et al. 2006, p. 312).[16] We will revisit the issue of relationships between the general multifactorial impulsivity construct used in these studies and the restricted concept of impulsivity as operationalized in behavioral economics, in chapter 8, section 2. For now, we point out that personality theory lacks a clear model in the economist's sense, rendering the concepts of impulsivity used in its precincts necessarily more diffuse and indefinite in behavioral implications. We thus doubt that it is reasonable to expect more than equivocal, and generally noisy, correlations between impulsivity as a personality trait and impulsivity in the more precise sense of PE.

4.6   Evidence of Cognitive Impairment

We now consider some results emanating from cognitive neuroscience. These are discussed in the present chapter, rather than in our chapter on the neuroscience of addiction to gambling, because of the light we think they shed on molar-scale reward-bundling problems. Our later extensive discussion of neuroscientific issues, by contrast, will be focused entirely on molecular-scale reward-valuation processes we believe to be responsible for full-blown addiction.

Cognitive psychology understands decision making as a process primarily focused on the acquisition and manipulation of knowledge and the control of action, largely independently of questions about what makes some outcomes desirable or what motivates agents at all. Cognitive psychologists are in general much more concerned than behaviorists with the architecture of the processing systems (the brain and its subsystems) involved in decision making, and in how the inputs to the decision process are represented and manipulated. Cognitive neuroscientists (and their precursors in neurology and other areas) regard the frontal lobes and especially the prefrontal cortex of the brain as important for a range of capabilities, including what is sometimes called "executive" or "goal-directed" cognition. Many of the defects associated with damage to or dysfunction in parts of the frontal lobes are clearly of interest to students of disordered consumption, including DG.

The prefrontal cortex (PFC) is an interconnected set of brain areas that together are richly connected with most sensory and motor systems in the cortex, and with a number of subcortical structures, including core parts of the midbrain reward system (the primary focus of chapters 5–7). The PFC also has extensive back projections to the same areas, allowing the modulation of sensory processing and motor control via influence on brain processes specialized for those tasks. (For a recent review, see Miller 2000; see also Fuster 2004.) There are various theories used to interpret cognitive neuroscientific results regarding executive cognition, including different models of working and semantic memory (e.g., Tulving 1972), dynamic filtering (e.g., Shimamura 2000), and global workspace processing (e.g., Dehaene, Kerszberg, and Changeux 1998). Subtle experiments have demonstrated that at least some sorts of tasks show the PFC to be organized as a cascade of processes progressively recruited as the informational demands of a task increase (Koechlin, Ody, and Kouneiher 2003). Promising computer models have replicated human-like performance on some standard tests of PFC function, such as the Wisconsin Card Sorting Task (WCST) (Rougier et al. 2005).

Resisting impulsive choice is the kind of task that requires integration of knowledge across multiple modalities, and evaluation of options about which relevant information is not cued by current sensory stimulation (e.g., a contribution to the children's college fund), in contrast to (for example) the current presence of a gambling machine with lighted prize possibilities flashing.

Among the deficiencies noted in subjects with frontal lobe damage are "loss of ego" in the form of loss of interest in longer-run projects, or in the future generally (Knight and Grabowecky 1995), and greater tendency toward "perseverative" errors. The WCST is designed to detect the latter. It has subjects sort cards according to their shape, color, or the number of symbols appearing on them. Experimenters do not tell subjects the rule, but provide feedback on whether or not they are sorting correctly. When subjects successfully follow one rule, the experimenter switches to another without announcing that fact. PFC-damaged subjects (who also tend to score normally on IQ tests and other measures) on average find the first rule as reliably as other subjects, but subsequently fail to abandon it when the rule changes (Milner 1963). Monkeys with PFC lesions perform badly at a task designed to be analogous to the WCST (Dias, Robbins, and Roberts 1996). It has been hypothesized by various researchers that failure to modify behavior allocation in the light of negative feedback from the environment could lead to disordered consumption. Some sorts of failure of memory, too, could manifest in allocation that fails to respect the longer-run plans of the subject, or amounts to loss of such plans.

Subjects with frontal lesions are indeed worse than controls at goal-oriented tasks, such as purchasing the items on a short shopping list, which require representations of simple goals to be maintained for a period (Shallice and Burgess 1991).[17] These subjects, who could perform individual subtasks ("buy a loaf of bread") effectively, tended to spend too much time on single parts of the set of subtasks required to meet their overall goals, or otherwise got distracted from pursuit of those goals. A variety of other results suggests that frontal lobe damage impairs ability to retain a representation of a response when that representation needs to be maintained over a delay, even when other tests of associative memory show no defect, or otherwise show greater susceptibility to distraction (e.g., Goldman-Rakic 1992; Chao and Knight 1995; McCarthy et al. 1994).

It is also increasingly clear that subjects with consumption problems show specific performance defects in Stroop paradigm tasks. (In the default Stroop task, subjects are asked to name the color in which a word is displayed. Some trials are "incongruous," in which, for example, the word "red" appears in green letters. Subjects typically take longer to answer on incongruous trials and make more mistakes.) For example, ˻ugle and Melamed (1993) and Regard et al. (2003) both found that ˻on-substance-dependent pathological gamblers were impaired at a ˻troop task compared to control subjects. Potenza et al. (2003a) failed ˻ find Stroop impairment, but did find decreased activity in the left ˻entromedial PFC among pathological gamblers. Brand et al. (2005) ˻ound that interference susceptibility measured in various ways, ˻ncluding by a Stroop task, was highly correlated with the rate of risky decisions made in a decision task. Kertzman et al. (2005) found that performance on the reverse Stroop task (where subjects are asked to read the word rather than name the color) in non-substance-dependent pathological gamblers was significantly slower and significantly less accurate than in control subjects.

Additional studies have found that subjects with consumption problems have specific or additional reaction time deficits when presented with cues associated with their problem, even if these cues are irrelevant to the task. (For example, the task might be to say of a word whether it is monosyllabic or polysyllabic; in this case a disordered gambler may take longer to respond when the word is "jackpot.") This effect has been found with, among others, regular cannabis users (Field et al. 2006), cocaine users (Hester, Dixon, and Garavan 2006), and disordered gamblers (Boyer and Dickerson 2003); for a recent review, see Cox, Fadardi, and Pothos (2006). Such results suggest that these subjects have specific difficulties with regulating their attention in general, and specific impairments in the presence of stimuli associated with the targets of their consumption problems. Recent brain imaging work, some of it discussed in chapters 5 and 6, gives some insight into the mechanisms of this, and their relation to other features of the reward system.

All of these phenomena can be directly related to reward bundling as discussed in chapter 3. To be effective a personal rule must be remembered, and the series of individually non-impulsive choices it describes must promise more reward than the series of impulsive choices starting with the current threat to the rule. This, like much executive cognition, requires reconstructing and maintaining representations of goal states including considerations that are independent from the immediate context. Failures of attention could manifest in lapsing into context-driven choosing even after recalling and being briefly motivated by the rule. Failures of memory could manifest in failure successfully to recall or reconstruct the considerations in light of which the rule promises any benefit at all. In general, as we discussed in chapter 3, both the maintenance and the collapse of personal rules are framing effects. Cognitive impairment is, in part, loss of capacity for sophisticated reframing. We distinguish this from the reduction of prefrontal control over midbrain motivational influence that we will discuss in detail in chapters 5 and 6 as a core aspect of the dynamics of addiction, including addiction to gambling. Of course, both aspects of compromised PFC functioning may be neurochemically and neuroanatomically related, and this may be a direct channel by which molar and molecular-scale processes exert reciprocal influence.

4.7   Situational Influences on Choice and Decision

Almost all of the work surveyed above is concerned with more-or-less stable and trait-like differences in performance on some discounting or other cognitive task that aims to reliably separate groups with impulsive consumption problems from groups without such problems. To the extent that such work yields robust results, we would hope to be able to predict the extent to which a person with high delay discounting or damage to PFC could reasonably be predicted to lose more money in a casino than an individual without those characteristics. A separate issue concerns how immediate features of the environment can influence choices regarding immediate and delayed rewards. That is, regardless of trait-like differences between people in discounting, are there environmental characteristics that can shift the entire distribution of persons toward making more (or less) impulsive choices? If such characteristics exist and are, at least sometimes, deployed in gambling settings, then those characteristics may be targeted by policies aimed at changing gambling behavior. Reasons to believe that vulnerability to DG is significantly under the control of environmental contingencies, and not just endogenous dispositions, are important to the case we will make in chapter 8 against general reduction of DG to a neurochemical pathology, even as we advocate reduction of full-blown PG to such a pathology.

There are a host of exogenous factors of different kinds that can induce temporary changes in how people make decisions. These factors include priming effects from seeing or thinking about something before making a choice, chemical effects arising from consuming various kinds of substances including alcohol, and factors like pain. It has been known for some time that simply seeing a smiling face, even if so briefly that it is not consciously noticed or remembered, leads to greater reported approval of what is observed shortly afterwards (Zajonc 1980, 1984). Some striking experiments in the early 1990s showed that the emotional content of sentences can have appreciable effects on behavior. This work found that people who thought about sentences mentioning age walked more slowly for a period afterwards than those who didn't, and that thinking about sentences relating in different ways to assertiveness and politeness also tended to make the test subjects measurably more assertive or polite. (In these experiments the subjects believed themselves to be engaged in a language test involving the sentences in question, and their rate of movement or propensity for assertive or polite behavior was measured in the corridor after they believed the experiment to have been concluded. See Bargh 1990, 1992.) A more recent study found that subliminal images of smiling faces presented before subjects were given the opportunity to pour themselves a drink led to subjects pouring and consuming more of the offered beverage, and to increased willingness to pay for more of the beverage. Subliminal presentations of frowning faces had the opposite effect (Winkielman, Berridge, and Wilbarger 2005).

Recent experiments have demonstrated the effects of situational priming on discounting. For example, Wilson and Daly (2003) hypothesized that attending to pictures of attractive women would put men into a "mating mindset," and that one feature of this would be temporarily steeper discounting for delay. Their reasoning was that unless the present was valued disproportionately, sexual opportunities would be sacrificed too often. The researchers found exactly what they predicted, and also (although to a smaller extent) that looking at pictures of expensive cars had a similar effect on female subjects.

Alcohol is ubiquitous in gambling environments. It is thus highly relevant to note that acute administration of alcohol leads to increased impulsivity in rats (Poulos, Parker, and Le 1998). (A reader who finds herself sarcastically saying "Thank goodness for science!" at this point is reminded that "impulsivity" here means something more specific than usual.) A study of electronic gaming machine players in a real commercial venue found that, according to the gamblers, alcohol consumption was a major contributor to diminished control over whether or not to continue playing (Baron and Dickerson 1999). Another study (Kyngdon and Dickerson 1999) in an experimental setting used real gaming machines and measured the extent to which subjects persisted in the face of losses. Half of the subjects drank an alcoholic beverage (equivalent to 30 grams of alcohol) before participating while half drank a non-alcoholic placebo beverage. It was found that subjects who had consumed alcohol were twice as persistent against losses as members of the placebo group. Half of the subjects in the alcohol group lost their entire original cash stake, compared to only 15 percent of the placebo group subjects.

An obvious question raised by this striking result is whether alcohol consumption leads to modification in discounting. In a study by Richards et al. (1999) all subjects were first assessed for delay and probability discounting, and then administered a beverage which in half of the cases was alcoholic while in the other half was a placebo, before being assessed again for delay and probability discounting. This study found that alcohol consumption had no effect at all on discount rates in the case of either delay or probability. This result is, at least initially, very surprising, given that alcoholics are known to be more impulsive in the specifically behavioral sense.[18] It is possible, though, that the absence of a change in discounting in this case is explicable by reference to peculiarities of the procedures used to assess discounting. Subjects were repeatedly asked which of two options they preferred, but did not experience wins and losses during the procedure. Sometimes, at the end of the procedure, one or more of the choices were randomly selected and the subject was paid whatever they said they preferred in the selected case. (This standard procedure in BE, often ignored in psychology, is intended to encourage subjects to attend seriously to their choices, since any given choice could turn out to be "real.") In cases where subjects chose chancy options, they might well have failed to earn anything, but their loss will have taken place only *after* the discounting procedure was concluded and hence would have had no effect on the procedure or its result. More simply, if there are no losses in a standard behavioral discounting task, one can hardly expect to see an effect of greater perseverance in the face of losses on the part of subjects who have consumed alcohol.

Following the failure of Richards et al. to find an effect of alcohol on delay discounting, Reynolds, Richards, and de Wit (2006) set out to remedy the experimental problem just described. They used the Experiential Discounting Task (EDT) (Reynolds and Shiffbauer 2004), in which subjects make repeated choices between very small rewards, some of which are very briefly delayed (by up to 60 seconds) or uncertain. All payouts were made in cash (collected by pressing a "bank" button) that subjects accumulated in a glass container next to the computer on which the questions were generated. The choices themselves followed a form of titration algorithm, and enabled indifference points to be estimated and discount curves approximated. (This is a clear advantage over the IGT, which does not permit such progressive refinement of measurement, and merely reports the proportion of "favorable" choices made in a series of blocks imposed over the 100 turns.) Consumption of alcohol significantly increased frequency of impulsive responses on the EDT, but *not* on a conventional question-based measure of discounting.

This latter result fits well with what is already known about the cognitive effects of alcohol consumption. Psychologists maintain that the effects of alcohol on social behaviors (at least) are more pronounced in situations containing both actual rewards and actual penalties,[19] and especially where more substantial rewards and penalties are occasionally incurred (Lau, Pihl, and Peterson 1995).[20] Moreover, consumption of alcohol outside the laboratory increases propensity to engage in various risky behaviors, including risky sex (Halpern-Felsher, Millstein, and Ellen, 1996) and aggression (Galanter 1997).

The findings that alcohol consumption leads to impaired decision making at gambling should be read in the light of additional work (Stewart et al. 2002) showing that gambling itself can lead to greater voluntary alcohol consumption (compared to a control activity of watching an action movie while alcohol was freely available), and that gamblers who were also drinking were more likely to undergo negative mood changes, even when gambling losses were factored in, than people who gambled but drank non-alcoholic beverages. This suggests that not only might people who drink and gamble be more likely to make bad decisions, they may also be made less happy at the time they are gambling by the fact that they have been drinking.

Judging from this brief survey of situational influences on choice, it is plausible to suggest that packing a gambling environment with images of smiling faces, messages of generosity, expensive cars, attractive floor staff, and alcohol may move the population of gamblers as a whole in the direction of making decisions on the basis of short-range rather then long-range interests. We suspect that neither regular gamblers nor industry participants or regulators will be set reeling in astonishment at this suggestion, and it is not surprising that typical gambling venues contain many of the features just listed. We have bothered to review careful evidence here mainly because the exciting work in neuroscience that will preoccupy us for the next three chapters has encouraged in some quarters the idea that all DG is "organic," in the sense discussed in chapter 1. We must be reminded that this is overreaching. That said, we turn now to the work that has motivated this idea, which indeed leads us to reach a good deal further in the direction of reductionism with respect to problem gambling than we would have expected a few years ago.

5

The Neuroeconomics of
Addiction

5.1 Four Theses about Addiction and Pathological Gambling

(In this chapter and thereafter we will use "PG," "DG," and "AG" to denote both pathological, disordered, or addictive gambling and pathological, disordered, or addictive gamblers. Good old English grammar will prevent this from causing confusion or ambiguity.)

In the previous two chapters we described the behavioral economics of impulsivity. Evidence from many countries indicates that, notwithstanding the tendency of clinical screens used in research to overestimate the prevalence of severe DG in populations, the majority of DGs fall short of the full battery of behaviors that have classically been associated with the concept of "addiction." On the basis of the science related to this point in the book, the question remains open as to whether the distinction between mere problem gambling and full PG has any non-arbitrary basis. As discussed earlier, an important part of the background to *DSM-IV*'s codification of PG was its symptomatic resemblance to the classical substance addictions. But, as noted in chapter 3, scientists in the behaviorist tradition have sometimes been skeptical as to whether substance dependencies represent a distinctive pathology with unambiguous internal markers that explain the main behavioral properties associated with addiction.

No one, as far as we know, has ever denied that some ingested substances create chemical dependency in the sense that dependent people experience aversive and sometimes even dangerous biochemical withdrawal syndromes on terminating use. Thus, addicts have often been conceptualized as those people who tolerate over-frequent (by their own lights) cognitive and behavioral impairment due to ingestion of substances because they fear the withdrawal costs. As we saw in chapter 3, this is the perspective of the first generation of BE models of addiction. However, it predicts that those drug-dependent people who *do* successfully withdraw should thereafter be less likely, now that they are fully acquainted with the relevant costs and benefits, to lapse back into dependency than people who were never addicted. But, of course, the reverse is true. Even many heroin addicts go through the trauma of withdrawal several times, returning to dependency each time after a dry period. Emphasis on this fact, common to all drug dependencies, led to displacement of biochemical dependence as an essential substratum for the behavioral patterns of classical addiction in much of the theoretical and clinical scientific literature. In consequence, some scientists came to doubt that "addiction" picks out anything more robust and determinate than people with extreme degrees of incompetence at legislating and maintaining personal rules (i.e., at bundling).

It is thus reasonable to wonder first whether addiction denotes a kind of state or process that science ought to recognize, and second whether problem gambling and PG as behaviorally characterized or operationalized (e.g., in the CGI and other *DSM*-based screens) are anything other than endpoints on a continuum of bundling difficulties, meeting at a fuzzy and indeterminate borderline rather than a well-defined point of discontinuity.

Beginning in this chapter, and continuing through the following two, we present the case for the following four theses concerning the two questions just posed:

(1) The substances that have traditionally been regarded as classically addictive—stimulants, alcohol, nicotine, and opiates—all, by different neurochemical mechanisms, trigger a distinctive pathology in a specific brain system, the so-called dopamine reward pathway. This provides a justification based on scientific values—that is, on our interest in grouping phenomena for maximal explanatory and predictive power—for the regimentation of "addiction" as a scientific concept. Specifically, "addiction" should be treated as the name of the reward system pathology that we will describe.

(2) Most, probably almost all, people who actually meet the *DSM* criteria for PG (i.e., excluding those who are misdiagnosed as false positives by insufficiently discriminating screens such as SOGS) demonstrate the same neurochemical disorder as drug addicts, even when they are not addicted to any drugs. Therefore, we should regard most currently diagnosed PGs as being addicted to gambling. Furthermore, behavioral analysis of PG should give way to neuroscientific analysis:

people who currently match the *DSM-IV* criteria for PG but who turn out not to be addicts should no longer be classified as PGs. We should adjust our behavioral criteria so that PG is coextensive with AG. In the language of philosophers of science (to be explained below), we should *locally reduce* PG to AG.

(3) Currently available studies comparing the reactions of PGs and drug addicts to pharmacological interventions support the thesis that most PGs are addicts. This provides a clinical justification for the reduction of PG to AG.

(4) Because AG does not compound the basic mechanism of addiction with subsidiary chemical influences on the brain, and because it triggers the distinctive reward system pathology directly, AG is usefully regarded as the template, or basic model, for addiction in general.

The statement of these theses might lead the reader to suppose that they amount to declaring the limits—and quite stringent limits at that—on economic theory as a potential contributor to the understanding of DG. Of course, we have acknowledged that the majority of DGs are not AGs, and so fall within the explanatory purview of PE regardless. However, we aim to show here that economics also plays a key role in framing the identification of PG as AG. It does so as an application of a new branch of neuroscience called "neuroeconomics." It is because PE provides our most powerful theoretical model of non-addictive DG, while NE best models AG, that we require a hybrid of PE and NE to understand DG as a whole. The general thesis that PE and NE are complements rather than rivals in the integration of economic theory with the cognitive and behavioral sciences is the main conclusion of Ross (2005). The demonstration of the applicability of this in the specific instance of DG can thus provide specific exemplification of the complementarity of PE and NE that is described, only in much more abstract terms, in Ross's earlier book.

Philosophically alert readers will wonder how and why DG should call forth a *hybrid* of PE and NE models if, as we have said, the boundary between non-addictive DG and AG is relatively sharp and clean. Consider an analogy. In physics, there is a standard boundary between the domains of applicability of quantum mechanics and general relativity. It is vacuous to say that physical theory in general is a "hybrid" of these two theories because, for any given phenomenon, physicists employ one theory or the other, not a mixture of both. (True hybrid models, theories of so-called quantum gravity, remain speculative at this time.) Thus, showing that PE integrates with cognitive–behavioral science to explain *part* of DG, and that NE integrates with a different part of cognitive–behavioral science to explain a *different* part of DG, does not, it may be objected, support Ross's philosophical thesis, except trivially insofar as it shows economic theory participating in the wider project of behavioral science in more than one way.

Underlying this kind of objection are, in part, philosophical issues around the individuation of scientific phenomena. If a class of phenomena, in this case DG, cleaves neatly into two subclasses for purposes of explanation and prediction, why should we go on regarding the original phenomenon as a proper theoretical kind? In this book we aim to shed some light on this question, as it specifically applies to DG, without attempting any purely philosophical assault on it or sweeping resolution of it. As the philosopher of science W. V. Quine emphasized throughout his career, there is no marked or stable boundary between naturalistic philosophy and science. We furthermore believe that philosophy should always be antecedent to science, and that scientific hypotheses typically get distorted when pressed into service as philosophical exhibits (Ladyman and Ross 2007). Therefore, in the final chapter of the book, when we seek to summarize the general state of our knowledge of DG, we will not lead with philosophical questions. Instead, we will directly discuss several models of impulsivity that have been put forward as rivals to the PE models described in chapter 3. As we indicated there, these models are all versions of what we call "opponent process" theories, and have their roots partly or wholly in NE. The question of whether these models are in fact rivals to PE accounts that are based on the matching law and hyperbolic discounting involves, we will show, inextricable conceptual and empirical aspects. We will try to help the reader organize her thinking about the conceptual side of the issues, but will leave her to settle on her own preferred philosophical stance after demonstrating the complications that the science exposes.

Before we put philosophical issues aside, however, we must deal with a related one that is otherwise apt to raise questions and confusion in some readers. Our theses together claim that one subvariety of DG reduces and another does not. This will raise objections of two opposite kinds, from rival philosophical perspectives. Some philosophers and scientists, so-called "holists," reject all reductionist theses, or at least all reductionist theses about human behavioral and cognitive phenomena. On the other hand, a small minority of philosophers and many scientists—especially many neuroscientists—take it as axiomatic that *all* behavioral and cognitive phenomena should ultimately be reduced to neurochemical and/or neurophysiological ones. In our view, scientists should be moved to avoid taking sweeping philosophical positions on the ontological status of vast classes of phenomena by observing the empirically unmotivated wastes of energy into which philosophers have been drawn by lining up on alternative sides of such positions. Yards of ink have been spilled in the philosophy of science literature over whether science in general progresses by *ontological reduction*—that is, by reducing more abstract types of objects and processes to less abstract (more "concrete," typically mechanical) types. Philosophers who believe in ontological reductionism generally hold that it is achieved by means of *intertheoretic reduction*—that is, by demonstrations that theories of more concrete types and processes explain and predict the contents of theories of more abstract types and processes. For example, it is a common idea about the cognitive and behavioral sciences that theories of mental processes should reduce to theories of neural processes (intertheoretic reduction); and this might in turn be taken to imply that the mind just *is* the brain (ontological reduction). What is at stake here is not necessarily "spooky" mind-body dualism— the popular spook that most scientists probably mean to reject when they side with across-the-board reductionism. We think that philosophers *have* successfully established that such reductionism is an unnecessarily strong response for seeing off dualism and supernaturalism.[1] Antireductionist philosophers, few of whom are traditional dualists, typically insist only that theories of the mental describe neural processes in interaction with environmental ones, at a level of abstraction that can't be cashed out in purely neural or neurocomputational terms. However, our opinion as relevant to this book is that *both* across-the-board reductionism and across-the-board antireductionism overgeneralize. The history of science, in our view, supports three conclusions about reduction: (1) *seamless* reductions of either the ontological kind or intertheoretical kind are vanishingly uncommon, (2) *effective* reductions allowing for some rough fits are not infrequent, but (3) many highly abstract types and processes are irreducible, so a scientific research program can be thoroughly successful without producing or promising any reductions (see Ladyman and Ross 2007 for details). It is because we believe (2) that we can argue for a reduction of PG to AG that may force reconsideration of some cases (the "rough fits"). The motivation for such reduction is pragmatic: it captures more powerful generalizations, facilitating both prediction and explanation. It is because we believe (1) that we can suppose that part of DG could effectively reduce to AG without this, as a matter of logic, sundering DG apart for all purposes. And it is because we believe (3) that we can argue for *local* reduction of PG in a wider context where we do not expect DG *as a whole* to reduce—and thus, where we are left with a class of phenomena over which PE, rather than neuroscience, will provide the general theory. Any successful argument for a local reduction, and any successful argument for the irreducibility of some other class of phenomena, must be based strictly on contingent empirical data. Nothing at all about what does or doesn't reduce to what can be established by philosophical reflection.

The discussion to come is organized as follows. The present chapter will not concern gambling directly; its job is to set the stage for those that follow. In the first section of the chapter we will describe the new subdiscipline of NE, and its role in the wider family of the neurosciences. The second section will outline the currently prevailing neuroeconomic model of the midbrain reward system, indicating where there is consensus and where there is continuing disagreement or uncertainty. Wider controversies over how to integrate this model with PE perspectives on impulsivity will be mentioned from time to time, but their details and evaluation will be postponed until the final chapter of the book, after we have completed our review of the evidence for and implications of a neuroeconomic theory of PG as AG in the two intervening chapters.

5.2   Neuroeconomics

To place NE in its context, we begin by introducing vocabulary for the various branches of the sciences that are relevant to the brain mechanisms and processes underlying PG. *Neuroscience* refers indiscriminately to all of them together. *Neuroanatomy* studies the structural components of the brain, their placement relative to one another, and the mechanics of their interactions. (This is the part of neuroscience most analogous to auto mechanics.) When the reader looks at figure 5.1 in section 5.3 below, the areas she sees labeled are neuroanatomical parts. Next: *neurochemistry* and *neurodynamics* study, respectively, the molecular and the electrical bases by which these parts of the brain handle and transform information and pass it from one part to another. This refers to the fact that the brain does its work in two main physical ways. The first is through chemical modulations that broadcast widely about *overall conditions* (e.g., "Things are good here," "Things are getting worse here," "Things are exciting here") and *generic responses* (e.g., "Let's fight," "Let's get away from this"). The second is through sending electrical signals that register *specific states* of affairs (e.g., "That is a red object," "That is Mom," "The capital of Zambia is Lusaka") and brain-region-specific responses (e.g., "I want you [another brain area] to stop talking to me").[2] Because the meanings of electrical signals are more fine-grained, they are more sensitive to individual variations in history, learning and context; two neuroelectrical events indistinguishable with respect to their general neuroelectrical properties may have very different implications for the cognitive and behavioral lives of two different people. Despite the fact that someone whose neurochemical states weren't targeted and refined by neuroelectrical signals wouldn't behave like a person at all, in this chapter, the details we'll get into will exclusively concern neurochemistry rather than neurodynamics. The next general branch of neuroscience we need to distinguish, *neuropsychology*, attempts to localize mental processes to particular brain or physiological processes by mainly focusing on disorders of language, perception, and action. Neuropsychology is, in effect, the part of neuroscience that coordinates the attention of neurologists, psychiatrists, psychologists, and neurophysiologists. Finally, *cognitive science*, including cognitive neuroscience, studies the ways in which neuroanatomy, neurochemistry, and neurodynamics interactively influence perception, motor behavior, decision, thought, emotions, mood, and consciousness. When you wonder about how your brain contributes to the production of your thoughts and actions, identified in terms you can present to yourself in everyday language, you're mulling on topics of cognitive neuroscience.

The disciplinary perspective from which we have written this chapter is that of a newcomer to the above set of neurosciences, the very existence of which might strike some readers as a bit bizarre on first encounter: *neuroeconomics*. We aim to demonstrate that this is the most fruitful organizing platform from which to provide an integrated account of (much or most) PG. However, NE is a sufficiently novel construct to most people's ways of thinking that we can't introduce it, as we did the neuroscience branches above, with just a few sentences. Several pages of explanation therefore follow.

The basic assumption behind NE is that humans, like all other learning agents, have goals among which trade-offs are required due to scarcity. How do people select appropriate means for achieving these goals, and how do they calculate the trade-offs among them? Part of the answer adverts to guidance from reinforcement signals. That is, with each decision a person makes, she receives information about at least the short-term consequences of that decision in the form of immediate reward, punishment, or the mere absence of reward. In addition, thanks to a combination of episodic memory and generalization through inference (in which social bookkeeping—that is, the monitoring and suggestions of other people—plays a key role), people can often interpret the consequences of their decisions with respect to those decisions' impacts on the likelihood of future rewards. As such, reinforcement signals act as advisers or counselors to the brain. They help us update knowledge about a certain behavior on the basis of experience in the course of enacting that behavior. In the reinforcement learning literature the guidance signal often gets referred to as "the critic," for reasons that will be evident.

When we talk about "valuation" of decisions or possible courses of action, we refer to the relative ranking by the critic of possible or actual states of affairs in terms of "better than" and "worse than."[3] Without such an evolved internal currency in the nervous system, a creature couldn't assess the relative value of events relevant to expected supplies of different things it wants. For example, suppose an organism encounters a mating cue and a food cue at the same time, using different sensory modalities (i.e., information processed through different sense organs). To which shall it respond? Or, if it can respond to both, how shall it trade off possible relative allocations of attention to them? An organism that could only compare them by first working out a new, speculative, once-off theory of the specific economic situation would likely fare very badly in any real environment. If an organism is to be guided by the evolutionary learning of its species—which is a very powerful source of information, because it's been going on for so long—then the neurochemical dispositions of its brain will need to play a role in informing its judgments. An organism that failed to make any use in its economic decisions of what its species had learned throughout its evolution would be badly adapted—indeed, impossibly badly adapted. This entails that the brain must directly compute over units that represent the value of mating or eating (or fleeing, or fighting, or sleeping, etc.) at some more abstract level—roughly as a person can weigh her house and her breakfast and the value of her life to her spouse in one currency, namely dollars.[4]

So, what is this internal currency? Just a few years ago, no one had a very clear idea. Now, thanks to fMRI[5] and other new technologies[6] that let us non-invasively peer into the living brain while people behave and think, we are beginning to gain an understanding of what this internal currency is that we use to make decisions (Glimcher 2003; Kable and Glimcher unpublished). Experiments performed with monkeys suggest that it consists of variations in firing rates in dedicated neurons in parts of the brain that collectively make up the so-called "reward system" (that is, the system for processing information about actual or potential valuations). An increase in spike rates in these neurons means that a stimulus seems to the brain to be "better than predicted," a decrease means it's "worse than predicted," and no change means it's "just as expected" (so, this signal says to the rest of the brain: "Don't pay more or less than the default level of attention to the stimulus").

Cognitive neuroscientists individuate "systems" in the brain by identifying generic functional responses with relatively encapsulated pathways by which specific brain chemicals, *neurotransmitters*, propagate their influence. By "relatively encapsulated" we mean only that it is possible up to some useful practical limit to model the pathway's influence on overall behavior in isolation from other groups of neurons. We have already indicated the functional specification of the reward system. As a neurotransmitter pathway, it is distinguished by its reliance on dopamine, now becoming popularly known as the "chemical of satisfaction" (see Berns 2005). Later, we will describe the neuroanatomy of this pathway. First, however, we will concentrate on the way in which the reward system dopamine signals constitute information processing about valuation. That is, we will indicate how the system is represented in models from computational neuroscience.

fMRI evidence (McClure, Daw, and Montague 2003) strongly suggests that the reward system implements what is called temporal difference (TD) learning (Sutton and Bartow 1998). TD learning is a rule—an *algorithm*—that describes the way in which the reward system estimates a *value function* V^* (that is, a principle for taking a stream of possible information as input and turning it into a stream of advance relative value estimates as output). More technically, the rule denotes a family of functions that relate a situation at a particular time s_t to a time-discounted sum of expected rewards (idealized as numeric measures r of received utility) that can be earned into the future. Suppose, following McClure, Daw, and Montague (2003), that t, $t+1$, $t+2$, and so on, represent times on some arbitrary measurement scale. Let γ be a discount parameter between 0 and 1, as discussed in chapter 3. Then the TD equation is

$$V^*(s_t) = E[r_t + \gamma r_{t+1} + \gamma^2 r_{t+2} + \gamma^3 r_{t+3} + \ldots]$$

which we close by writing

$$V^*(s_t) = E[r_t + \gamma V^*(s_{t+1})]$$

This describes the procedure by which the reward-system learning algorithm continuously inputs new information to keep refining its estimate of V^* to get a particular stream of actual temporal valuations V. From this we can define a measure δ of the extent to which the value estimates of two successive states and a reward experienced by the system are consistent with one another:

$$\delta(t) = r_t + \gamma V(s_{t+1}) - V(s_t),$$

where δ is an error signal that pushes $V(s)$ toward better estimates as it gets more data. If $V(s_{t+1})$ turns out to be better than expected, then $\delta(t)$ will be positive, thus indicating that $V(s_t)$ needs to be adjusted upward. If $V(s_{t+1})$ turns out to be worse than expected, $\delta(t)$ will be negative and $V(s_t)$ will be adjusted downward. If $\delta(t) = 0$ then no learning occurs (as it shouldn't, since the system has received no new information).

The TD algorithm presupposes substantial advance knowledge by the system of the structure of its learning space. But the reward system is not flummoxed by unfamiliar learning contexts. To model learning in situations where there is not yet a rich representation of the relationships between possible actions and values, computational learning theorists have developed a variant of TD learning called "Q-learning," which models a family of algorithms for learning value functions over state-action pairs (Sutton and Bartow 1998, pp. 148–151; Montague, King-Cassas, and Cohen 2006). In this book we will ignore this complication, because we assume that the highly structured environments provided by commercial gambling environments facilitate direct implementation of the simplest TD learning model (above) following short periods of initial familiarization.

That the dopamine reward system implements TD learning is not generally considered controversial. However, there are different views among researchers as to the wider role of this learning. The reward system appears to integrate all of the following functions: (1)

perception of expected reward, (2) perception of risk, (3) learning environmental cues that predict reward, (4) learning comparative values of rewards, (5) focusing attention on cues that predict rewards, and (6) motivating the system to act on the basis of these cues (thanks to projection from the dopamine system to motor neurons). Two considerations make it unlikely that TD learning is the source of this integration. First, recent evidence due to Preuschoff, Bossaerts, and Quartz (2006) strongly indicates that functions (1) and (2) are performed independently of (3)–(6) in the dopamine system (and (2) might initially occur elsewhere in the brain). Second, in its basic form—the form presented above—TD learning does not predict a discovery due to Gallistel (1990), that conditioning outcomes in animal learning are timescale-invariant. This means that responses from a given animal will be the same in two otherwise identical learning conditions if the interval durations between cues and rewards in one condition are a constant multiple of the durations of the other. In general, TD learning has been framed as a model of classical association conditioning, after Rescorla and Wagner (1972). By contrast with association models, scalar expectancy theory (SET) (Gibbon 1977) and rate estimation theory (RET) (Gallistel 1990), as unified by Gallistel and Gibbon (2000), are *timing* models of conditioning phenomena. According to such models, animals represent the durations of intervals and the rates of relevant events, and conditioned responding occurs as a function of the comparison of rates of reinforcement. Animals are drawn to environments with higher such rates by gradient climbing, rather than forming explicit associations between stimuli and conditioned responses. For ease of reference, we will call the unification of SET and RET "G-learning."

G-learning is naturally compatible with melioration as modeled by Herrnstein and described in chapter 3, since melioration is just optimization of current reward rate. This should not be read as suggesting that melioration as a molar model *implies* G-learning as a *molecular* theory. Unless a molar model reduces to a molecular model, it will be compatible with multiple molecular models. However, because PE is not in the first place a learning theory, G-learning offers an enlightening framework for thinking about the prospective unification of molecular accounts of learning with PE. Sanabria and Killeen (2005), commenting critically on Ainslie's model of molar appetite, note that "a key property of signals of reinforcement is that they become both conditioned reinforcers, or CRs, and conditioned stimuli, eliciting approach"

(p. 661). This leads them to ask: "Is this the behavioral substrate of desire, of appetite? If so, then Ainslie's hyperbolic interests, Skinner's CRs, and Pavlov's CSs are the same entity. A theory of one is a theory of all" (ibid.). Ainslie (2005, p. 667) responds favorably to the suggestion and expands on it, commending Sanabria and Killeen for

mentioning the opportunity [raised by PE] to revise "the hoary study of CRs [conditioned responses]." I judge such a revision to be among [my theory's] most important implications. . . . [F]or the selection of responses, the potential of brief temporary preferences to lure organisms into responses that are aversive overall, could let us do without the *deux* [*sic*] *ex machina* of a second, "conditioned" selective principle that is so often invoked to explain aversive, involuntary or maladaptive processes. . . . The model of aversion as a rapidly cycling addiction comprising reward and inhibition of reward lets us add conditioned processes to the marketplace of rewarded processes.

In this perspective, G-learning, to the extent that it applies directly to the reward system, would suggest a natural way of unifying the molar and the molecular accounts of entrapment by addictive targets. Ainslie's "rapidly cycling addictions" would simply be conceptualized as high-reward-rate "environments" that lure organisms' attention and approach, unless the dopamine reward system is opposed by other neurotransmitter pathways and thereby prevented from completely dominating molar behavior. Here might also be the molecular substrata for Ainslie's personal rules: cognitive dispositions that strengthen the effectiveness of such hypothetical opponent systems. Later, we will present some neuroscientific evidence for exactly this picture. Gallistel anticipates this idea by likewise arguing that classical and operant conditioning amount to the same thing. In impulsivity studies there has been a long-running and unresolved debate over the relationship between supposedly classically conditioned cravings and apparently instrumentally conditioned preparations for consumption of addictive or pseudo-addictive targets. Perhaps the debate has been inconclusive because these are one and the same process. But if G-learning is sufficient to provide neurocomputational foundations for Ainslie's molar account, then what is the role in impulsive choice, if any, of TD learning in the dopamine system?

A recent computational model of the reward system by Daw (2003) makes the two kinds of learning complementary. In this model G-learning is taken to precede, and indeed to enable, TD learning.

Suppose an animal has learned a function that predicts a reward at t, where the function in question decomposes into models of two stages: one applying to the interval between the conditioned and the unconditioned stimulus, and one applying to the interval between the unconditioned stimulus and the next conditioned stimulus. Then imagine that a case occurs in which at t nothing happens. Should the animal infer that its model of the world needs revision, perhaps to a one-stage model, or should it retain the model and regard the omission as noise or error? In Daw's account the animal uses G-learning to select a world model: whichever such model matches behavior that yields the higher reward rate will be preferred to alternatives. Given this model as a constraint, TD learning can then predict the temporal placement of rewards (call this "when"-learning). This hybrid approach allows Daw to drop two unbiological features of the original Montague, Dayan, and Sejnowski (1996) model of TD learning by the dopamine system: tapped-line delay timing and exogenously fixed trial boundaries, which are plausible only in the sparse and controlled setup of the laboratory. This is surely progress, as it is doubtful that anyone ever took these two properties for anything other than modeling conveniences. But at this point it can no longer be said to be clear what, if anything, is the "canonical" model of the role of TD learning in the dopamine system.

Fortunately for present purposes, at a slightly higher level of abstraction this uncertainty about molecular mechanisms becomes less important. As noted above, there is increasing consensus that the reward system integrates reward prediction, valuation, salience and approach, whether it does so by bolting together two learning algorithms, as in Daw's model, or by implementing a single more complex one, as in the predictor-valuation (PV) model of Montague and Berns (2002). Given the possibilities left open by present empirical knowledge, we can treat PV either as a direct molecular account of one learning process, or as an account one level up in the molar direction of a function implemented by G-learning and TD learning together.[7] The PV model is characterized as follows. Suppose $R(x,n)$ estimates the value of a reward distributed at various possible times $x, y, z, \ldots, n$ in the future, scaled according to the uncertainty attending to the intervals between the estimation point and each time, as in:

$$R(x, n; D) = \int_{-\infty}^{+\infty} dy\, G\left(x-y, (x-n)D\right) r(y)$$

where $G(z,b) = (2\pi b)^{-1/2} \exp\{-z^2/2b\}$ and D is a constant. Then the value $F(n)$ the brain attaches to getting a particular predictor signal at perceptual time n is given by:

$$F(n) = \int_n^{+\infty} dx\, e^{-q(x-n)} \int_{-\infty}^{+\infty} dy\, G\left(x-y_1\left(x-n\right)D\right)\rho\left(y\right)$$

$$= \int_n^{+\infty} dx\, \left\{e^{-q(x-n)}\right\} \bullet \left\{R\left(x, n; D\right)\right\}$$

$$= \int_n^{+\infty} dx\, [\text{discount future time } x \text{ relative to perceptual time } n] \bullet$$

$$\left\{\text{diffused version of reward estimate } \rho(x) \text{ for some } x \text{ and } n\right\}.$$

Learning that these molar and molecular functions describe the value-learning processes of the brain amounts to discovering the brain's economics, since we can use these processes to quantitatively model the opportunity costs the brain implicitly pays—in its own terms—for attending to one stimulus over another or issuing one motor response rather than another.[8] Economics, as noted earlier, is the study of trade-offs among goals of systems given scarce resources available to the systems in question for achieving the goals in question. In NE, the systems that bargain with one another to trade off among scarce resources are subsystems of the brain. The scarce resources over which these subsystems compete and cooperate are the restricted opportunities for attention, learning, and action by the whole nervous system. Hence the coinage "neuroeconomics."

fMRI work has suggested that there are levels of discrimination in value-coding structure in the reward system from which the PV model abstracts. (That is, the model averages over some of the details of reward representation at the molecular level.) Some neurons encode expected value (magnitude × probability) of rewards, while others encode a reward's subjective utility in context (i.e., its *opportunity cost* in terms of its cardinal ranking relative to other possibilities). It is likely that as NE develops further over the coming years, it will call forth application of the full set of technical resources of mathematical microeconomics in understanding the principles by which the brain relates perception to the allocation of attention and preparation for action. The discovery of Preuschoff, Bossaerts, and Quartz (2006) that the distinction drawn in financial valuation theory (and in BE, thanks to Bossaerts and Plott 2004) between expected reward and risk measured by variance is directly implemented in midbrain is a striking case in point. One would not have imagined that financial economics would turn out to be brain science at a highly aggregated level; that it has represents scientific unification at its most thrilling.

We recommend NE as the framework for integrating the neuroscience of (much or most) PG, and addiction-like behavioral phenomena in general, because, as we will argue in the sections and chapters to come, these phenomena have turned out to be pathologies of the reward system. As we discussed in chapter 3, they are patterns wherein the system *locally* values rewards that cause the *global* welfare of the person the system regulates to drop over time, and to regret her earlier choices despite the fact that she could (at least from some past point) have foreseen her own regret. Under what circumstances does $V(s_t)$ keep pushing the valuation of another gamble, or another hit of cocaine, higher than the available alternatives, even when some other aspect of the person—either some other system in her brain, or her whole self in aggregate—would prefer that she choose one of the alternatives? Just a few years ago the answers to this question were speculative. Now we know a good deal—though very far indeed from everything—about them on the basis of neuroscientific evidence.

Having now explained our neuroeconomic perspective, our next task is to introduce the neuroanatomy, neurochemistry, and neurodynamics of the dopamine reward system.

5.3   The Reward System

The reward system integrates aspects of both an old, interior part of the brain that we share with vertebrates in general, and the prefrontal cortex (PFC) whose dramatic growth (along with that of the frontal cortex) in hominids was a salient feature of our evolution and a necessary factor in our unique form of adaptive intelligence. For years it was standard practice to refer to the older structure as the "limbic system" and the newer brain as the "cognitive system," based on the idea that emotional responses are primitive and rational ones are an adaptive refinement. Over the past decade or so, it has become clear that this is misleading; the older part of the brain performs many "rational" calculations, and emotional judgments and motivations are crucial to the functioning of the frontal cortex. However, it remains true that the two parts of the brain developed under different evolutionary pressures. Furthermore, a core aspect of the old limbic/cognitive dichotomy remains particularly relevant where the reward system's role in overall behavioral control is concerned. As we will later discuss in detail, the reward system requires supervision from frontal circuits to avoid leading the organism as a whole down impulsive paths. However, this is not because the reward system's evaluations are distinctively "emotional" or "limbic"; it is because they are specialized.

Whenever evolved structures must co-opt the functional outputs of other structures that evolved much earlier, we should have our eye out for characteristic pathology patterns that result from the fact that the older structure was not selected for its capacity to serve the newer one. Natural selection typically cannot yoke together different systems evolved under different pressures and with different available building blocks, and avoid what engineers call "kludges"—that is, incipient vulnerabilities that are patched around when the system is running under optimal conditions, but that expose predictable bugs when circumstances degrade in characteristic ways. The widespread and relatively standardized pathologies of addiction may well be kludges stemming from the imperfect adaptation of the midbrain to its new role as a service department for newer cortical systems.[9] We will revisit this idea in the concluding chapter of the book.

The figures below show the brain regions that play leading roles in the neurobiology of reward. In the old interior part of the brain we have the striatum, which is itself part of the basal ganglia and includes the nucleus accumbens (NAcc), a small part of the brain that will play a large role in the coming account of addiction. The striatum interacts intimately with the "emotional center," which is composed of the hypothalamus, amygdala, and hippocampus. Below them are the "basecamp for reward," the ventral tegmental area (VTA), and, flush beside the VTA, the pars compacta of the substantia nigra (SNpc). Just exterior to these, and separately evolved, is the anterior cingulate cortex (ACC).[10] In front and outside we have the recently expanded PFC, divided into ventromedial and dorsolateral regions. At the bottom of the PFC is a dedicated site of cortical reward processing, the orbitofrontal cortex (OFC). Reward processing and response patterns in people are functions of the ways in which these structures interact.

To help fix the idea of the various circuits and directions of influence we'll be describing, we begin with a series of images of the brain with areas of interest highlighted. The brain is structured, layered and folded in all directions, so no single image can do the job of showing what we need here.

In figure 5.1 the exterior of the brain is shown from the side, with the motor cortex, the dorsolateral PFC, and the OFC labeled. The

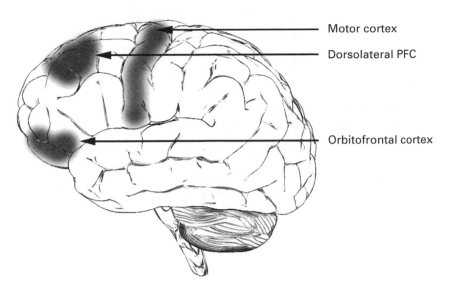

Motor cortex

Dorsolateral PFC

Orbitofrontal cortex

Figure 5.1

ventromedial PFC (VMPFC) borders the dorsolateral PFC, but lies on the insides of the two hemispheres of the brain and so would not be visible from this orientation. The areas highlighted in this figure occur on both sides of the brain.

The main parts of the set of reward-specialized brain systems we will be discussing are deeper within the brain. Figure 5.2 is also a side view, but in it the one hemisphere has been removed, so that the middle of the brain ("facing" in the same direction as the image in figure 5.1, so that were the eyes included in either image they would be looking to the left) is being viewed. The SNpc is located close to the VTA appearing on this figure.[11]

Figure 5.3 shows the brain in a more roughly three-dimensional view, as though it was facing in the direction of the thick black arrow. Note that the hypothalamus borders the thalamus, and does not appear on this figure because it is obscured by the dorsal striatum.[12]

The final figure, figure 5.4, is schematic, sacrificing fidelity to anatomical proportions in order to represent a system of connections.[13] (One new term occurring in this figure, "GABA," denotes another neurotransmitter discussed later in this chapter.)

It has been recognized for many years, mainly on the basis of work with animals, that the VTA and the SNpc are the two structures that

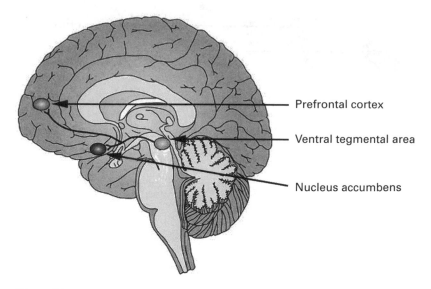

Figure 5.2

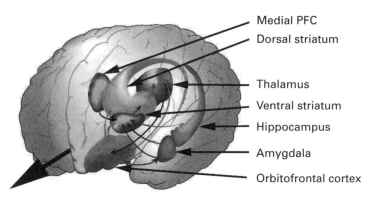

Figure 5.3

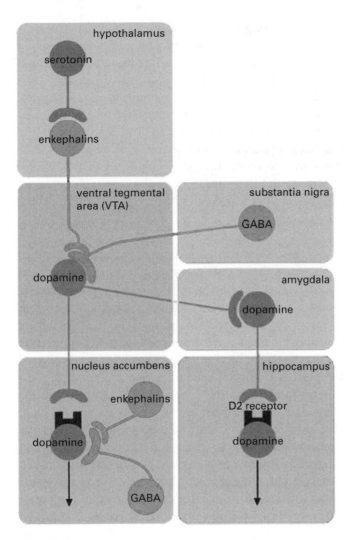

Figure 5.4

send reward signals out through the rest of the brain. Their role was revealed in a series of experiments whereby rats who were supplied with levers they could press to directly stimulate these areas through implants would do so repeatedly and relentlessly, ignoring less direct reinforcers like food and water to the point of death (Niesink et al. 1999, chapters 5 and 6). In this pattern researchers immediately recognized the prototype for substance abuse. The discovery of the underlying neurochemistry and neurodynamics of obsessive substance ingestion has therefore constituted a main part of the history of reward-system research. Relevant facts based on animal work have been under assembly for decades, but development of the integrated neuroeconomic model had to await fMRI investigation since 2000.

We distinguish VTA and SNpc from one another mainly by reference to the different neurotransmitter pathways through which they feed reward signals forward. It is through variance in dopamine-releasing rates that VTA and SNpc implement the PV model described in the previous section.[14] To reiterate that account in the context of neurotransmission, above-baseline dopamine release is interpreted by the rest of the brain as meaning that a reward has been received that was better than expected, disappointment relative to expectations is indicated by below-baseline dopamine release, and baseline dopamine release is the default state meaning that reward levels are as predicted. It will be crucial to our understanding of addiction and PG that the brain is generally more responsive to *changes* in the environment than to absence of change. The brain signal derived through fMRI is much larger for surprisingly good and surprisingly poor rewards and tends to be associated with low signal change for conditions that don't alter the status quo. The large human brain is primarily an organ adapted for learning, to which status quo conditions make little contribution. Therefore, brains do not waste resources on them. The reward system is no exception to this principle.

As described in the previous section, communication within brains occurs by both neurochemical and neuroelectrical signals. On the neuroelectrical dimension, brain cells are wired together in circuits through which varying electrical pulses are passed along connecting cables called dendrites. Different brain cells participate in different neural pathways partly by means of their various specific dendritic connection patterns. However, neurons don't transmit the signaling pulses from one to another by implementing an electrical switchboard. Instead,

they influence one another's probability of receiving signals by emit-
ting chemicals at synapses. How likely it is that a given signal will cross
the space between the synapse of one neuron and the synapse of
another neuron is a function of the level of that synapse's chemical of
interest—i.e., the neurotransmitter to which it distinctively responds—
in the fluid of the brain at the site in question.

Neurons are sorted into types on the basis of which neurotransmitters their synapses release and respond to. There are three neurotransmitters of particular importance in reward processing. Thanks
to the recent popularity of antidepression agents like Prozac that
modulate serotonin levels in different parts of the brain, serotonin
has become the best-known neurotransmitter among the general
public. We then group all the parts of the brain that communicate
with one another by releasing and taking up serotonin as together
comprising the serotonergic system. Similarly, the pathways through
the brain created by linked dopamine releasers and receivers are
referred to as the dopaminergic system. The third is the noradrenergic
system.

The reward system is the set of processes in the brain that computes
the outputs broadcast as dopamine pulses by VTA and SNpc. We will
begin our tour of it with the hypothalamus. This directly monitors basic
bodily states, such as blood sugar and temperature levels, that are
direct proprioperceptive (i.e., inwardly but unconsciously perceived)
indicators of changes relevant to the overall system's present and
expected utility. Hypothalamic information serves as fundamental
input to the reward system, and *connects* reward to representation of
hedonic pleasure, which also involves the ACC.[15]

We have emphasized "connects" here to stress that although reward and pleasure are related, they are not the same thing. This
may be the single most important point on which neuroscience calls
for a revision in popular "common sense" about targets of addiction
and compulsive behavior. When reward and pleasure are muddled
together, as they are in everyday thought and talk, we're led to think
that (e.g.) a heroin addict must pursue heroin "because she likes it."
Her attempts to kick her habit then seem to require us to say that
she simultaneously *doesn't* like it—and now we find that it's hard to
say anything coherent about the whole matter. Neuroscience forces
us to separate not just two but three kinds of psychological state:
(1) the extent to which a state is hedonically pleasurable; (2) the extent
to which a change of state is treated by the brain as a reward; and

(3) the extent to which a person *judges* a change of state as improving or reducing their immediate or longer-term welfare. It turns out from the study of the brain—this is not something one settles by appeal to philosophical opinion on the concepts of "pleasure" and "reward"— that (2) and (3) are more intimately associated with one another than either is with (1).

A landmark fMRI study suggesting this was performed and reported by Berns et al. (2001). They found that subjects' subjective reports of pleasure discrimination between fruit juice and water were correlated only with activity in cortical areas associated with sensory processes, whereas responses to unpredictability were correlated with activity in the NAcc, thalamus, and medial OFC. These areas have in common that they are involved in dopamine-regulated input to attention allocation and (through connection with motor neurons) to preparation for action. Thus, pleasure response seemed to be occurring outside the direct reward-response loop.

A wave of subsequent experiments building on this classic investigation has established as a basic principle of NE that people (behaviorally and neurally) "want" many things they don't (hedonically) "like."[16] Furthermore, they can readily learn not to want things that they like, if the latter become predictors for other things they don't want or like. For example, people who successfully lose weight often do so by learning to find fatty foods that they formerly enjoyed disgusting to consider. Of course, many targets of impulsive appetite induce hedonic pleasure while they're being consumed, and this is often crucial to their initial attractiveness. However, just as many smokers actually find the sensations of at least many of the cigarettes they smoke (e.g., the 30th of a long night) mainly unpleasant (while smoking them, anyway), so we should not assume that a PG *must* experience a warm subjective thrill while she's rolling the dice.

There is an obvious reason why most people don't clearly distinguish between pleasure and reward, even though they play distinct roles in the brain. Consciously experienced pleasure is one (only somewhat reliable) proxy for, or predictor of, reward. Precisely *because* it is the consciously experienced signal of probable reward, it's one we notice when we introspectively reflect on the motivations for our behavior. (We also notice some motivators programmed into us by socialization, such as injunctions to moral duty; these get coded in public language and we notice them by literally talking to ourselves as if we were other people, not by directly "looking inside.") However, most of what goes

on in our brains is not consciously accessible in itself, while nevertheless contributing to our interpretations of what we think we're experiencing. Hedonic pleasure signals evolved in primitive ancestors of ours
that had much less complicated reward systems than we do, and the
pleasure system we've inherited from them probably responds unequiv-
ocally—that is, in a way not strongly mediated by reward signals—only
to some very basic cues, such as air temperature, sexual contact, and
whether we are damp or dry. The rest of what we loosely interpret as
pleasure is probably built out of second-order associations between
pleasure signals and reward signals (e.g., getting into bed predicts
warmth and sex, so getting into bed comes to be experienced as directly
pleasurable). As creatures whose main evolutionary adaptation has
itself been adaptive intelligence, however, we have reward systems that
were precisely selected so as not to give pleasure signals priority over
our curiosity about changes in environmental reinforcers. This is why
pleasure is not a strongly reliable proxy for reward in people. More to
the point, as emphasized at the end of the preceding paragraph, it isn't
as important to behavioral motivation as is generally and casually
imagined. People who suffer catastrophes to their anterior cingulates
and report losing hedonic color from their subjective worlds remain
susceptible to reinforcement learning (Berridge and Robinson 1998;
Schroeder 2004, pp. 121–122). By contrast, lesions to the components of
the reward system typically produce profound breakdowns, ranging
from Parkinson's disease to total motivational disintegration. Rats
whose reward systems were trained to respond positively to terrible-
tasting food ate the food while making facial expressions characteristic
(in rats) of unpleasant experiences (Berridge and Valenstein 1991). The
fact that we are evolved to pursue what stimulates our reward system
more diligently than what makes us feel good will turn out to be a
fundamental part of the neuroscientific explanation of addiction and
PG.

As predicted by the PV model, unpredictable stimuli produce stronger responses in the VTA, NAcc, and ventral striatum than do familiar
ones (Berns et al. 2001). It is clear from empirical study that the stronger
NAcc response is a direct function of an elevated surge of dopamine
from the VTA. This response specifically signals *positive* surprises;
dopamine neurons show only minor, probably indirect, response to
aversive and neutral stimuli (Mirenowicz and Schultz 1996; Schultz
2002). In particular, the NAcc is unresponsive to such stimuli (Knutson
et al. 2001). Thus, contrary to what common sense might have expected,

reward and punishment are not coded along a single continuum to which a single, modular brain system responds. This will prove important to understanding why adverse consequences of addiction and AG are notoriously ineffective, at least by themselves, in reconditioning afflicted people. Dopamine neurons do not discriminate with respect to the sensory modality through which stimuli are delivered; they "care" only about the extent to which a stimulus is relevant to the difference between the prediction and the delivery of its associated reward (Schultz 2002). This is relevant to explaining why, in drug-dependent people and PGs attempting recovery, *anything* that has been a characteristic part of the person's habitual environment for drug taking or gambling is an equally strong potential trigger of relapse. As learning proceeds, the system stops responding to administration of the reward itself and responds instead to its predictors (ibid.). Furthermore, dopaminergic neurons show depressed response when rewards are smaller than what learning would have led the system to predict; thus the dopamine neurochemistry converges qualitatively with the PV model that quantitatively describes the fMRI data (Martin-Soelch et al. 2001).

A major barrier to the understanding of behavior by common sense is that everyday psychology misleadingly separates—or, at least, fails to strongly connect—the passive, perceptual aspect of reward and the active response to rewarding prospects. This partly stems from everyday psychology's overly direct connection of pleasure with reward; pleasure, as we have seen, *is* relatively passive and weak as a response motivator. But natural selection did not build massive learning systems for us so that we could *contemplate* complex attractions; in the brain, learning is for doing. Note also (a point to which we will return in more detail shortly) that thinking about something (as opposed to thinking about other possible things) is not (as in *Hamlet*) the opposite of acting. It is a kind of action, since it involves the brain neurochemically and neurodynamically *doing something* (i.e., using resources for this rather than that). We should thus not think of reward learning as akin to a kind of perception, even though dopamine does subserve reward perception in addition to learning (Preuschoff, Bossaerts, and Quartz 2006). The learning function of dopamine is, fundamentally, a mechanism for allocating neural resources and prompting behavior. The VTA and SNpc directly project to the motor anterior cingulate and motor PFC. By this pathway, dopamine signals entrain motor habits that can proceed with minimal mediation after learning. This includes both "bodily" behavioral habits and "thought" habits in the sense of automatic associations we make when presented with familiar stimuli. (Schroeder [2004] reviews experiments from the 1990s that we can now, in light of what we've since learned about the dopaminergic system, recognize as showing this.) The portentousness of this for addictive and compulsive phenomena, in which people feel that they have lost deliberate control, will be evident. Where the reward system is concerned, paying attention to something and doing something about it are more or less the same thing—it can't, as it were, tell the difference between caring about (e.g.) gambling and getting busy preparing to gamble.

The most dramatic indication of the intimate relationship between the reward/dopaminergic system and motor behavior, and one that will turn out to be profoundly important to our understanding of PG/AG, is the range of consequences attached to impairment of the system's capacity to send adequate dopamine signals. Parkinson's disease is a degenerative disorder of the dopamine system as vested in the SNpc. Its symptoms are loss of motor control (expressed in movement inability or difficulty [akinesia], tremors, and rigidity), impaired cognition (difficulties with concentration, planning, and learning) and motivation (Schultz 2002, p. 247). Lesser compromises of the system due to lesions or chemical antagonists produce subsets of these same symptoms to varying degrees.

Identifying dopamine as underlying reward processing was not a simple process. As recently as 2003 there was still disagreement on the interpretation of the relevant findings. In the most complete survey of reward system science that had been done to that time, Berridge and Robinson (1998) argued that dopaminergic response does not mediate reward learning in the sense of that phenomenon as it was then modeled (as "capacity to predict rewarding events based upon associative correlations," p. 313). Rather, they suggested, the system mediates "attribution of incentive salience to otherwise neutral events" (ibid.). By this they mean that dopamine response to a stimulus is the basis for the organism focusing and maintaining attention (both perceptual and behavioral) on that stimulus. As Schroeder (2004, p. 116) explains, "experiments in which the dopamine-releasing cells of the VTA projecting to the motor PFC were destroyed found that this impaired monkeys' abilities to keep a prior intention in mind long enough to execute it after a delay." Schroeder cites Durstewitz, Kelc, and Güntürkün (1999) as suggesting that the primary role of dopamine in the motor PFC is precisely to stabilize its goal-serving motor intentions against interference by other possible motor intentions that would be counter-productive. That is, information about expected reward is used to keep people and other animals like us focused upon our reward-directed intentions, to prevent us forgetting them or going off to do something else before carrying them out. (Schroeder 2004, p. 116)

Part of the reason it was natural for Berridge and Robinson to frame this idea as a *rival* to the reward-learning model of the dopaminergic system stems from the fact that reward still had not (in 1998) been fully disassociated from pleasure. Their 1998 survey devoted substantial critical attention to establishing that dopamine projections to the NAcc and neostriatum are not needed for "normal hedonic evaluations, for hedonic modulation, or for learned adjustments in hedonic value." They noted that incentive salience attribution corresponds roughly to what behavioral economists had dubbed "decision utility," defined as "the degree to which a goal is chosen or sought" (p. 334). They recognized, of course, that decision utility— "wanting"—and hedonic appreciation—"liking"—are related; thus they suggested that once decision utility is associated with a stimulus, "on each subsequent encounter . . . its capacity to support wanting is maintained or strengthened by associative reboosting of the incentive salience assigned to its representation. Reboosting happens when a wanted incentive is followed again by activation of hedonic liking" (ibid.).

In retrospect, this critical quarrel—as is usually the case with apparent scientific disagreements—was really a step along the road to completing consensus on the conceptual clarification of "reward" and its distinctions from related phenomena. "The compatibility of specific reward learning models," declared Berridge and Robinson,

hinges on precisely what . . . authors of reward learning hypotheses for dopamine function . . . mean by "expectation of reward." If these reward learning hypotheses posit that dopamine mediates Pavlovian learning about *incentive value alone* (not stimulus-reward association per se, not hedonic value, not cognitive expectation of outcome) and that anticipatory neuronal responses to conditioned stimuli occur because those stimuli carry *incentive motivational* qualities, such as incentive salience, separately from mere association or from hedonic qualities, then those reward learning hypotheses are compatible with our incentive salience hypothesis. . . . If, however, dopamine neurons are posited to mediate any other sense of "expectation of reward" . . . then either the reward learning hypothesis or the incentive salience hypothesis must be wrong. (Ibid., p. 336)

We think the concluding sentence above is mistaken. Dopamine neurons *do* mediate "expectation of reward" in the most elementary sense of perceiving and tracking expected reward (Preuschoff, Bossaerts, and Quartz 2006). However, it does *not* follow from this that one or the other model of dopamine's role in integrating learning, attention, and preparation must be wrong, since the perceptual functions of dopamine appear to be independent of this integration. Berridge and Robinson's invitation to proponents of the reward-learning hypothesis to refine their concept of reward met, ultimately, with a favorable response. The first paper to state the mature model of dopaminergic learning, by McClure, Daw, and Montague (2003), essentially fused Berridge and Robinson's incentive salience hypothesis with Berns and Montague's PV model. All recent theories of dopaminergic learning, they pointed out, "agree on the singular principle that dopamine function is causally located between the identification of a potential future reward and the generation of action to pursue it" (p. 425).[17] However, the incentive salience hypothesis "leaves off after the identification of a goal" (ibid.). What McClure, Daw, and Montague mean by this is that Berridge and Robinson's hypothesis is a theory of the behavioral meaning of dopamine signals, but incorporates no account of learning except for the imprecise talk of "reboosting" that they associate with it. This won't do, since even if an initial dopamine response is taken to strongly bias selection of a goal, the system must still choose an action sequence, and choice in this context can't be separated off from reward valuation as expressed in relative motivational response. TD learning, as described earlier, is precisely an algorithm for this, nudging the system toward actions that lead to better-than-predicted rewards. Here is where the PV model can take up the slack: if the rate of dopamine neuron spiking encodes a prediction error signal, where incentive salience is then taken to be a function of the magnitudes of these errors, then the gap in Berridge and Robinson's model is closed. "We propose," say McClure, Daw and Montague, "that the concept of incentive salience is the expected future reward. . . . In addition, we propose that the role of dopamine in learning to attribute such expectations to situations that are predictive of reward . . . and in biasing action selection toward such situations . . . serve[s] as the formal counterpart to the ideas of Berridge and Robinson . . . about the role of dopamine in attributing and using incentive salience" (ibid.).

As previously stated, here we have the current model of reward system learning and behavioral control that has been confirmed by numerous experiments conducted over the past two years, several of which will be discussed below, and which will provide the basis for our later claim that PG/AG may become a pharmacologically manageable health problem. The power of the model is nicely illustrated by application to a study—one directly relevant to gambling behavior—in which the interpreters under-exploit it. Zink et al. (2004) compared skin conductance and blood-oxygenation-level dependent (BOLD) responses—the signals measured by fMRI—in two groups of subjects. One group earned amounts of money as a function of their success at performing a task, while the other performed the same task but received equivalent expected quantities of money independently of task performance. As expected, significantly greater activity in the dopaminergic reward pathway (NAcc and caudate nucleus) was observed in the first group. Zink et al. interpret this as showing that dopaminergic activity mediates salience *rather than* expected future reward. This dichotomy appears to be false: both interpretations are correct. For the first group of subjects in the Zink et al. experiment, the money was an incentive to action and therefore was salient. If the current full synthesis of reward system models as described above is correct, then we should surmise that this produced additional and more sustained dopamine response with later onset than in the second group. We will argue over the sections and chapters to come that dopamine's function in integrating reward learning, attention, and seeking behavior is the basis of gambling's capacity to trip the circuit into runaway self-amplification. That dopamine also mediates reward perception adds to the power of the midbrain system to push alternative behaviors aside when special circumstances and the neurochemical reaction to them frees it from cortical management.

5.4   The Neurochemistry of Addiction

Section 5.3 explained the basis for the neuroecomic hypothesis that at the basis of reinforcement (perhaps facilitated by a G-learning of world models) lies the PV model of the reward system as an implementation of TD learning. On this account, all decision making behavior is to some extent reward-dependent. Next, we presented evidence that a midbrain dopaminergic circuit projecting to the OFC and PFC is the site of reward valuation and primary response. In the present section we will ask: can we understand in neurochemical terms how substances on which people become dependent might trip the reward system so as to generate the behavioral patterns classically associated with addiction? A crucial requirement for such understanding is that the neurochemical facts, interpreted through the neuroeconomic model, explain why disposition to relapse, rather than fear of withdrawal, is the great bane of addicts who try to achieve more stable lives.

We have pointed out on several occasions that "addiction" has been used in loose and varying ways in different everyday, clinical, and scientific contexts, so much so that many behavioral scientists have avoided serious use of the concept. Economists (at least those who follow the leading "revealed preference" approach to attributing utility functions) group motivational phenomena together by reference to their outward behavioral properties. Setting off "addicts" as those who are allegedly chained to certain behavioral patterns by fear of withdrawal costs, as once was standard in psychology and psychiatry, rested on assuming the behavioral centrality of this property in advance of careful evidence for it. Then the evidence, when it came in, went the other way, in the sense that most traditionally so-called "addicts" turned out to be more capable of withdrawal than of avoiding relapse, despite their knowing that relapse implies facing the pain of withdrawal all over again at some point. As noted above, if fear of withdrawal were the dominant and decisive factor for addiction, then this would make no sense. Because, prior to recent strides in understanding the brain, there was not an alternative consensual basis for drawing a sharp line between addicts and non-addicts, the ultimate scientific value of this concept, with its folk origins, could be called into question in some precincts (especially behavioristic ones).

The clinical research community, by contrast with more theoretically focused behavioral modelers, never stopped referring to "addicts" as a special class of patients. We think that recent discoveries in neuroscience show that they were right. We are persuaded that there are, after all, distinctive neural properties in a subset of people who abuse substances that are very strongly correlated with substance-abuse dispositions markedly more severe and intractable to various interventions than occur in other people. The main features of this pattern are robust across particular personal and cultural circumstances. Behavioral properties classically associated with addiction, along with proneness to relapse after successful withdrawal, seem well explained by the PV model of the reward system, which in turn has an underlying neurochemical model that also explains why the leading agents of drug dependence can lock the system into hysteresis (self-amplification).

Then, as we'll see in chapter 7, the behavioral patterns typical of addiction are highly responsive, in detail, to certain neuropharmacological interventions that the neurochemical model of the neuroeconomic effects predicts. There are no better grounds for thinking one has isolated a real phenomenon than having a cluster of robust causal regularities tied together by a quantitatively paramaterized model that generates testable predictions, and which continues to prove applicable to new phenomena. To which new phenomena have the neurochemical and neuroeconomic models turned out to apply? One answer is: PG. PGs, we argue in chapter 6, appear to manifest distinctive neurochemical properties when these are individuated according to a certain model inspired by the PV account of reward, and these then explain the behavioral phenomena that originally confounded the folk view of addiction. If PGs turn out to be both neurochemically and behaviorally distinctive in ways common to them and to drug-dependent people, and if the unification of models at these levels suggests that this is no coincidence, then it is hard to imagine how the claim that PGs are genuine addicts could receive clearer justification.

We begin the argument by quoting a representative clinical operationalization of addiction, formulated by a group of researchers in 1998 who had their eyes on the neuroscientific data that were beginning to accrue: "Addiction, also known as substance dependence . . . is a chronically relapsing disorder that is characterized by three major elements: (1) compulsion to seek and take the drug, (2) loss of control in limiting intake, and (3) emergence of a negative emotional state (e.g., dysphoria, anxiety, irritability) when access to the drug is prevented" (Koob, Paolo Sanna, and Bloom 1998). Note that all of these aspects can be identified and induced in laboratory animals. As a result, when Koob, Paolo Sanna, and Bloom stated this operationalization, they already knew that it described a behavioral complex that was strongly correlated with unusual profiles in animals' dopaminergic systems. These systems are composed of two major projection pathways: one from SNpc to striatum and one from VTA to NAcc, frontal cortex, and amygdala. Stimulant drugs such as cocaine and amphetamines inhibit reuptake of dopamine after it has facilitated synaptic transfer, so that it accumulates in NAcc. Opiates recruit additional mechanisms (mu-opioid receptors) in VTA and NAcc, while alcohol inhibits GABA neurons throughout the brain. Since GABA neurons inhibit dopaminergic neurons in VTA, the second-order result of GABAergic inhibition is the same flood of dopamine into NAcc that is characteristic of cocaine.

Alcohol additionally promotes serotonin and mu-opioid receptors. Similarly, nicotine affects functioning in both the mesolimbic dopamine pathway and the opioid peptide circuit.

Given what we have learned about the reward system, we should be able to see quickly how modified dopamine flow and concentrations are correlated with some of the familiar properties of addiction. Dopamine, after all, facilitates focus on salient reward predictors and primes the system for motor action in response to such predictors. A key part of addiction is clearly obsessive concentration on the target of abuse, coupled with a relentless tendency to pursue it in action. But this is still a long way short of explaining the molecular mechanisms of addiction. Why do dopamine concentrations pair with obsessive pursuit of certain *specific* rewards, namely stimulant drugs, opiates, alcohol, nicotine . . . and gambling? That is, why don't people with elevated dopamine levels in NAcc just impulsively consume whatever happens to be to hand in good supply? In chapter 3 we drew attention to George Loewenstein's observation that no one impulsively consumes purely instrumental goods like petrol or writing paper. That truth is so obvious when pointed out that one can easily miss the further question it invites: what is it about some rewards, such as cocaine and nicotine, that makes the brain treat them as *not* mainly instruments (for pleasure, utility, or fitness, depending on the modeling context)? A related series of puzzles arises around the question of what it is about dopamine concentrations that leads to the characteristic *dynamics* of addiction, in which addicts become *sensitized* to their object of addiction.[18] That is, why does an addict show heightened behavioral effects to stimuli that predict the objects of her addiction—and consume steadily more of it even while her reported hedonic pleasure from it drops?

As with all products of natural selection, the brain is not designed in the way that an engineer would assemble a machine. That is, there are no simple one-to-one relationships between neurotransmitters or other chemicals and styles of behavior. A first complication is that interesting behavior types result from interactions among different neurotransmitters (and other brain chemicals, such as peptides). In the case of addiction, the key interacting neurotransmitters, in addition to dopamine and GABA, are glutamate and serotonin. A second complication is that some neurotransmitters—e.g., glutamate—enhance synaptic activity, while others—particularly GABA—inhibit it. And a third complication is that even for a given neurotransmitter within a single neuroanatomical region (e.g., dopamine in the VMPFC), one finds different classes of receptors that behave differently from one another in the same chemical context. Thus, for example, in the PFC there are four kinds of dopamine receptors (referred to as D1, D2, D3, and D4 receptors) distinguished by response properties.

We can best illustrate the extent of this complexity with an example. Dopamine interactions with GABA and glutamate play the key role in causing sensitization in addicts (Steketee 2002). The specific ways in which they do this, however, vary in detail from substance to substance, due to the ways in which different substances variously modulate overall balances of neurotransmitter levels at specific brain sites. Dopamine synapses with both glutamate and GABA neurons in the VMPFC. But GABA neurons synapse on these same cells. Then, whether dopamine excites or inhibits a given cell depends on whether that cell is or isn't also receiving GABA transmission (Gulledge and Jaffe 2001; Yang, Seamans, and Gorelova 1999). Indeed, it is also sensitive to the neuroelectrical state of the cell membrane (Yang, Seamans, and Gorelova 1999). In general, whether dopamine release in the VMPFC stimulates or inhibits GABA and glutamate release depends on whether it is taken up by D1 or by D2 receptors. In the same chemical context, D3 receptor activity seems to *oppose* D1 and D2 activity. And then we must remember that GABA release inhibits (among other things) glutamate neuron response. Notice, then, that to determine a prediction of whether a given boost of dopamine will produce a net increase or decrease in glutamate activation will require both exact knowledge of which receptors are triggered and quantitative measurement of relative, dynamic neurotransmitter levels at the start of the process.

The nonspecialist reader might be dizzy now—our point was to make her so—and perhaps also a bit dismayed. In terms of physical articulation, the brain is the single most complex functional system studied in all of science. If understanding its responses to stimuli requires, for each stimulus, a complete molecular pathway model, then it seems that all molecular-level neuroscientific explanations will be hard to achieve, will be highly specifically complicated, and will be difficult to integrate into generalizable knowledge—or, where pathologies are concerned, general treatment strategies. For example, we have several times made reference to the effect on the brain of "stimulant drugs," citing as examples the standard cases, cocaine and amphetamines. These substances indeed act in the same way at a high enough level of abstraction—e.g., that of the PV model. But Steketee (2002) shows in a review of research that, in fact, the ways in which they influence VMPFC, and then influence VMPFC's effect on subcortical regions in processes of sensitization, are quite different. They also differ in the ways in which they increase dopamine concentrations in NAcc to begin with: cocaine blocks reuptake, while amphetamines stimulate efflux from synapses.

Does this imply that we should expect different pharmacological treatments for cocaine and amphetamine addiction? Well, yes and no. As we'll see in chapter 7, these drugs have enough in common in the way they act (i.e., both increasing dopamine in NAcc) that scientists can already synthesize a single sort of agent that works powerfully to reduce their addictive hold. Because their neurochemical actions are different at a deeper level of detail in the way just indicated, this therapy will likely be considered crude after further research leads to a later generation of drugs, so that ultimately we will probably have one improved therapy for cocaine and another for amphetamines. At present, to cite another example we will review in chapter 7, pilot studies are testing drugs developed for relief of cocaine addiction on PGs. While there is good reason to think these drugs will make a difference, and while this contributes importantly to our argument that AG is the basic form of addiction, it will be surprising if agents specifically sculpted for use against cocaine addiction turn out to be our *ultimate* best response to AG.

The underlying point here is that the scientific study of a phenomenon never reaches a final resting point. At any given time we will know just so much about specific addictions, and there will be more we're about to know still waiting around the corner. Thus, for all addictions our scientifically based treatment strategies will go on indefinitely improving with our understanding. At present, we can rank our knowledge of the neurochemistry of the major substances of abuse, from greatest to least, roughly as follows:

• Cocaine
• Amphetamines
• Alcohol
• Nicotine
• Opiates

The contention about gambling we'll defend is that it has an interesting status in terms of the list above. Just a few years ago, it would have belonged at the bottom of the list. It was an open question, indeed, whether there even is such a phenomenon as "addiction" to gambling in the sense of a distinctive type of neurochemical and neurodynamic processes associated with severe and chronic DG behavior. Now, however, there is strong evidence that not only is there such a thing as AG, but that it resembles the better understood substance addictions, those at the top of the list above, more than it does those at the bottom. In fact, we'll present reasons for thinking that AG may be *the* most basic and fundamental form of addiction, the form around which can be built a general template for addiction models; models of targets with more specific and complex causal effects, such as heroin, will then be (considerable) complications to this template. We can summarize this claim, one of the central theses of the book, as follows: *in studying AG we come as close as possible to studying the generic form of addiction.*

In working up to this claim, the first thing we need to do is indicate the *general* properties of stimulant drug addiction, abstracting from details that *separate* special pathways among the stimulant drugs. In reviewing leading data, we will add explicit notes drawing attention to aspects that are suggestive where AG is concerned. Though we will discuss some data on subjects addicted to other substances, especially nicotine, we will confine ourselves to aspects of these data that reflect on neurochemical patterns that all addictions have in common— namely, those directly associated with learning in the dopaminergic system.

Enhanced dopamine release into striatum contributes to the promotion of action from representation. Enhanced dopamine release into NAcc, specifically, promotes focus, attention and learning in accordance with the reward learning/PV model. This provokes urges to engage in exploratory behavior centered on the target of attention. Stimulant drugs act directly to increase dopamine in NAcc, thus causing effects that mimic behavioral response to novel stimuli (Chambers, Taylor, and Potenza 2003). In addition, dopamine activity acting on D3 receptors interacts with glutamate and GABAergic neurons in *both* NAcc and VMPFC to alter the firing potentials of synapses in subcortical regions and thereby causes behavioral sensitization—that is, heightened motor response to learned cues for the rewards associated with the substance (Everitt, Dickinson, and Robbins 2001). In particular, it causes so-called "long-term potentiation" at synapses, an implementation of memory. We know that D3 receptors in striatum are particularly coupled to movement control, because—and this will later emerge as important in research on AG—animals given agents that block D3 receptors develop Parkinson's symptoms (Baik et al. 1995). Serotonin (5-HT) release inhibits excitatory effects of dopamine on subcortical areas, and so low serotonin is correlated with both addiction learning and probability of relapse.

It is well known that younger people, especially adolescents, are much more prone to develop addictions, and to be less able to avoid relapse during recovery attempts, than older people. The large majority of addictions begin in adolescence, and adult occurrences of addiction can be predicted to some extent from adolescent behavior.[19] It is therefore indirect confirming evidence for the general model above that, as Chambers, Taylor, and Potenza (2003) describe, adolescent mammals have heightened dopaminergic responses and diminished inhibitory 5-HT systems. Furthermore, PFC, which plays an inhibitory role in the development of addiction and which dopaminergic action must hijack during potentiation for addiction to occur (see below), is not yet fully mature in adolescent humans. Their brains adapt faster and more permanently to stimuli in general. Thus, it is not surprising that since addiction is a variety of adaptive learning, young people are more vulnerable to it (Gray 2004).

There is direct evidence that the neural learning of addiction requires active exploration by subjects. That is, brains don't adapt to drugs by simply "soaking them up"; they adapt by forming new patterns of active response to make receipt of drugs more likely. "Plasticity" is the term for the disposition of a learning unit (anything from the whole brain to a single synapse) to adapt to new input. At the excitatory (glutamate) synapses implicated in addiction learning, a measure of plasticity is the ratio of two types of glutamate receptors, AMPA and NMDA. Dumont et al. (2005) performed an experiment which revealed that self-stimulation by means of cocaine and food pellets by rats changes this ratio, whereas passive administration of the same quantities of these rewards doesn't. This is consistent with some venerable puzzles about addiction, such as the fact that hospital patients given high doses of morphine for extended periods don't generally develop addiction. The result vividly underscores the way in which the reward learning/PV model, as an account of the learning of salient *relationships* between environmental cues and actions, captures addiction. This feature will emerge as central in the account of AG.

Bechara and Martin (2004) found that human substance addicts suffer from measurable impairment of working memory relative to controls. In general this probably does not reflect any structural compromise of brain areas (though specific forms of such damage do occur following years of alcohol abuse), but is instead a function of the focusing effect of dopaminergic learning, which inhibits attention to anything other than the addictive target. A number of the performance differences between substance abusers and controls on the Iowa Gambling Task, as reviewed in chapter 4, may be explained by this aspect of the neurobiology of addiction. It may be especially relevant to AG in light of the well-known fact that PGs' behavior while gambling is less sensitive than other people's to shifts of odds against them. The greater motivation of AGs to gamble may be complemented by the greater difficulty they have in cognitively processing the implications of changing odds. This evidence is supported in another recent study by Garavan and Stout (2005). In their experiment, human addicts showed poorer than normal performance at cognitive learning (in attention-switching, Stroop,[20] and inhibitory control tasks) based on positive and negative feedback from other people. Interestingly, during processing of these cognitive tasks, addicts under fMRI showed strongly enhanced activity in ACC, another direct site of projection from VTA and SNpc, relative to controls. Addicts' cognitive performance improves when they take a shot of their drug, which is consistent with the reward learning/PV model: drug reward temporarily reduces the distance between predicted reward state and actual reward state, and so dampens the mesolimbic noise that interferes with cognitive processing. Smokers are all aware of the greater pressure they feel to reach for their drug while trying to concentrate. Of direct relevance to AG, in the Garavan and Stout experiment, hypoactivity of anterior cingulate in addicts is correlated with lower response to losses during cognitive learning.

A suggestive study of the relationship between addiction and attentional gating is reported by Martin-Soelch et al. (2001). They conducted a PET neuroimaging study involving four groups performing cognitive tasks for monetary and nonmonetary rewards: (1) normal controls, (2) smokers, (3) opiate addicts, and (4) Parkinson's sufferers. Group (1) showed diverse neural responses to both sorts of rewards, in all the brain regions that our knowledge of the reward system would lead us to expect. However, smokers showed response only in OFC, right cingulate gyrus, and left midbrain—nothing in striatum (or thalamus). Opiate addicts showed less response than controls in dopaminergic areas to all rewards, and no response in dopaminergic areas to nonmonetary rewards. Group (4) matched group (1) except with respect to their lack of OFC and striatal responses. Thus we have another illustration of the extent to which addiction focuses the reward system to the exclusion of targets other than the object of addiction. It is interesting, as the researchers note, that nicotine appeared to be a more powerful agent in this regard than opiates. If this initially seems surprising to our intuitions, we might use the occasion to reflect on why we find it so. Our everyday idea of "impulsiveness" incorporates reference to stereotypical socially disruptive behavior that indicates impaired judgment. In this respect, smoking will seem the least dangerous of addictions (aside from its impact on organs other than the brain). However, the relevant concept of impulsivity in the neurochemistry of addiction is the neuroeconomic, not the everyday one. The impact of nicotine on smokers' *molar* patterns of judgment appears to be relatively profound. For example, Bickel and Johnson (2003, pp. 431–434) review evidence that smokers discount the future at generally lower rates after they quit, a correlation also found for other drug addicts.[21] A similar confusion between everyday and neuroscientifically grounded psychological concepts probably contributes to some of the prevailing skepticism about gambling as a target for genuine *addiction*. The facts about nicotine, however, show that cognitive and motivational impairment resulting from addiction need not be straightforwardly manifest as socially inappropriate behavior (or intoxication as the folk understand it).

Another important study showing the effects of dopaminergic attentional gating in addicts, by Garavan et al. (2000), demonstrated that cocaine addicts demonstrate significantly less activation in the projection from VMPFC to NAcc than normal controls on being shown sexually evocative pictures.

Kalivas, Volkow, and Seamans (2005) report work that refines our understanding of behavioral attentional gating in addicts by separating its two underlying neurochemical substrates. Activation patterns in recovered rat cocaine addicts presented with cocaine-associated cues suggest that dopamine release in the projection from PFC to NAcc is responsible for strongly cuing the learned expectation of reward in response to the cues, while adaptations in glutamate synapses in NAcc reduce plasticity and impair the animals' abilities to learn to respond to alternative rewards. Since the drug in this case is cocaine, which has turned out to be the closest drug model to gambling (see chapter 6), our interest in AG motivates attention to some molecular details. Kalivas, Volkow, and Seamans appeal to a neurochemical model of dopamine action due to Seamans and Yang (2004). On this model, dopamine action gives rise to two possible states in VMPFC depending on whether influence at D1 or D2 receptors predominates. If D2 reception predominates, then multiple excitatory inputs promote VMPFC output to NAcc. If D1 reception predominates, then all signals below a high threshold are inhibited. In cocaine withdrawal, protein signaling to D2 receptors is reduced, thus inducing the animal to seek stimuli that can clear the high D1 threshold—namely, stimuli associated with cocaine. Here, then, is a neurochemical model of the mechanism by which withdrawal gives rise to cravings.

Further details have come to light on the way in which dopamine and glutamate neurons complement one another in subserving reward learning and in generating addiction (Kelley 2004). Cells in NAcc and VMPFC on which their dopamine and glutamate neurons jointly synapse act as coincidence detectors in associative learning; essentially, an animal or person is motivated to act when dopamine and glutamate signals agree with one another in sending positive signals. Glutamate responds to specific sensory information and "teaches" the system to respond to new information with a similar profile (as with any other neurotransmitter system, by modifying synaptic potentials). It thereby lays down episodic memories that are guides to subsequent actions. Dopamine neurons, by contrast, are alert for global states of the world that suggest reward prospects. But how can something as simple as a neuron respond selectively to an abstract property like reward? The basic molecular neurochemistry of dopaminergic influence is now understood. Ventral striatum and VMPFC neurons are normally held quiet by negative resting membrane potentials (called "K+" currents) unless pushed into depolarized states by inflow from cerebral cortex and thalamus. This inflow probably represents changes in perceptual and/or proprioperceptual streams. Following Dennett (1991), one can reasonably think of this detection activity as constituting initial, semi-automated "judgment" about stimulus significance; we say "*semi*-automated" to emphasize that this is not simply reflexive response of the classical (Sherringtonian) type, but involves both computational and interneural competition from the earliest parts of the process (Glimcher 2003). When the neurons are depolarized, dopamine excites them; when they're polarized, it dampens them further. However, the reward system is designed to both amplify these initial judgments and make them difficult to behaviorally revise; natural selection decided, as it were, that we should not waste precious cognitive resources reconsidering judgments. Where these judgments concern contingencies that are relatively resistant to the organism's direct manipulation, this is a sound design principle.

However, if the organism happens to find a lever in the environment with which it can reliably surprise itself, then dopamine's disposition to take initial positive responses to stimuli and reinforce them so long as learning continues can become an hysterical cascade of self-reinforcement. To be "reliably surprised" may sound paradoxical, but it is really just the familiar idea that you might know just where in town you can always go to see peculiar people. The neurochemistry of drug addiction is a crucial part of the explanation as to why *these* rewards (i.e., cocaine, nicotine, etc.), but not petrol or writing paper[22] or most other things, trigger this hysteresis. The dopaminergic self-reinforcement is the first part of the addictive response, the aspect that produces obsessive focus on the addictive target. A second aspect of the syndrome becomes operative as glutamate "stamps in" the dopaminergic response by modifying synapses to be alert to distinctive sensory predictors. Thus a pattern of salience cues is established, so that "opportunities" to consume the addictive target (opportunities which the organism itself has discovered the power to create to a greater extent than uncontrolled contingencies) are always detected and then, by virtue of the dopaminergic amplification, crowd out other potential objects of attention and attractors for behavior. Thus the smoker cannot bear to finish a meal without lighting up, the drinker cannot pass the bar without going in, and, as we will see in the next chapter, the gambler experiences a compulsive rush when she hears jangling coins. It is for this reason that vulnerability to relapse, rather than fear of withdrawal, is the true bane of the addict.

Powerful though the reward system is in regulating behavior, however, it is not in charge. Though dopamine concentration in NAcc is necessary for addiction, it is not sufficient for it; after all, stimulant drugs produce high concentrations of dopamine in NAcc of non-addicts, and most people who are exposed to addictive substances or gambling do not become addicts. In animals with frontal cortex, and especially in humans, cognitive judgment plays a standing regulative role in behavior. Addiction, however, specifically neurochemically limits this role. To say "subverts" in place of "limits" appeals to an irresistible—and appropriate—metaphor. Goldstein and Volkow (2002) review a substantial body of evidence that addictive targets do more than hijack the mesolimbic reward system; they also impair inhibition of subcortical responses by PFC circuits. One of the ways that some drugs do this is as directly as possible: stimulants, alcohol, and opiates physically destroy some frontal circuitry. More subtly, consumption of addictive substances appears to cause reformation of dendritic links, as a result of which normal cortical inhibition of amygdala is reduced (Robinson et al. 2001; Rosenkrantz and Grace 2001; Miller and Cohen 2001). In effect, addiction first hijacks the reward system below decks, then commits mutiny on the bridge by sabotaging the cognitive systems that would otherwise check its influence.

Adding this evidence to that which we have already reviewed on the dopamine-glutamate mechanism in midbrain, Goldstein and Volkow construct an integrated model of addiction that they call "impaired response inhibition and salience attribution" (I-RISA). This model is a specific instance of a general family of similar models, which, collectively, now dominate the neuroscience of addiction. I-RISA links the neural processes underlying four distinct aspects of addiction to substances: intoxication, craving, compulsive drug administration, and withdrawal. The main distinctive general feature of intoxication is dopamine concentration in NAcc. Craving then arises from the learned association between the drug reward and various stimulus contingencies, based on modified synaptic potentials in amygdala, hippocampus, thalamus, anterior cingulate, and OFC. (The basis of subjective experience of cravings presumably lies somewhere other than within the reward system. Very recent evidence as of this writing tentatively implicates insula. See Nasqvi et al. 2007.) Compulsive drug administration is then the consequence of the mesolimbic reward system that has learned to treat the addictive target as an overwhelmingly salient reward acting semi-autonomously in controlling behavior. Strong dopaminergic and serotonergic responses support withdrawal, symptoms of which include dysphoria (sadness), anhedonia (hedonic discomfort), impaired cognition, and irritability. To stress the point again, fear of withdrawal is almost certainly not the main factor in maintaining addiction. Instead, as a result of the resculpting of prefrontal circuits that reduces cortical inhibition of midbrain governance of behavior, the cravings induced by the addiction-trained reward system, against which alternative rewards have difficulty competing, are often sufficient to provoke relapse after periods of abstinence. Because of the way in which the reward system learns, cravings are induced by any of the cues with which the target of addiction was associated during learning.[23]

Most aspects of the I-RISA model are anticipated in a general account of the neural learning and maintenance of addiction given by Everitt, Dickinson and Robbins (2001). They add further details on the functional neuroanatomy of the process that we have not yet mentioned. In particular, they distinguish between NAcc *shell* and other NAcc subregions. Animals with lesions to nonshell subregions of NAcc show impaired learning of addictions; this does not apply to NAcc shell lesions. Addictive learning is also impaired by lesions in the central nucleus, but not the basolateral area, of the amygdala. This is initially puzzling, since basolateral amygdala, but not amygdala central nucleus, projects to NAcc. The answer Everitt and colleagues suggest to this puzzle is that amygdala central nucleus regulates the dopamine neurons of VTA, thereby affecting NAcc response. NAcc shell regulates its own dopamine innervation via projections to VTA and NAcc core. We consider some neuropharmacological implications of these findings in chapter 7.

The I-RISA model does not, however, address two further questions about addiction. Without answering these, a full etiological understanding of PG/AG will remain elusive. They are: (1) What distinguishes things that can be targets of addiction from things that aren't?; and (2) What distinguishes those who become addicts from those who don't?

On the second question, genetic factors seem to tell at least part of the story. Laakso et al. (2002) report early work on the search for a genetic basis of vulnerability to addiction. The obvious first place to look is at genes that regulate the dopaminergic system. Unfortunately, there are many of these. A basic technique for trying to isolate culprits for addiction is by selectively knocking out dopamine-regulating genes from animals and then searching for differences in susceptibility to addictive substances that correlate with these knockouts. A main result so far is that "[o]f the many knockout mice tested to date in paradigms of drug addiction, the mGluR5 mutant mouse is the only line that fails to self-administer psychostimulants" (p. 221). For an alternative technique for isolation of addiction-related genes, based on breeding of so-called "congenic" animals, see Wise 2000 (p. 31). A third approach is to rear twin animals and selectively alter genes or suppress gene activation in some twins but not others. We return to the more specific question of possible genetically based predispositions for AG later.

Stress from the environment has been clearly identified, both in folk experience and by science, as causally significant for addiction. In the brain, stress is manifested when hypothalamic corticotropin-releasing factor releases adrenocorticotropic hormone from the pituitary-adrenal system, which in turn releases glucocorticoids. Stress also activates the sympathetic nervous system and emotional systems. When stress persists through failure of attempts to relieve it, it recruits a range of neural systems and can ultimately affect most of the brain (Koob and Le Moal 2000). Even mild stress has direct implications for neural activity throughout the brain, so it is no surprise that stress and reward system pathologies are closely linked. Obviously, however, in the overwhelming majority of cases where people are stressed, including cases where they are stressed for prolonged periods, no addiction results. Nor does stress seem to be a necessary condition for addiction onset, since drugs that relieve stress are themselves potentially addictive. It will not surprise any researchers if addiction's developmental etiology turns out to lie in complex interactions between genetically based predispositions and contingent sources of stress from the environment, perhaps with a small subset of people whose genetics are such that they are almost sure to develop addictions regardless of their life circumstances. While developing an effective medical *preventative strategy* against addiction would require us to know more than we do now about its ultimate predisposing conditions, development of effective medical *interventions* in addiction need not wait upon such knowledge; our rapidly expanding knowledge of proximate mechanisms, as reviewed in this section, ought to be sufficient.

The other open question identified above, why certain reward sources are regular targets of addiction and others aren't, is fundamental to our concern with PG/AG. To this we turn in the next chapter.

6

Addictive Gambling as the Basic Form of Addiction

6.1 Gambling as Reward System Manipulation

Tradition has taken drugs (including alcohol) to be the core addictive targets for a number of reasons. First, all of the leading drugs except nicotine produce vivid episodic "highs" in which judgment is impaired and hedonic pleasure is enhanced (at least for a time). This means that for most drugs there is a strong distinction between sober and intoxicated states. Furthermore, it is straightforward to comparatively measure any given person's quantity and rate of consumption of drugs. Folk wisdom therefore doesn't usually need to distinguish between addiction to drugs and very heavy or frequent use of them. Given social disapproval of intoxication (based on its significant social costs), this is a reasonable approximation. A person who is very often drunk probably *is* addicted to alcohol. The majority of other recreational drugs are illegal, so once again the rough assumption that regular users are addicts is sustained by high imposed costs: a few very wealthy people aside, who but an addict would keep anteing the cash and running the risks to maintain a constant supply and intake of cocaine?[1]

In the context of this popular wisdom, it is not surprising that talk of addiction to nondrug rewards is often regarded as metaphorical. It is common for people to be referred to as "addicted" to television or sex or shopping, but all that is typically meant by this is that the activity in question consumes an unusual proportion of the "addict's" time—a proportion the attributor regards as socially, psychologically, or morally inappropriate. How many of these popularly regarded "addictions" involve objectively attributable pathologies is unclear. Recall from chapter 3 that a behavioral economist can consistently define someone as having a problem with the consumption of some kind of good just in case the person both systematically invests in the good and invests in unsuccessful efforts to consume less of it. Clearly, consumption problems in this sense can arise for almost anything and can be highly idiosyncratic. On the other hand, it is doubtful that just anything has the intertemporal utility dynamics necessary to trip dopaminergic hysteresis and adaptation of glutamate and serotonin circuits. We have previously cited Loewenstein's point that purely instrumental goods like writing paper don't appear to be targets for addiction to anyone. In light of the previous chapter, we can promote this from a folk observation to something more like a scientific fact, because we can see why it holds. Such understanding of addiction as we have now achieved depends on the idea that an addictive target has to be the consumption consequence of pursuing a *reliable* cue for *surprise*. We emphasized that this is only *apparently* paradoxical. Nevertheless, such a relationship is not one into which most consumption streams can enter. Drugs pull off the trick by directly interfering with the brain's expectations about its own microprocessing—and reliably doing so every time, so long as dosages are adequate and (in the case of nicotine) appropriately spaced. It would be baffling to this understanding of addiction if people could become addicted to consumption streams that are easy to access, highly uniform in their downstream behavioral and hedonic effects, and lack capacities to directly manipulate neurotransmitter levels. Consider, for example, everyday drinking water. According to the PV model, the reward system would not go on loading dopamine in response to the cues for this sometime reward unless water were scarce in someone's environment, or access was restricted as a standing condition, or the hypothalamus registered a distressful level of deprivation which, for some reason, was not turned off by drinking. (Note that a person might suffer from cognitive or hypothalamic disorders that caused them to drink water obsessively in consequence of misperception; then, we would say, the point of modeling addiction as a reward-system pathology would be vindicated through showing that, and why, it would be misleading to say that the person in question was addicted to water, their "addictive-seeming" behavior with respect to it notwithstanding.) Of course, this purely qualitative implication of the model leaves us with a large range of cases that must be regarded as undecided in advance of the necessary neuroscientific research.

Among nonsubstance foci of impulsive behavior, there is evidence that problem shopping, as per the PE operationalization, is a recurrent pattern, at least in contemporary affluent societies (Müller et al. 2004);

according to one prevalence study, it afflicts 1.1 percent of French adults (Lejoyeux et al. 1996). However, we are aware of no follow-up neuroscience research that sheds light on the extent to which inconsistent investment by problem shoppers is correlated with neurochemical phenomena resembling those associated with addiction. The fact that some impulsive shoppers (or impulsive copulators or television watchers or stamp collectors) display some of the phenomenological and behavioral properties typical of drug and alcohol addicts should not be regarded as clear evidence. "Addiction" in the popular sense of the term is a familiar, culturally tagged syndrome that some people adopt as a norm around which they and others can structure expectations (after the fashion described by Hacking 1999); this norm can in principle be constructed around any perceptually and socially salient consumption pattern.

We stress the importance of caution here for one main reason. We are about to argue that evidence strongly indicates PG to be not only a distinctive neurochemical disorder but also the core addictive phenomenon on which others, specifically substance addictions, should be modeled. This is portentous in light of the popular polarization between behavioral concepts of addiction, which tend to be a priori liberal about what can and cannot be genuine objects of addiction, and reductionist concepts organized around physiological withdrawal symptoms as the addictive tethers. Promoters and users of the latter concept of addiction are often skeptical concerning the appropriateness of regarding anything other than an exogenous chemical as a possible object of addiction. Arguing, as we do, that (1) PG/AG is the basic form of addiction and that (2) addiction should be conceptualized as a neurochemical phenomenon implies direct rejection of the popular disjunction of conceptual alternatives. It thus also invites a casual slide into supposing that anything bearing the behavioral and phenomenological properties that gambling shares with addictive drugs must turn out to be an addiction in the neuroscientific sense that we advocate. For reasons we will discuss in chapter 8, the conjunction of the PE and neuroeconomic perspectives lead us to strongly doubt that most behavioral habits popularly called "addictions" are true cases. As we will argue there, the prospects of new pharmacological interventions against addiction based on current neuroscientific discoveries attach high ethical importance to this question, and motivate a principle according to which a variety of impulsivity should be treated as non-addictive until proven (by neuroscience) otherwise.

For the moment, the task before us is to assemble the evidence that PG resembles, indeed constitutes the elementary model for, the classical substance addictions with respect to its neuroscientific profile. We must note in this context that science has not been uninfluenced by popular ambivalence over whether gambling is the sort of thing that can be a proper object of addiction. Since the dawn of the medical model of addiction, the overwhelming bulk of careful investigation it has inspired has been investigation of impulsive substance use. For that reason alone many scientists have joined the general public in being undecided about literal gambling addiction. This situation has been altered by an explosion of scientific research into PG over the last decade. Shaffer, Stanton, and Nelson (2006), in documenting and discussing the contents of and motivations for this activity, emphasize that a main contribution of the recent work has been to demonstrate that PGs can be reliably distinguished from other gamblers on a variety of demographic and behavioral variables. But it was not until the advent of contemporary neuroscience that we began to find a basis for firmly distinguishing between objectively literal and constructed addiction, in the sense of having a qualitative basis for dividing people into those who are appropriate potential targets for neuropharmacological interventions and those who are not. Behavioral studies certainly provided preliminary evidence for the scientific value of the construct of addiction. However, one need not be in the grip of general ideological reductionism to acknowledge that when a diathesis and associations with fundamental abnormalities of a biological nature can be demonstrated for a psychopathological construct, the way in which the construct is used should be reconsidered in light of new medical and policy prospects.

The I-RISA model of addiction and the underlying PV model of the reward system motivate such reconsideration. The models we have presented allow detailed characterization of relationships between particular people's brains and particular sources of reward for those people. One can distinguish a nicotine and a cocaine addict from one another, and from a non-addict, by examining their brains under fMRI or other scanning technologies, as they are cued to anticipate different experiences. In principle at least, we could pick out addicts, provided they have sufficient history of use, by examining details of the connections between cells in their cortices and subcortices.

Genetic research adds additional promise here. Researchers are starting to identify some of the genetic determinants of how reward systems develop, including the early response genes and postsynaptic density proteins involved in reward learning. Some of these proteins are altered in long-term ways by even single exposures to the classically addictive drugs. Exposure of recovered rat morphine addicts (but not normal rats) to drug-paired environments produces expression of a particular gene (*c-fos*) in several brain areas: medial prefrontal, ventrolateral orbital, and cingulate cortex (Kelley 2004). There are similar findings for cocaine, amphetamine, nicotine, beer, and palatable food (ibid.) (at least when the animals are in novel environments [Wise 2000]). There is evidence that all of this applies to some people with respect to gambling (Ibáñez et al. 2003).

From recognition of gambling as a genuine target of addiction in some people, we will now argue for a stronger point. This is that AG emerges under the combination of the reward leaning/PV neuroeconomic model and the I-RISA neurochemical model as the template of "basic" addiction, the form on which all other addictions are complications. This has been obscured by the cultural accident discussed above, that scientific study of addiction began by focusing on drugs. However, there is now a neuroscience of AG. Furthermore, this neuroscience is visibly beginning to force open the door to effective neuropharmacological interventions against the disorder, as we will discuss in the next chapter. This is as we should predict if AG is basic addiction. In general, addictions will prove more difficult to treat the larger the number of different brain circuits they implicate; alcohol addiction, for example, is likely to prove a more stubborn treatment target than cocaine addiction because cocaine affects the reward system in a simpler way than alcohol. It is because gambling most closely resembles cocaine in the relatively unmediated way in which it triggers reward system hysteresis that we are optimistic concerning the prospects for neuropharmacological management of AG. This also lies at the core of our claim that AG is *basic* addiction. Cocaine directly causes the reward system to be surprised, while coming paired with reliable cues. Other drugs produce the same end state indirectly. Gambling is the fundamental case because here the reward system stumbles on a way to *naturally* pair reliable cuing with surprise. AG demonstrates what it is *about the brain itself*—as opposed to the brain plus a special exogenous chemical—that gives rise to the potential for addiction. Thus AG is the window to the heart of the general addictive syndrome.

The fact that models from neuroscience identify distinctive properties that allow us to distinguish drug addicts, and then to associate AGs with them, still leaves us with puzzles about the developmental etiology and onset of addiction. The possibility of gambling addiction is bound to seem unlikely under any account of addiction that *begins* with drugs producing long-term changes in the brain as a consequence of the chemical properties of those drugs. As Wise (2002) argues, this includes not just traditional accounts that focus on chemical dependence and withdrawal, but also careless applications of current science that identify the onset of addictions with neuroadaptations. Wise emphasizes that the rewarding properties of direct stimulants are learned extremely quickly; after as few as two or three electrical stimulations to the hypothalamus in their brains, rats will begin frantically pressing levers for more and ignoring food and water. Obviously, neuroadaptations cannot yet have occurred at the first point at which pursuit of the reward appears to be compulsive. "While it is clearly the case that brain changes associated with tolerance and dependence and brain changes associated with sensitization can develop under the right circumstances," Wise points out, "what remains to be determined is the degree to which either of these changes is necessary for motivational habits to become compulsive. The rapid onset of compulsive self-stimulation [in rats and primates] would seem to preclude any of these drug-induced long-term neuroadaptations as a necessary condition for compulsive drug-seeking" (pp. 233–234).

AG is the wild (as opposed to laboratory-constructed) phenomenon that establishes the applicability of Wise's point to humans. If drugs were the only possible targets of addiction in humans, then it would be open to us to identify addiction with the causal consequences of sensitization to drugs. In effect, that is just what the folk model of addiction did by making fear of withdrawal the definitive mark of addiction, before the discovery that sensitization is a product of neuroadaptation. It is entirely implausible, however, that sensitization to gambling causes compulsive gambling; clearly, if there is such a thing as neuroadaptive sensitization to gambling, then it is compulsive gambling that is a causal factor for sensitization rather than the other way around. Neuroadaptation (of the relevant sort) is reliably diagnostic of addiction and important to its course, but not part of its etiology.

For these reasons we see the intrinsic chemical properties of drugs as special-case *distractions* from the fundamental structure of addiction. The special cases are of course important in their own terms, and we should expect that their distinctive features will introduce crucial complications into the development of a suite of optimal neurophar-macological therapies for addictions. But sound method in both pure and applied science directs us to write our general theory around basic manifestations of phenomena, adding special parameters for special cases. These considerations suggest that AG should move to a position of central focus in the development of BE and neuroeconomic modeling of impulsivity and addiction. In their summary of the I-RISA model, Goldstein and Volkow (2002) anticipate this point when they say "a paradigm that simulates compulsive behavior (such as gambling when it is clearly no longer beneficial) might offer invaluable insight into the circuits underlying loss of control in addiction" (p. 1645).

In an addiction science that takes AG as the template instance, neu-robiology does not reduce away insights from psychology and NE, but complements them. Our attention is directed, in the first place, to understanding reward as a general but also sui generis process. Common sense is unfamiliar with the second idea, since common sense identifies reward with receipt of any kind of tangible benefit (a nutri-tious meal, a monetary ticket to further consumption, a status-enhancing social acknowledgment, etc.), often including shots of hedonic delight. As Wise stresses, however, rewards, as neuroscience requires us to understand them, are "unsensed incentives." The point of this phrase, in the context of reflections on targets of addiction, is that although people sense the hedonic consequences of drugs, they are not directly conscious of their rewarding properties. (This is most obvious in the case of nicotine, which is strongly addictive despite the fact that its episodic hedonic properties are not vivid to experienced smokers.) In the case of AG, we are apt to wonder what it is that the gambler is getting that keeps attracting her to gamble more. Is it thrills, or money, or relief from boredom, or what? It now seems that this is the wrong question to ask. Once we understand reward in the neu-roeconomic sense, there is enlightenment in saying that *what leads some people to have a problem with gambling is that it is rewarding in itself.*

This statement will likely appear trivializing rather than illuminating if the reader does not yet appreciate how different the neuroeconomic concept of reward is from folk conceptions. As Wise points out, in neuroscience the distinction between a reward and a predictor of a reward is subtle, perhaps non-existent. Rewards are units of informa-tion that "by association establish otherwise neutral stimuli as things to be approached" (p. 233). The reward system is a device for leading animals to approach certain things rather than others, and it encodes no distinction between what is of ultimate benefit and what simply happens to predict an experience the animal is conditioned to seek. In the case of animals that must adapt to changing environments, the system has a bias for—takes as rewarding—any predictor of novel experiences that are not aversive. People, furthermore, are the ultimate novelty seekers, our freakishly large brains signifying our status as the only animals in whom exaggerated drive for cognitive exploration is the basic species-specific adaptation. This emerges directly in the dopaminergic system's design: dopamine is released not by familiar stimuli, but by positive surprises. New, direct experimental evidence for this has recently been furnished by Bunzeck and Düzel (2006). Furthermore, as Wise reminds us, since the sensed properties of the reward in the folk sense (i.e., the food in the mouth, the orgasm, the drug high, the receipt of the winnings at the window) are not typically surprising, the learning functions of the system (in distinction from the purely perceptual functions identified by Preuschoff, Bossaerts, and Quartz [2006]) become unresponsive to them. So saying as we do that dopaminergic learning responds to *predictors* of reward implicitly identifies the relevant economic agent as being the whole person—the agent to which (e.g.) orgasm counts as a reward. By contrast, insofar as we regard the relevant economic agent as the reward system itself—that is, insofar as we assume the neuroeconomic perspective—what we've been calling "predictors of reward" *are* (when positively surprising) the system's rewards. Thus the very name of the PV model incorporates a residue of the folk conception; no wonder we must struggle to truly displace it. But this is what we mean in saying that it is a mistake to ask what further value—entertainment, profit, or something else—gambling serves. The reward system is built for gambling, so gambling serves it.

We think that this perspective largely lifts the veil of mystery from AG. What gambling fundamentally consists in is paying for the possibility of a surprise. This requires that odds in one's favor not be *too* high, and it may even be important to the reward process that they're negative. This doesn't imply that the gambler doesn't prefer winning to losing. Recall from chapter 4 that PE frees us from the limitation that to make sense of the behavior of whole people in economic terms we must suppose that all of a person's choices can be explained by reference to a single preference schedule. All people who like gambling, and not just DGs, want two things at once that they can't have both of: to win every bet, and to participate in processes where there's a high risk of losing. Should this really surprise us? How many people want, in general, exciting lives but in which nothing truly seriously threatens them? In paying to be surprised, the gambler is paying to engage his or her reward system in the most direct and straightforward possible way. In light of this insight, is it still surprising that when people discover that there are institutions where one can buy such direct manipulation of the dopaminergic system, hysteresis is induced in some of them? We suggest that the real surprise should be that *anyone* who gambles can *avoid* doing so pathologically. That is, if parts of us really are built to seek out surprise, and gambling produces opportunities for surprise with such convenience, it is perplexing that we don't all end up like the rats pressing levers that lead to stimulation of their hypothalami to the neglect of food and water.

The reader might still think we're making a lot of noise about the obvious. So for the precise sense in which puzzles arise for neuroeconomists *before* the insight, consider a sophisticated discussion by Ahmed (2004). Reviewing a neuroeconomic model of cocaine addiction developed by Redish (2004), Ahmed points out that the model depends on the fact that cocaine directly causes dopamine release in NAcc, and so predicts strong reward regardless of any other contingencies. But then, Ahmed wonders, what about "addictions to ordinary rewards, such as fatty foods, which, unlike cocaine, produce a dopamine signal that can be accommodated" (p. 1902)? We do not know whether people become addicted to fatty foods—that many overindulge in them is not automatically evidence for addiction—but in the clearest case of an ordinary reward to which people *do* become addicted, gambling, the answer to Ahmed's question is straightforward. Given what reward *means* in the mesolimbic system, and given what gambling *is* from this point of view, it, just like cocaine, is guaranteed to predict strong reward come what may. In many people the resulting dopamine signal *cannot* be accommodated.

We hope it is now clear what we mean when we say that AG is the basic template of addiction. We mean more than just that it is the one stereotypical form in which there is no accompanying intrinsic chemical complication. We are alluding also to the fact, as explained immediately above, that gambling simply *is* direct stimulation of the midbrain reward system. We thus suspect that the syndrome of AG is relatively simple. We will now review preliminary evidence that we think bears this out. If our hunch is right, the prospect of managing AG pharmacologically looms as a realistic ambition.

6.2   The Neuroscience of Pathological Gambling

In this section we will summarize results from the empirical neuroscientific research that has been done on PGs. This work comes from a variety of branches of neuroscience, each with a slightly different tradition of interpretation. We have pulled them together under *our* principles of interpretation, those of NE as described in the preceding section of this chapter. Thus the authors of the studies we cite might not always agree with our take on them, though there should of course be no disagreements about the factual results.

One problem that may have occurred to the reader is that all of the studies we will review gather their samples by reference to *DSM*'s behavioral operationalization of PG. We are proposing to replace this operationalization with one based in neuroscience. How, then, can we rely for our argument on studies that recruited subjects by reference to criteria we believe to be only rough proxies? In fact, there is an underlying logic there that serves our case nicely. As we will document, strong correlations have been found between neurochemical properties of the reward system that have been identified with drug addiction, as reviewed in the previous chapter, and tendencies to PG. The subjects in these studies were identified using SOGS and similar screens. As we discussed in chapter 2, we know that these screens over-select for PG as operationalized by *DSM*. Therefore, most samples almost certainly contained people who, not being PGs, were not AGs (assuming there are, as we are about to argue, AGs). But in that case, the proportion of *non-addicted* PGs in the samples that would have been consistent with finding strong correlations between signatures of neural addiction and PG has a low upper bound, because of the interference with statistical significance, the "noise," already coming from the screening errors. Thus, the tendency of SOGS to make errors in one direction when used as a screen for research purposes actually helps us make a useful inference. No one would have designed the science this way on purpose. Ex ante there was a strong probability that the presence of the false positives picked up by the screens might have either hidden AG from detection entirely, or left us unsure whether we should conclude that there is a non-AG version of PG that is still worth distinguishing from mere problem gambling. However, the application of conservative significance criteria to the studies we will review, *given* our prior knowledge that the screens err toward false positives rather than false negatives *by reference to the DSM criteria*, is our basis for concluding that

PG should be identified with—in the language of philosophy of science, "locally reduced to"—AG.[2]

The first and most basic question to ask about the empirical neuroscience of PG is: do we have clear and recurrent evidence of abnormal subcortical and prefrontal dopamine response in PG subjects? Until very recently the answer was "no," but positive findings have been arriving at an accelerating rate since 2005. This has been a consequence of two developments: new interest based on availability of new investigative methods, and serendipitous discoveries among Parkinson's Disease patients. We contend that this evidence is much more compelling than it would otherwise be when it is integrated by reference to the I-RISA and underlying PV models.

Early investigations of dopamine and PG relied on measurement of levels in cerebrospinal (CSF) and other body fluids. Shinohara et al. (1999) found elevated peripheral dopamine levels in PGs relative to controls following gambling episodes. Similarly, Bergh et al. (1997) reported evidence suggesting increased CSF dopamine turnover in male PGs. However, this was called into question by a replication that corrected for flow rate of cerebrospinal fluid (Nordin and Eklundh 1999), giving renewed credence to earlier results due to Roy et al. (1988), who had found no differences in CFS or other fluid dopamine levels between PGs and controls. With respect to this means of investigating the dopamine-PG relationship, note that the neuroeconomic model does not predict that PGs will have higher levels of dopamine in their general nervous systems; it predicts higher concentrations of dopamine in the striatum and specifically in the NAcc, and even then only when PGs are experiencing stimulation by gambling cues.

Two studies have found correlations between dopamine circuit activity and gambling in healthy subjects (Koepp et al. 1998; Breiter et al. 2001). In the context of general knowledge about the reward system, this represents not so much positive evidence for PG as AG as it does for a failure to confute the hypothesis at the first step. Any model of PG based on properties of reward-system processing would be in serious trouble if gambling did not appear to stimulate the reward circuits in the first place.

In a 2004 review of neuroscientific and other biobehavioral studies of PGs, Goudriaan et al. (2004b) mention some scattered evidence implicating reward-system pathology. A sample of PGs had lower average baseline systolic blood pressure while gambling in the lab than controls. In contrast, skin conductance measures were more aroused by gambling cues in PGs than in controls. In general, however, psychophysiological studies of PGs until very recently could not measure effects capable of discriminating among neural pathways or processes. In addition, earlier behavioral studies were often compromised by a factor that behavioral economists tend to stress more than psychologists: experimenters frequently offered no real stakes, or very small stakes. This generic economist's worry has special force where the reward system is concerned, in light of what our model suggests about the way it works: small or absent stakes are unlikely to arouse a particular dopaminergic system that has protracted experience of gambling. This is part of the background to our having said that in the absence of research reported in the past two years, we would not be in a position to say whether there appeared to be any such phenomenon as AG. (In this connection, we should also note a further methodological concern, which applies as well to many fMRI studies. Studying subjects gambling in abnormal environments might easily lead to misinterpretation of heightened reward system activity. The problem here is that if there are novel associations to be learned between strange environments and gambling, the reward system will have work to do just for that reason.)

The first neuroimaging study of PGs that yielded data of direct relevance to the hypothesis that PG is AG (in our sense) was conducted by Stojanov et al. (2003). They compared the prepulse inhibition (PPI) of PGs to that of controls. PPI is a measure of the reduction of brain activation to a stimulus S2 when a distracting stimulus S1 (a noise tone) is presented immediately before it. Researchers examine the acoustic startle reflex, which is an indicator of "sensory motor gating" that inhibits processing of S2 so that S1 may be properly interpreted by the brain. Dopamine is the neurotransmitter mediating PPI. In Stojanov et al.'s experiment, PGs showed reduced PPI relative to controls. This is evidence of one of increased endogenous dopamine activity, higher serotonin response, or higher glutamate response. As explained in the previous chapter, all three of these possible explanations are consistent with what we see in the neurochemistry of substance addiction. Stojanov et al. argue that the explanation most consistent with other evidence is that reduced PPI results from enhanced endogenous dopamine activity rather than reduced dopamine neurotransmission. However, they mainly appeal in this connection to the conclusion of Bergh et al. (1997) cited above, which, as noted, was subsequently undermined.

Recent fMRI work by Reuter et al. (2005) and Potenza et al. (2004) provides direct evidence for reduced VTA activity in PGs during performance of rewarded tasks, echoing a similar finding with alcoholics. We will consider these last two studies in greater detail shortly.

In most of the other neuroimaging studies reviewed by Goudriaan et al. (2004b), sample sizes were small, comorbidity factors were not assessed, and more PG subjects than controls had suffered brain traumas or taken psychotropic drugs. These are all severe compromising factors in efforts to compare PG with drug addictions.

Neurochemical evidence is also available. Five studies have shown deficiencies in 5-HT (serotonin) levels in PGs, and two studies have shown noradrenergic dysfunction. A further pair of studies measured higher peripheral NE levels and blood levels of epinephrine in PGs than in controls while subjects gambled and on days when gambling activity was concentrated (ibid., p. 133). This is significant because Steketee (2002) cites evidence that epinephrine promotes dopamine flooding in the VMPFC. In a study too recent for inclusion in the review by Goudriaan et al., Meyer et al. (2004) found that PGs showed higher heart rate, norepinephrine, and dopamine levels than controls during a session of casino blackjack.

In chapter 4 we discussed the literature on performance of conventionally regarded addicts and PGs in the Iowa Gambling Task that is intended to measure cognitive bookkeeping as relevant to discounting. In one such experiment, Cavedini et al. (2002) scanned PGs and controls performing the IGT and other cognitive decision tasks using fMRI. PGs performed as well as controls on tasks that depended on generalized effective functioning of the frontal lobes, but performed worse on the IGT. The authors suggest that this implies specific impairment of the VMPFC. They argue that "[t]hese data seem to suggest the existence of a link between PG, OCD and drug addiction, all having diminished ability to consider future consequences, which may be explained, at least in part, by abnormal functioning of the orbitofrontal cortex" (p. 338). They note that "the literature suggests that deficit on decision making may reflect altered neuromodulation of the orbitofrontal cortex and interconnected limbic-striatal system by both the ascending 5-HT and mesocortical dopamine projections . . . and that the functioning of the dopaminergic system, possibly mediating positive and negative reward, and the noradrenergic system, possibly mediating selective attention, is altered in pathological gambling" (p. 339). The first suggestion is consistent with the I-RISA model's mechanism for impaired response inhibition in addicts. The second, more general, suggestion points directly at the reward system.

In a 2004 study, Zack and Poulos used a novel methodology to investigate the extent to which stimulant drugs and gambling cues elicit common neural responses. They fed 30 mg of D-amphetamine to four groups of subjects: (1) PGs, (2) PGs comorbid for alcohol dependence, (3) alcohol-dependent subjects who were not comorbid for PG, and (4) healthy controls. They then assessed subjects' subjective motivations to gamble and measured comparative reading rates under conditions where subjects were presented with cuing words from motivationally distinct semantic fields (gambling-related, drinking-related, positive affect, negative affect, neutral). Amphetamine, a drug whose stimulant properties are mediated by the dopaminergic system, increased self-reported motivation to gamble in PGs but not in controls. Furthermore, increased severity of PG predicted increased motivation under stimulant influence. By contrast, alcohol, as discussed earlier, exercises its drug effects by means of a different pathway, primarily involving GABA-A activation and glutamate inhibition and working only indirectly on dopaminergic function. It is therefore noteworthy that amphetamines did not prime for drinking motivation in nongambling alcohol abusers, suggesting that PG resembles stimulant drug action more than either resembles alcohol response, including in alcohol addicts. By the reading speed measure, stimulant drugs uniformly increased speeds across conditions in nongamblers, while elevating attentiveness to gambling-related stimuli and reducing attentiveness to neutral stimuli in PGs. The authors relate this to a study by Kischka et al. (1996) indicating that reading speed differences are modulated by dopaminergic signals. These results are consistent with previous suggestions that AG neurochemically resembles stimulant drug dependence, and does so to a greater degree than it resembles alcohol dependence.

In related work, and using a novel and complex experimental design, Potenza et al. (2003b) investigated the hypothesis that PG brain responses to gambling cues more closely resemble cocaine addicts' responses to cocaine cues than they do the responses of subjects with obsessive-compulsive disorder (OCD) to triggering stimuli. The motivation for this is the traditional interpretation of PG as a compulsive disorder, as contrasted with the recent evidence that paints it as an addiction. The expression of the hypothesis in the experimental setting was that PGs would show elevated mesolimbic responses, rather than elevated cortico-basal-ganglionic-thalamic responses, compared to controls. The subjects (all male) were shown videotapes of sad, happy, and casino-gambling scenarios. They were instructed to push buttons to signal the onset of emotional and motivational episodes, and were asked to rate peaks and intensities of these episodes. The groups did not differ significantly in subjective responses to sad and happy scenarios. However, all PGs, but only a minority of non-PGs, reported gambling urges while viewing gambling scenarios. Before subjective response in the gambling scenarios, PGs showed decreased activity, and controls increased activity, in the OFC, basal ganglia, and thalamus. Sad and happy scenarios elicited no significant differences. At time of subjective response, PGs showed increased activity relative to controls in the OFC for gambling scenarios, and in the ventral striatum (VS) and OFC for happy scenarios. During the final period of viewing, after presentation of the scenarios, PGs had decreased activity in some regions for sad scenarios relative to controls, and decreased activity in the ventral ACC for gambling scenarios. Other studies have associated this with positively valenced mood. So, on the one hand, anticipatory cue responses in PGs differed from those of OCD subjects (who went the opposite way), but on the other hand, the later decreased activity in the ACC distinguished PGs from cocaine abusers. With respect to the role of the reward system, the first result associates PG with addiction. Since the ACC as been implicated in decision making relevant to control of impulses, the second result has PGs conforming *better* to the I-RISA model than cocaine addicts.

Of interest following on from the first result above is an fMRI examination by Crockford et al. (2005) of male PGs and controls while they watched alternating video images of gambling scenarios and of nature scenes. This study was motivated by the expectation that if mesolimbic processing of motivation associated with reward expectancy in PGs activates the OFC, this should be accompanied by elevated activity in the dorsolateral PFC (DLPFC) so as to recruit working memory to track the expected gambling-relevant information. In the experiment, PGs indeed showed elevated DLFPC activity relative to controls while watching the gambling videos, but not while engaged with the nature videos. In addition, PGs showed elevated activity relative to controls in the right parahippocampal region and left occipital cortex during the gambling presentations. These elevated activations correlate with subjective reports of cravings to gamble by the PG subjects. The results are interesting in light of a finding by Dorris and Glimcher (2004) that the posterior parietal cortex (PPC) encodes transformations of

representations into generation of movement, since the DLPFC is recip-
rocally linked with the PPC. Subjective cravings may in part be the
experience of preparation for action. (Tentative evidence suggests that
the *experience of*, as opposed to the causal trigger for, cravings may be
based in the insula; see Nasqvi et al. 2007.)

In a study shedding further light on impairment of response inhibition, Potenza et al. (2003a) scanned PGs and controls under fMRI while
they performed a Stroop task (see chapter 5), on which separate studies
by Rugle and Melamid (1993) and Regard et al. (2003) had reported
impaired performance by non-substance-dependent PGs compared to
control subjects. (As noted in chapter 4, Kertzman et al. [2005] found
similar results for PGs' performance on the functionally equivalent
"reverse Stroop task.") In Potenza et al.'s experiment PGs differed from
controls only in showing decreased activity in the VMPFC—once again
suggestive of reduced capacity for impulse control and conforming to
the prediction of the I-RISA model of addiction.

A related result was found by Reuter et al. (2005) when they scanned
PGs and controls under fMRI while the subjects were engaged in a
guessing game for prizes. PGs showed decreased activation in the VS
on wins, just as drug addicts do. They also failed to show the increased
VMPFC activity demonstrated by controls, complementing some of
the results described above (those of Cavedini et al. 2002 and Potenza
et al. 2003a) and predictive of impaired response inhibition in accordance with the I-RISA model. Reuter et al. interpret their data in a
way consistent with the I-RISA model as applied to PGs, but go
beyond it in also offering a hypothesis about the causal background to
development of addiction:

Drug self-administration experiments have suggested that organisms try to
maintain a homeostatic baseline level of dopamine in the ventral striatum,
which in normal volunteers can be maintained by weak reinforcers found in
everyday life. In contrast, in PGs (who have reduced striatal activation), natural
reinforcers are not strong enough for dopamine to reach and maintain this
homeostatic baseline level. At this stage organisms seek additional, stronger
reinforcers, such as drugs of addiction or gambling, to compensate for the lack
of activation. (Reuter et al. 2005, p. 148)

This hypothesis rather outruns available data in our opinion, though
it has some qualitative basis in the general neuroscience literature on
addiction (e.g., Koob and Le Moal 2000).

Earlier in this chapter we described evidence for a more modest
speculation on the developmental basis of addiction, stemming from

Chambers, Taylor, and Potenza's (2003) work on correlations between age-related vulnerability to addiction and the stages of development of the human brain. As we saw, the adolescent brain, which is selected for relative emphasis on exploration, has underdeveloped cortical response inhibition machinery compared to the typical adult brain. In follow-up work, Chambers and Potenza (2003) reviewed the relationship between this correlation and data on PG. As we've noted, PG rates are higher among adolescents than among adults, despite less convenient access to gambling venues and less disposable income in the former. Furthermore, PG in adolescence is a predictor of PG in adulthood (Winters, Stinchfield, and Fulkerson 1990) (though most heavy adolescent gamblers do not become PGs). Thus it seems significant that, as the authors say, "[I]n adolescents as compared with adults promotional mechanisms [i.e., the dopaminergic system] are relatively hyperactive and inhibitory mechanisms [i.e., the OFC and 5-HT circuits] relatively hypoactive" (p. 76). Unfortunately, no direct fMRI studies of adolescent PG subjects have yet been reported. However, Bjork et al. (2004) carried out a study on typically developing children that suggests a different neural basis for special vulnerability to PG in adolescents. They compared the BOLD responses of 12- to 17-year-olds with those of 21- to 28-year-olds on a delayed monetary reward task. Their results do not support the hypothesis that adolescents have increased reward cue-elicited anticipatory VS activation. They indicate an adolescent VS activation deficit rather than a VS activation surfeit as a factor for risky behavior. According to this account, adolescents may seek more extreme incentives as a way of compensating for low VS activity levels (Spear 2000). Either way, the risky behavior observed in adolescents appears to be due to faulty reward processing of some sort. Regions and time-courses of reward-related activity have also been shown to be similar to those observed in adults, as evidenced by condition-dependent BOLD changes in the VS and lateral and medial OFC in response to positive versus negative feedback (May et al. 2004).

To the extent that we have grounds for looking for the developmental etiology of PG in preadulthood (including in prenatal genetic background), we may be interested in "twin data" on PG. "Twin studies," in which fraternal twins who grew up in the same household are compared with fraternal twins raised separately with respect to a dependent variable, have long been employed in developmental psychology as a way of exploring the relative causal strengths of genetic and environmental influences. Such a study has been conducted for PG by Eisen et al. (1998) on 3359 twin pairs. The authors find that inherited factors explain between 35 and 54 percent of reports of five *DSM* symptoms of PG that could be estimated statistically. Familial factors explain 56 percent of reports of three or more symptoms, and 62 percent of PG diagnoses.

Of interest as evidence for the basis of PG in the dopamine system is preliminary work examining the genetic characteristics of PGs. Pioneering studies have been carried out by Ibáñez et al. (2003). There are, in general, two approaches to trying to isolate genes for specific properties or pathologies. Linkage studies, which are typically the most powerful, look for marker alleles within families that distinguish affected from unaffected family members. Very often, however, samples of related people that are large enough relative to expression rates of the pathology for statistical power cannot be found. Genetic detective work thus more often relies on association studies, which look for statistically significant correlations between polymorphic alleles (sites on the DNA molecule where different possible expressions have been identified and statistically estimated) and expression of the pathology in an affected group relative to a control group from the same population. We cannot find any reports on linkage studies of PGs as of this writing. However, Ibáñez et al. describe seven association studies, of which all but one were conducted by their research group. A helpful property of these authors' work is that they motivate their hypotheses by efforts to provide separating evidence between conceptions of PG as an obsessive-compulsive disorder mainly implicating the noradrenergic system and the family of addiction models (including I-RISA) we have defended here that direct attention to the dopaminergic pathways. In light of the latter model, as they say, "genes relevant to the function of serotonergic, dopaminergic and noradrenergic systems could be considered as candidate genes in PG" (p. 16). Ibáñez et al. found a DNA sequence (a promoter polymorphism) for expression of a protein known as MOA-A, which has been associated with control of neurotransmitters found in the reward system, to be significantly increased in male PGs as compared to controls. "Interestingly," they comment, "although serotonin is a preferred substrate for MOA-A, MOA-A is expressed in the brain mainly in dopaminergic neurons, raising the question of whether these allele variants are more likely to result in changes in serotonergic or dopaminergic transmission" (p. 18). The group also studied a polymorphism in the D2 dopamine receptor gene and found "significant differences in allele distribution in PGs with as compared to those without co-morbid psychiatric disorders" (ibid.). In female but not male PGs, the same team (Perez de Castro et al. 1997) discovered the DRD4 7-repeat allele, coding for less efficient receptors, to be significantly more frequent than in controls.[3] Finally, they cite a report due to Comings, Rosenthal, and Lesieur (1996) of "statistically significant association between the Taq-A1 allele of the D2 dopamine receptor gene in pathological gamblers compared to controls," and note that the Taq-A1 allele "has also been found to be associated with other impulsive-addictive-compulsive behaviors, leading some researchers to propose a *Reward Deficiency Syndrome* as an underlying genetic foundation for these disorders" (Ibáñez et al. 2003, p. 18).[4] This interpretation of the results has aroused some controversy, especially as the Taq-A1 polymorphism is now known to be located in a nearby kinase gene where it causes a Glutamate ⑧ Lysine substitution (Neville, Johnstone, and Walton 2004), thus obscuring its functionality.[5]

Additional evidence for comorbid heritability of PG has been furnished by Potenza et al. (2005), who show a matched genetic contribution with near-perfect overlap to PG and major depression. Very strikingly, Slutske et al. (2000) found common genetic vulnerability to PG and alcohol dependence in male subjects. They explicitly interpret this as suggesting a genetic basis for disposition to addiction as a generic pathology.

Thus the prospect looms that genetics could explain vulnerability to the dynamics described by the I-RISA model, and some or perhaps even most AG could turn out to have a genetic etiology. This would of course have portentous implications for prevention possibilities, as we stand at the dawn of the age of genetic screening and therapies. It should be noted that more than one genetic syndrome will likely turn out to be implicated, since genetic correlations with AG found to date have tended to be sex-specific. This might, indeed, explain why AG prevalence among males is reliably higher, in all countries where statistical evidence has been carefully collected, despite the fact that differences in testosterone levels do not appear to be related to dispositions to AG (Blanco et al. 2001).

On its own, none of the evidence reviewed in this chapter would be decisive for the hypothesis that most PG is AG (in the sense of I-RISA). As many recent philosophers of science have emphasized, however, what is taken to license a so-called local reduction (i.e., specific reduction in a context where across-the-board reductionism is denied) is the co-presence of two factors: (1) convergence to the reduction from multiple, independent *kinds* of evidence, and (2) *unification* of this converging evidence by means of a general, testable model. Factor (1) provides inductive warrant for a local reduction, and factor (2) explains the local reduction. Explanation is essential for reduction because, where philosophical or across-the-board reduction*ism* is denied, explanation becomes the justifying *point* of proposing a local reduction: one reduces for the sake of generalizing power. We think that the evidence we have reviewed in this chapter goes quite far toward establishing factor (1) for the local reduction of PG to AG. The I-RISA model of addiction and the underlying PV model of reward learning, attention, and motivation give us factor (2).

In the case of a branch of science with direct engineering (including medical, clinical, or policy) applications, a further motive for local reduction can be facilitation of diagnosis and treatment. Successful treatment based on the assumption of an underlying unity among apparently diverse syndromes such as (in this case) PG and the various drug addictions also amounts to further evidence supporting factor (1) motivations for local reduction. The next chapter will review recent discoveries that PG responds to clinical—especially pharmacological—interventions that would be mysterious if the I-RISA and underlying PV models were not approximately true. In our opinion, this additional evidence, when added to that surveyed in the present chapter, boosts factor (1) considerations for local reduction "over the top." Within the wider context of generally irreducible DG, PG should be locally reduced to AG. We postpone discussion of the implications of this to chapter 8.

7   Clinical Evidence and Implications

7.1   General Considerations

Chapters 5 and 6 reviewed evidence, respectively, for viewing addiction as a reward system pathology, and for viewing PG as the simplest and most straightforward instance of this pathology. The primary goal of this chapter is to review clinical evidence, especially regarding the treatment efficacy for PG, of pharmacotherapies that affect the dopamine reward system. Collectively, in our view, this evidence is sufficient to warrant replacing the behaviorally derived concept of PG with the neuroscientifically anchored concept of "addictive gambling." We'll postpone the bulk of this argument until the end of this chapter, however, because all the studies reviewed here had individuals diagnosed with PG as participants.

A debate continues within the psychiatric community as to the appropriate classification of PG. *DSM-IV* classifies it as an impulse control disorder, along with kleptomania, pyromania, intermittent explosive disorder, and trichotolomania (American Psychiatric Association 2000). However, given the phenomenally compulsive quality of PG, a small but significant literature has argued for classifying it as an obsessive-compulsive disorder, which is among the anxiety-spectrum disorders in *DSM* (American Psychiatric Association 2000). A third approach to the classification of PG, the one for which we surveyed evidence in the previous chapter, understands PG as an addiction. We are not alone in our preference for including PG with other addictions. Potenza (2006), for example, reviewed evidence of similarities between PG and substance use disorders (SUDs), a major *DSM-IV* category, with an eye toward having them classified together in *DSM-V*. He found that PG and SUDs are quite similar with respect to qualitative diagnostic criteria, clinical characteristics and social factors, co-occurring disorders, personality features and behavioral measures, biochemistry, neurocircuitry, and genetics.

An additional similarity between PG and SUDs is high rates of natural recovery (i.e., significant improvement without formal treatment) relative to other psychiatric disorders. Some estimates of natural recovery rates in SUDs are as high as 50 percent (Robins, Locke, and Regier 1991). Slutske (2006) studied natural recovery in PGs using two national surveys in the United States. In the two surveys, of those individuals with a lifetime history of *DSM-IV* PG, in the past 12 months 38.9 percent and 36.9 percent had no PG symptoms, and 84.8 percent and 63.0 percent no longer met the PG diagnostic criteria. Clearly, many PGs can recover from the condition, although little is known about the processes through which this improvement occurs. More is known about the processes of natural recovery in SUDs, especially concerning variables of relevance to BE. For example, Tucker, Vuchinich, and Rippens (2002a) found that individuals who recovered from alcohol dependence had experienced a distinct constellation of negative life events during the year prior to the quit attempt *plus* a constellation of positive life events in the year after. Apparently, negative events motivate a serious attempt to quit drinking, which must then be reinforced by positive events. Also, Vuchinich and colleagues (Tucker, Vuchinich, and Rippens 2002b; Tucker et al. 2006) developed an income- and expenditure-based measure of degree of preference for short-term rewards (e.g., drinking) relative to long-term rewards (e.g., saving money) and found that it predicted successful natural recoveries better than more traditional measures, such as drinking behavior, problems caused by drinking, and alcohol dependence. Finally, Granfield and Cloud (2001) demonstrated the importance of "social capital" (collective interpersonal relationships) to natural recovery from SUDs, which is consistent with Rachlin's relative theory of impulsivity discussed in chapter 3.

We have argued that the act of gambling is by nature an economic behavior in which decisions between different rewards are made by assigning relative values to them. We have shown this economic behavior to have neural correlates by reviewing neuroeconomic findings from functional neuroimaging. Such studies have revealed neural reward pathways associated with human economic decision making. We have reviewed literature suggesting drug addiction to be a condition in which the neurobiology of reward processing has gone awry, establishing the I-RISA model as the most comprehensive and scientifically sound model to date. Given that gambling is by nature an economic behavior, it follows that PG should also, like drug addiction, be viewed as reward processing (economic behavior) gone awry. And so indeed we have reviewed a burgeoning literature demonstrating that dysfunctional economic behavior with associated neurobiology in PG serves as the template for modeling all addiction by exhibiting addiction's core properties in a more basic and less noisy form. In line with the psychiatric view, we believe PG to be a disease of the brain reward centers. In certain people, gambling may activate and dysregulate endogenous midbrain processes, thereby hijacking brain circuits that normally implement more forward-looking behavioral scheduling. Despite catastrophic financial, interpersonal, occupational, and even legal consequences, the hijacking of reward centers leads to continued and progressive loss of control over gambling behavior in the minority of sufferers who are unable to arrest the process.

In this chapter, we strengthen this argument by reviewing evidence that pharmacological treatments acting on neurotransmitters involved in reward processing (serotonin and dopamine) show increasing promise of efficacy as treatments for PG.

7.2   The Pharmacological Treatment of Pathological Gambling

Two recent reviews (Grant, Kim, and Potenza 2003; Hollander et al. 2005b) show that, compared to other psychiatric disorders, there has been a paucity of studies investigating the pharmacological treatment of PG. At present there are no medications for PG approved by the U.S. Food and Drug Administration (which can be expected to set the precedent for the rest of the world because the majority of the relevant research occurs in the U.S.). The "gold standard" for approving a medication is whether the drug has been assessed through double-blind randomized controlled clinical trials (RCT). Such studies require random assignment of PGs to either active treatment or placebo groups, where both investigators and patients are blind to group status. With a few exceptions, RCTs are yet to be conducted for PG and most of the studies reviewed here should therefore be regarded as preliminary.

Table 7.1 summarizes the pharmacological treatment studies carried out to date for PG. They include five classes of agents: mood stabilizers, serotinergic agents, post-synaptic 5-HT antagonists, opioid receptor antagonists, and atypical antipsychotics.

Table 7.1
Pharmacotherapy trials for the treatment of pathological gambling.

Authors	Drug	Type of Study	Sample Size	Findings
Mood Stabilizers: Lithium, Carbemazepine and Valproate				
Moskowitz (1980)	Lithium 1800 mg/day	Case report	3 PGs	Complete cessation of gambling
Haller and Hinterhuber (1994)	Carbemazepine 600 mg/day	Single case report, double blind (12 weeks placebo; 12 weeks active)	1 PG	1 complete remission, sustained for 30 months
Pallanti et al. (2002)	Lithium, Valproate	14-week single blind	42 PG patients (23 Lithium; 19 Valproate)	Symptoms decreased one-third over 14 week period in all patients regardless of whether Lithium or Valproate was taken
Hollander et al. (2005a)	Sustained release lithium (300–900 mg/day)	10-week double-blind placebo-controlled	40 PGs with comorbid diagnoses of Bipolar spectrum disorders	Significant improvement in the 29 completers with regard to gambling symptoms
Serotonin and Serotonin Reuptake Inhibitors (SRIS)				
Hollander et al. (1992)	Clomipramine 125 mg/day, 175 mg during open label period	Single case report, double-blind (10 weeks placebo) followed by open label for 28 weeks	1 PG	Significant improvement in gambling symptoms sustained through open label period
Hollander et al. (1998)	Fluvoxamine 207 mg/day	Single-blind (8 weeks placebo; 8 weeks treatment)	16 (no severe psychiatric comorbidity)	7 of 10 subjects who completed showed significant improvement

Study	Drug/dose	Study design	Sample	Results
De la Gandara (1999)	Fluoxetine	Open label treatment for 6 months plus supportive psychotherapy vs. supportive psychotherapy alone	20 PGs	Significantly more reduction in symptoms in fluoxetine plus psychotherapy group
Hollander et al (2000)	Fluvoxamine 207 mg/day	7-day single-blind placebo followed by a double-blind crossover	15 PGs (no severe psychiatric comorbidity)	Improvement for fluvoxamine significantly greater than for placebo
Blanco et al. (2002)	Fluvoxamine 200 mg/day	Double-blind, 6 months	34 PGs	Improvement only in young male PGs
Zimmerman and Breen (2002)	Citalopram 34.7 mg/day	Open label 12 weeks	15 PGs	4 of 7 completers showed decrease in gambling symptoms
Kim et al (2002)	Paroxetine 20–60 mg/day	1 week single-blind placebo followed by 8-week double-blind paroxetine or placebo	41 PGs (no severe psychiatric comorbidity)	Significantly more reduction in symptoms in treatment group
Grant et al. (2003)	Paroxetine 10–60 mg/day	Multisite, double-blind placebo-controlled trial with 1-week placebo lead in followed by randomization for 16 weeks.	76 PGs	No statistical differences between treatment and placebo groups for study completers
Saiz-Ruiz et al. (2005)	Sertraline 50 to 150 mg/day	6 months in a double-blind, flexible-dose, placebo-controlled study	60 PGs	Sertraline was not statistically significantly superior to placebo in the overall sample

Table 7.1
(continued)

Authors	Drug	Type of Study	Sample Size	Findings
Dannon et al. (2005a)	Fluvoxamine (200 mg/day) vs. topiramate (anti-convulsant; 200 mg/day)	Patients randomized in 2 groups to receive either fluvoxamine or topiramate for 12 weeks in a parallel fashion.	15 PGs received topiramate; 16 PGs received fluvoxamine; no other Axis I or II disorders	Both drugs appeared to be efficient in reducing gambling symptoms
Grant and Potenza (2006)	Escitalopram 10–20 mg/day	12-week open-label trial followed by an 8-week double-blind discontinuation phase	13 PGs with co-morbid anxiety	Significant reduction in both gambling and anxiety symptoms
Post-Synaptic 5HT Antagonists				
Pallanti et al. (2002)	Nefazodone 50 mg/day titrated upward to max 500 mg/day	Open label 8 weeks	12 PGs	Significant improvement in 9 of 1 2 completers
Opioid Receptor Antogonists: Naltrexone				
Crockford and El-Guebaly (1998b)	Naltrexone 50 mg/day	Single case report, open label	1 PG and alcohol dependent	Reduction in symptoms compared to treatment period of 20 mg/day fluoxetine
Kim and Grant (2001a)	Naltrexone 157 mg/day	Open label	17 PGs (no severe psychiatric comorbidity)	Significant reduction in symptoms

Kim and Grant (2001b)	Naltrexone 188 mg/day	1-week single-blind placebo followed by 11-week double-blind placebo or treatment	83 PGs (no other Axis I disorders)	In 44 completers significant improvement in symptoms
Kim et al. (2001)	Naltrexone 250 mg/day	Double-blind placebo control	83 PGs	In 45 completers significant improvement in all outcome measures
Grant et al. (2006)	Nalmefene (either 25 mg/day, 50 mg/day, or 100 mg/day)	Multicenter, 16-week, randomized, dose-ranging, double-blind, placebo-controlled trial	207 PGs	25 mg/day Nalmefene group had significantly reduced gambling symptoms. Higher dosage groups experienced intolerable side effects
Atypical Antipsychotics				
Potenza and Chambers (2001)	Olanzapine	Single case study: olanzapine after trial of haloperidol (typical antipsychotic)	Schizophrenic patient with co-morbid PG	Cessation of gambling behavior
Black (2004)	Bupropion (up to 300 mg/day)	Open-label 8 weeks	10 PGs with ADHD features	Significant improvement to resist gambling and reduction in symptoms
Dannon et al. (2005b)	Bupropion vs. Naltrexone	Patients randomized in 2 groups to receive either naltrexone or sustained-release bupropion for 12 weeks in a parallel fashion	19 PGs received naltrexone; 17 PGs received bupropion; no other Axis I or II disorders	Similar findings for both types of drug with around 75% of PGs rated as full responders

7.2.1   Mood Stabilizers

Mood stabilizers have been sporadically used to treat PGs since the 1970s, because of shared features with bipolar disorder. Bipolar I and II disorder are associated with high impulsivity, which at face value seems to be responsive to mood stabilizers. Moreover, one of the symptoms of the manic phase of bipolar I disorder is impulsive and irrational financial behavior (*DSM-IV*).

Although studies of mood stabilizers have shown promise in reducing gambling behavior, they are few and methodologically limited in scope. In particular, it is unclear in the studies summarized in table 7.1 whether the comorbidity of bipolar disorder was considered in the description of sample characteristics. It may be that PG was not the primary diagnosis in these studies, and that when the primary (bipolar) disorder was treated, gambling symptoms decreased. Moreover, mood stabilizers like lithium, Topamax, carbamazepine, and Depakote are not understood to act on the mesolimbic reward systems (or dopamine). They are therefore not typically the drug of choice for substance abuse disorders, which, as we have demonstrated in chapter 5, target the neural reward circuitries. Moreover, the "impulsivity" associated with a manic phase of bipolar disorder is clinically conceptualized primarily as stemming from the grandiosity and excess of a manic mood, rather than "pure" impulsivity. Similarly, mood stabilizers seem to be wholly ineffective in treating attention deficit/hyperactivity disorder (ADHD), which is primarily seen as an impulsive disorder.

7.2.2   Selective Serotonin Reuptake Inhibitors

As shown in table 7.1, there is some evidence that selective serotonin reuptake inhibitors (SSRIs), such as clomapramine, reduce PG symptoms, particularly in males. This is intuitive in the light of the I-RISA model, since one of the two main neurochemical mechanisms it posits as underlying PG is 5-HT deficit, which expresses impaired cortical response inhibition of the amygdala. Furthermore, 5-HT agonists have been found to modulate dopamine release in the NAcc (Boulenguez et al. 1996). Several small single-blind and double-blind trials of the SSRI fluvoxamine (Prozac) showed it to be effective in controlling PG behavior, at least in the short term. Fluvoxamine has specifically been demonstrated to reduce extracellular dopamine levels in the NAcc

(Ichikawa and Meltzer 1995). Interestingly, in light of the role of sero-tonin in the I-RISA model, these effects seem to be independent of symptoms of depression, and doses for PG treatment efficacy are higher than standard doses for treating depression. This is supported by Hollander et al. (1998).

A challenge facing the above research on treatment efficacy of SSRIs is the fact that studies do not typically screen for comorbid depression and/or anxiety. The issue of comorbidity with depression was explored by Grant et al. (2003). They examined the efficacy of paroxatine on PGs with comorbid axis I disorders screened out. As indicated in table 7.1, they found no evidence of efficacy in comparison to placebos. As several gambling researchers (Grant et al. 2003; Dell'Osso, Allen, and Hollander 2005) point out, there seems to be much more information available on how to pharmacologically treat PGs by reference to some of their typical comorbidities than on managing PG per se. If a patient is comorbid for depression or anxiety, there are clearly grounds for treatment with an SSRI. In a PG with comorbid alcohol dependence, naltrexone therapy is an option favored by some evidence. However, the successful pharmacological management of PG would require our knowing what generally works against PG symptoms in the first place.

Another challenge facing investigators studying the efficacy of SSRIs in the treatment of PG is that some comparison studies have shown significant short-term response to placebos. For instance, Hollander et al. (2000) showed that in the first phase of one study there were no differences between the medication and the placebo groups, though such differences emerged later in the trial. But it remains a problem that most cited studies of SSRI trials with PGs (e.g., Zimmerman, Breen, and Posternak 2002; De la Gandara 1999; Blanco et al. 2002) have not been placebo-controlled. Moreover, there have been some interesting functional neuroimaging results (e.g., Wager et al. 2004) that indicated that placebo analgesia (a deadening or absence of the sense of pain without loss of consciousness) was related to decreased brain activity in pain-sensitive brain regions—some of which overlap with reward processing areas. Wager et al. (2004) demonstrated placebo association with decreased activation in thalamus, insula, and ACC, and increased activity during anticipation of pain in PFC, thus providing evidence that placebos alter the experience of pain. In speculating on the possible significance of this for reward-system modulation, however, one must bear in mind that, by contrast with assumptions of early conditioning models, it is now known that appetitive and aversive stimuli are coded as such in distinct, though overlapping, brain areas.

7.2.3 Post-synaptic 5-HT Antagonists

An antagonist for a given neurotransmitter blocks receptors for that neurotransmitter. Nefazadone (also called Serzone) is a phenylpipera-zine antidepressant with mixed adrenergic/serotonergic reuptake inhibitor effects. Despite the seemingly positive effects of Nefazodone, as shown in table 7.1, the drug was taken off the market in Europe and is, as far as we know, not being produced in the US. Liver toxicity was the reason for market withdrawal.

7.2.4 Opioid Receptor Antagonists

Interesting results have been obtained with opioid receptor antago-nists, in particular with naltrexone (Kim and Grant 2001a). Naltrexone antagonizes the mu-opioid system, activity of which is associated, according to the I-RISA model, with diminished GABA in the meso-limbic system that, in turn, contributes to dopamine concentration in the NAcc. Naltrexone is currently the drug of choice for most drug addictions, especially alcohol addiction, since it is known that alcohol addiction is predominantly affected through the GABAergic system. Naltrexone directly modulates GABA input to dopamine neurons in the mesolimbic pathway. Until the first recent trial of naltrexone (see the discussion of atypical antipsychotics below), which compared its action in non-alcohol-dependent PGs with controls (Dannon et al. 2005b), there wasn't yet strong reason to regard it as a supported approach to PG per se. Note that there is a small window between the minimum dosage indicated as effective and dosages that impair liver function (e.g., 188 mg/day). At a slightly lower dosage (150 mg/day), Kim et al. (2006) demonstrated the long-term efficacy and safety of naltrexone. Despite these grounds for caution on viewing opioid recep-tors as mainstream therapy for PG, the evidence of their efficacy sup-ports the I-RISA model of addiction, and its specific application to PG.

Recently, nalmefene hydrochloride, a long-acting opioid antagonist, has demonstrated efficacy in the treatment of alcohol dependence (Grant et al. 2006). Like naltrexone, it is obviously consistent with the I-RISA model of addiction, but is without associated liver toxicity. As listed in table 7.1, Grant et al. (2006) conducted a large (N = 207) double-blind, randomized, multicenter trial of nalmefene for PG. They showed that nalmefene reduced gambling symptoms (urges, thoughts, and behaviors) in subjects with PG, thereby offering for the first time a safer alternative to naltrexone.

7.2.5 Atypical Antipsychotics

Atypical antipsychotics (e.g., risperidone, olanzapine, quetiapine, and ziprasidone) are typically used, in relatively high dosages, for treating schizophrenia and other psychotic disorders. They are understood to antagonize dopamine D2 receptors along with serotonin 5-HT2A and/or 5-HT2C receptors. One study that investigated the effect of atypical antipsychotics on PG behavior centered on a single case, in which the patient had a primary diagnosis of schizophrenia (Potenza and Chambers 2001), while in another, 10 PGs were comorbid with ADHD (Black 2004). In the latter, the 10 PGs were treated with up to 300 mg/day of bupropion for eight weeks. Although there was significant improvement for all 10 subjects, the absence of a placebo control group and the comorbidity with ADHD are significant methodological limitations.

In the most methodologically careful study to date, Dannon et al. (2005b) compared bupropion (an atypical antipsychotic) and naltrexone (an opioid receptor antagonist) in a group of PGs with no axis I or axis II comorbid disorders. Each group was treated for 12 weeks. "Full response" was defined as absence of gambling for two weeks following treatment, combined with improved score on the global functioning scale. "Partial response" was defined as a decrease in the frequency of gambling and a decrease in the stakes wagered. Seventy-five percent of the bupropion-treated group and 76 percent of the naltrexone-treated group showed full response, and 100 percent of each sample showed a partial response. This study is particularly promising in the light of the argument advanced in chapter 5, suggesting that PG is a direct disorder of the dopaminergic system, with subsequent implications for PFC 5-HT circuits.

7.2.6 Summary of Pharmacological Treatment Evidence

No generalizations are warranted regarding treating PGs with mood stabilizers, because of small samples, ambiguous comorbidities among treated patients, and poor study designs. The research on SSRIs and atypical antipsychotics is more promising, and is conceptually consistent with the I-RISA model of addiction, but these studies also are plagued by comorbidity and methodological issues. Although promising in one study, post-synaptic 5-HT antagonists proved to be unsafe and are no longer being studied. The strongest evidence for efficacious pharmacological treatment comes from studies of opioid receptor antagonists. Grant et al. 2006 is perhaps the most impressive study, with a large sample, multiple sites, multiple doses of nalmefene, and double-blind placebo-controlled design. Moreover, Grant et al. screened out individuals with comorbid psychiatric conditions and used a community sample rather than a clinical sample. The latter is quite important where generalization is concerned, because only about 8 percent of PGs receive treatment (Committee on the Social and Economic Impact of Pathological Gambling 1999; National Gambling Impact Study Commission 1999). Tamminga and Nestler (2006) were enthusiastic enough about the Grant et al. study that they devoted their editorial to it in the issue of the journal in which it appeared. They summarize the applicability of the I-RISA model of drug addiction to PG, and note that the "underlying hypothesis about pathological gambling . . . is that the disorder is not about the gambling but about the addiction" (p. 180), and that "drugs that treat one addiction would be expected to treat another" (p. 180). This, of course, is exactly what Grant et al. found, and what we have argued is predicted by a consilience of several kinds and sources of other evidence.

Apart from opioid receptor antagonists like nalmefene there is another class of pharmacological treatment, as yet untested for its efficacy in the treatment of PG, that shows great promise for the reasons discussed in the next section.

7.3   D3 Dopamine Agonists and Partial Agonists

Some recent clinical observations of Parkinson's disease patients are most intriguing for the view that PG is an addiction. Dodd et al. (2005) reported on 11 Parkinson's disease sufferers, without histories of even mildly disordered gambling, who developed severe PG after stabilizing on courses of a dopamine agonist (pramipexole in nine cases and ropinirole in two cases). In all cases, PG symptoms resolved rapidly after the medication was discontinued. On the basis of this discovery, Dodd et al. performed a literature search that revealed six published reports collectively indicating 17 Parkinson's patients who developed PG after beginning courses of dopamine agonists. Most of these patients had also been taking a dopamine stimulant, levodopa. However, none of Dodd et al.'s sample developed PG while on levodopa alone, and three of the sample were not taking levodopa. The literature search sample implicates all of the commonly prescribed dopamine agonists, but specifically pramipexole (82 percent in Dodd et al.'s sample and 59 percent in the search set). Dodd et al. comment: "Pramipexole is a unique drug that is highly selective for the dopamine D3 receptor, with an affinity at least two orders of magnitude greater than for other receptors" (p. 5). Pramipexole plus pergolide and ropinirole, which are also selective (though less strongly so) for D3, account for 93 percent of the 28 induced PG cases. Dodd et al. note that "this makes intuitive sense in view of the localization of D3 receptors to limbic areas of the brain" (p. 5). Similarly, Grosset et al. (2006) reported that overall 8 percent of Parkinson's disease patients on dopamine agonists developed PG, with those on pramipexole showing the highest rate of PG.

Looking back on older data in light of this suggestive discovery, we find D3 receptors specifically implicated in some other work on addiction as a mesolimbic reward-pathway disorder. Pilla et al. (1999) found that targeting mesolimbic D3 receptors with a dopamine partial agonist "greatly" diminished cocaine-seeking behavior. This may seem paradoxical in light of what has just been said regarding Parkinson's disease patients on dopamine agonists developing PG, but it is only apparently so. Dopamine receptor agonists stimulate the receptor. The action of dopamine receptor partial agonists is more complex, as they appear to act as agonists when dopamine levels are depleted, as in Parkinson's patients (see Orsini, Koob, and Pulvirenti 2002), but to act as antagonists when dopamine levels are normal, as in Pilla et al.'s subjects (Harinder, Sokoloff, and Beninger 2002; Pulvirenti and Koob 1994). The underlying mechanism for this is not yet understood.

The I-RISA model as applied to PG of course predicts that treatments against cocaine seeking should be suggestive models for PG therapies. Everitt, Dickinson, and Robbins (2001) note, apropos of Pilla et al.'s study, that "it remains unclear whether this effect is mediated by blockade of D3 receptors within the NAcc, the amygdala or autoreceptors on the mesolimbic [dopamine] neurons themselves" (p. 134). However, they add that "[o]ne advantage of drugs acting at the D3 receptor is that its distribution in the brain is restricted to these few sites . . . and so unwanted side effects of such drugs are minimal." In addition,

Chiamulera (2004), in line with Andreoli et al. (2003), developed an
I-RISA-style model of nicotine addiction as a reward-system disorder,
and reports that "[d]opamine D3 receptor antagonist SB-277011 inhibited reinforcement of responding in a model of relapse to nicotine
where responding was induced by the sequential presentation of CX/
CS and then of a single nicotine injection" (p. 84).

The significance of the above for our purposes is, first, that it further
solidifies our argument that PG is an addictive disorder, and, second,
that the D3 receptor may be a viable target for the treatment of PG,
perhaps without leading to side effects of reduction in general motivation, concentration, and motor control. Indeed, a major challenge for
efforts to manage PG pharmacologically, if it is wholly or mainly a
reward-system pathology, is identified by Baunez et al. (2005). Because
drugs of abuse and "natural" reinforcers (of which, we argued in
chapter 6, PG is the template) exert their effects via the same neural
pathways and processes, one of the main challenges in treating addictions is to eradicate the pathological motivation for the drug without
impairing the general affective state of subjects. This is an especially
troubling concern when our treatment target is itself a natural reward.
Will it be possible to manage PG pharmacologically without inducing
general motivational apathy in patients? In this context, it would be
greatly encouraging if it turned out that anti-PG therapy could focus
on a sparsely distributed receptor such as D3.

All of the above is of course still merely suggestive. Only 8 percent
of Parkinson's disease patients on dopamine agonists developed PG
(Grosset et al. 2006), so we do not have evidence of a simple switch
that, turned too far in one direction, produces Parkinson's disease, and
turned too far in the other produces PG. Nevertheless, the prospects
for managing PG with *some* dopaminergic pharmacology, even if it
doesn't turn out to be as uniformly specific as a D3 reuptake inhibitor,
look increasingly promising.

7.4   The Comorbidity of PG with Other Psychiatric Disorders

It is important to consider the comorbidity and heterogeneity of PG.
In clinical practice, patients often show no response or only partial
response to pharmacotherapies and/or psychological interventions
that have worked well on others, which raises the question of heterogeneity of PG. Especially with regard to pharmacological interventions,
and since no data-driven taxonomy of PG is currently in clinical use,

clinicians cannot make treatment decisions a priori regarding PGs, and so tend to add other agents to their therapeutic approach when a patient appears to be treatment-resistant. For instance, if a serotonergic agent was initially prescribed but response is disappointing, an opiodergic agent may be added that can have positive clinical effects (Grant, Kim, and Potenza 2003). The same holds for adding a mood stabilizer to an SSRI or naltrexone. Finally, adding an atypical antipsychotic to an already established regime of serotonergic treatment ensures the targeting of both the dopamine and serotonin systems.

The heterogeneity of treatment response in PG may be accounted for partly by the fact that PG is a highly comorbid disorder. A recent review of trends in gambling studies research has shown that approximately 30 percent of research on gambling has contained the keyword "comorbidity" (Shaffer, Stanton, and Nelson 2006). Of these studies, the National Institute on Alcohol Abuse and Alcoholism's *National Epidemiologic Survey on Alcohol and Related Conditions* is the largest comorbidity study ever conducted, and most comprehensive in its assessment of comorbid diagnoses (Ladd and Petry 2002). This study ratifies conclusions of several earlier ones in showing that PG is highly comorbid with some axis I psychiatric disorders, and gives unequivocal evidence for the association between SUDs and PG. Virtually no negative findings have been reported for this association, which has furthermore been reported for both community-based and treatment-seeking samples. Recently, special attention has been paid to comorbidity with bipolar spectrum disorders and ADHD (Hollander et al. 2005a).

Axis II disorders, most notably antisocial personality disorder, also seem to be highly comorbid with PG. It has often been proposed that the high rates of comorbidity between SUDs and PG are explained by common personality variables (believed to be closely tied to neurobiological underpinnings). These may include impulsivity, sensation-seeking, risk-taking, problems in limit setting, negative emotionality, and neuroticism. A growing literature is now devoted to describing the neurobiological correlates of personality disorders as well as personality traits (Bohus, Schmahl, and Lieb 2004). In the framework of BE, personality differences are modeled as systematic differences in qualitative properties of cardinal utility functions: shapes, slopes, attitudes to risk, and so forth. They appear to be exogenous and unlearned, and to characterize all animals with central nervous systems including creatures as cognitively unsophisticated as guppies and garter snakes (Gosling and Vazire 2002). It remains to be determined whether this BE modeling assumption will be borne out by NE; we know of no research to date that begins the task of integrating neural correlates of personality, on the one hand, and reward-system response, on the other hand.

7.5 Nonpharmacological Interventions for PG

A PG psychological treatment literature based on scientific evidence is only in the nascent stage of development. A review of PG treatment studies published in 2003 (Toneatto and Ladouceur 2003) included just 11 studies, while a similar review published in 2005 (Pallesen et al. 2005) included 22 studies. The 2003 review concluded that cognitive behavioral therapy (CBT) seemed to have the most promise, while the 2005 review concluded only that "psychological treatments" were better than no treatment. Both of these reviews excluded a large number of other studies because they contained critical methodological flaws. Working out the numerous methodological kinks is quite common in the incipient states of any scientific literature. Among the most common methodological problems in the surveyed investigations were lack of random assignment to treatment and control conditions, inadequate or inadequately specified assessment procedures, inadequate or inadequately specified treatment protocols, ill-defined and/or poorly measured treatment outcomes, and insufficiently lengthy follow-up periods (Blaszczynski 2005; Nathan 2005b). Clearly, strong recommendations for specific nonpharmacological or extrapharmacological PG treatments would be premature, given the current state of knowledge.

7.5.1 Cognitive Behavioral Therapy

CBT currently is the dominant psychological treatment approach and has been successfully applied to various disorders, including depression, aggression, SUDs, fears and phobias, ADHD, pain, eating disorders, bipolar disorder, and learning disabilities. In general, CBT employs performance-based and verbal-based interventions to help patients change their thinking styles, which, in turn, brings about changes in emotions and behavior. A prevailing tactic is to critically examine the content of patients' thought patterns that are understood to underlie the experience of subjective distress and problem behaviors. For instance, many depressed patients believe "I am a total failure." In fact, of course, when the evidence for that cognition is examined, it turns out to be at best a gross exaggeration. The patient may have failed in some respects, as have we all, but her literal claim surely misrepresents reality. CBT focuses on changing such cognitive distortions to more accurately reflect the reality of a patient's life; for example, CBT can assist in changing the content of the attribution from "I am a total failure" to "I may have not been successful in passing my exams, but that does not mean I am a total failure." In addition to a focus on cognitive distortions, CBT also employs a range of behavioral techniques, including self-monitoring, behavioral rehearsal, behavioral contracting, daily activity schedules, and response prevention to assist in developing more constructive behavior patterns.

It is important to point out that although CBT interventions have been developed to target PG, they are for the most part not based on specific cognitive theories of *pathological* gambling. Existing cognitive theories of *gambling* are supported by studies showing that gambling is associated with a range of cognitive distortions (see Petry 2005 for a review), but it is unclear if such distortions are specific to PG. In fact, because most studies that investigated cognitive distortions have relied on college student samples, they may testify only to the fact that cognitive distortions are inherent in *any* gambling situation. Until these cognitive theories of gambling are thoroughly investigated in PG samples, they cannot shed light on whether PGs engage in specific cognitive distortions at higher frequency or with more intensity than other individuals. The results of studies including both PG and normal control groups have shown mixed results (Griffiths 1994; Gaboury et al. 1998; Hardoon et al. 2001).

Cognitive distortions apparently related to gambling include illusions of control, distorted representativeness and availability heuristics, ignorance of large-number statistics, and confusions of correlation and causation (Petry 2005, pp. 230–252). Thus, gamblers tend to believe that a given gambling event will predict or even influence subsequent gambling events, thereby failing to realize that gambling events are random and therefore independent. Many gamblers also think they have some control over gambling event outcomes, often on the basis of superstitious causal beliefs such as that blowing on the dice three times will result in a win. They also tend to selectively remember large wins while forgetting the majority of losses. Gambling environments inevitably exploit these cognitive distortions, if for no other reason than that they beset the majority of humans in all circumstances involving chance and probability and are extremely tenacious against reform in even the most motivated and least disturbed subjects (Bishop and

Trout 2004). Although a gambler who comes to better understand the unreliability of her natural beliefs might thereby gain a reduced disposition to gamble, CBT interventions based on such theories would not target reward processing, which as we have argued lies at the basis of PG.

Of the several CBT approaches developed to target PG, none, with the exception of Ladouceur and colleagues (Ladouceur, Boisvert, and Dumont 1994; Ladouceur et al. 1998, 2001, 2003), can be described as anything other than a "boutique" approach—that is, none has been assayed on more than a small and almost certainly unrepresentative number of subjects in a few distinctive treatment contexts. In consequence, rigorous measures of efficacy for such approaches are rare.

The group to which this complaint does not apply, Ladouceur et al. (2001), compared the efficacy of their CBT treatment with a waiting list control group. Subjects in the CBT group were first taught the concept of randomness (i.e., that each "throw of the dice" is independent), that there is an overall negative expectation of gain, and that it is impossible to control the game. Subjects were made aware of their miscalculations by having them "think out loud" while gambling. Outcome measures included *DSM-IV* PG symptoms, self-efficacy expectations (i.e., the degree to which subjects could refrain from gambling), perception of control over the gambling problem, and the desire to gamble. Results showed that 86 percent of the CBT subjects showed improvement on at least some of the outcome measures, a significantly greater percentage than the control group, and these therapeutic gains were maintained at six- and twelve-month follow-up points.

Ladouceur et al. (2003) used the same treatment approach in a similarly designed randomized trial. Again, a significantly larger percentage of PGs in the treatment group showed improvement in outcome measures compared to waiting list controls, and the gains were maintained at follow-up. In both these studies, the findings would have been more compelling had the study design included an attention placebo or an alternate treatment group (to show that the treatment is specific to gambling problems). Nevertheless, this work suggests that a gambling-tailored CBT may be efficacious in reducing DSM symptoms of PG.

While studies such as the above target the content of cognitive distortions, other CBT treatment approaches have focused more on the behavioral aspects of PG. For instance, imaginal desensitization (e.g., McConaghy et al. 1983, 1988; McConaghy, Blaszczynski, and Frankova

1991) is based on the notion that compulsive types of behavior are driven by increased arousal and tension produced by neurophysiological "behavior-completion mechanisms," which come into play when the compulsive behavior is stimulated but not actually completed. Patients are therefore systematically exposed to increasing levels of imagining the experience (and discomfort) of giving up gambling. Similarly, stimulus response prevention programs such as the one employed by Echeburúa, Baez, and Fernandez-Montalvo (1996) teach patients to inhibit a learned response (gambling) to a stimulus (e.g., casino advertisements) by exposing patients to the stimulus in a systematic way, thereby aiming at extinction of the gambling behavior. Both these treatment approaches are employed in the treatment of OCD, and are not motivated by attention either to reward processing mechanisms or to altering cognitive distortions inherent in gambling.

7.5.2 Future Possibilities

Chapter 6 argued that PG is a pathology of the midbrain reward system—reaching out to afflict circuits in other brain areas—equivalent to the core mechanism underlying drug addiction. The current chapter has strengthened this case by showing that pharmacological treatments that target midbrain reward processing are promising for the efficacious treatment of PG. The CBT approaches discussed above focus on altering the *content* of cognitive distortions associated with gambling, without targeting the core pathology of reward processing. The present section addresses the possibility of future psychological treatments that target the latter rather than the former.

Although CBT is currently the psychological treatment of choice for PG and most other psychiatric disorders, a new wave of cognitive therapies has emerged over the last decade to challenge CBT's dominance. These "third-wave" therapies are so called because they are a reaction to CBT, which was in turn the "second wave" of cognitive therapy following disenchantment with a "first wave" of behavior therapy in the 1950s. Clinical psychology and psychiatry in the first half of the twentieth century were dominated conceptually by Freudian psychodynamics and took little interest in the empirical evaluation of their treatment procedures. The early behavior therapists (e.g., Lindsley, Skinner, and Solomon 1953; Wolpe 1952) sought to improve that situation by applying discoveries in the Skinnerian and Pavlovian behavioral science laboratories to address human behavior problems, and to evaluate the results empirically. Importantly, the behaviorists wanted to constrain the language of therapists to comport with the scientific language of the behavioral laboratory, analyzing clients' problems in terms of conditioned and unconditioned stimuli, responses, and reinforcement, instead of in terms of unobserved unconscious motives or drives. Although the emphasis on empirical evaluation of interventions was a lasting contribution, the conceptual restrictions proved to be poorly suited to dealing effectively with intact adults. The early cognitive behavior therapists (e.g., Mahoney 1974; Meichenbaum 1977) argued persuasively for relaxing these restrictions and legitimized the analysis of clients' problems in terms of thoughts, beliefs, expectations, and desires. The development of third-wave cognitive approaches was motivated by the fact that CBT approaches focused on a limited range of cognitive phenomena in analyzing psychological disorders and were never well aligned with scientific cognitive psychology (Wells and Purdon 1999). In particular, the CBT focus was typically on the *content* of thoughts and beliefs rather than cognitive *processes*.

Third-wave cognitive therapies such as metacognitive therapy (Wells 2000) and acceptance and commitment therapy (Hayes, Strosahl, and Wilson 1999) are based on the notion of "metacognition," a construct introduced by Flavell (1979) in the context of developmental psychology to describe the processes and structures that monitor and control aspects of cognition. In short, metacognition refers to thinking about thinking, and is the aspect of the information processing system that monitors, interprets, evaluates, and regulates the contents and processes of its own organization (Wells and Purdon 1999).

There are two general components of metacognition: metacognitive knowledge and metacognitive regulation (Baird 1998; Flavell 1979). The first refers to knowledge or beliefs about the factors that affect the course and outcome of cognitive enterprises. For instance, a depressed patient may have a metacognitive belief that "If I believe that I am a total failure, I will not be motivated to try harder." This metacognitive belief might govern and influence her primary cognition. Once such a metacognitive belief is activated, that metacognitive knowledge is likely to influence the course of the individual's thought processes. This brings us to the second component of metacognition, metacognitive regulation. This refers to processes governing a number of executive functions, including planning, resource allocation (i.e., selective attention), monitoring, checking, and error detection and correction (Wells

2000). The monitoring process tracks ongoing cognition, whereas the control process modifies ongoing cognitive processes (e.g., by shifting attentional focus). To continue the example of the depressed patient, we would observe that she fully attends to negative feedback from others while allocating no attentional resources to positive feedback. Of course, she will not be aware of the fact that she displays such an attentional bias. However, through metacognitive therapy, we can facilitate reflection on the process by which she thinks, and thereby bring the unconscious cognitive process of attention allocation into conscious awareness.

The third-wave cognitive therapy literature has focused on attentional processes, and reward processing has not yet explicitly been considered as a metacognitive regulation agent. In chapter 5 we discussed the notions of "internal currency" and "valuation" that underlie behavioral allocation and choice. The reinforcement learning algorithm updates its reward predictions via errors in prediction (i.e., the critic), and learning stops when received rewards converge on predicted rewards for a given situation. This process can go awry in the case of drugs and gambling, for somewhat different reasons, because in these instances the algorithm can produce perpetual positive prediction error. As with the depressed patient's attentional allocation processing, reinforcement learning of course occurs outside conscious awareness. Would it be possible, however, and might it help combat impulsivity, to give voice to unconscious error detection (or lack thereof) through a metacognitive therapy approach?

By employing a "think aloud" paradigm during therapy, this may be achievable. Ladouceur et al.'s (2001) CBT intervention had gamblers verbalize their thoughts while gambling in order to challenge their beliefs about gambling events. If procedures were instead developed to make patients aware of the fact that they cannot "trust" the reinforcement learning in their brains in gambling situations, it may be possible to give the "critic" a voice, and for the patient to "talk back" at the critic as gambling proceeds. Talking back to the critic would imply that the reinforcement learning algorithm is adjusted by the gambler himself. Through such therapy, faulty error detection by the critic may be revealed, brought into conscious awareness, and altered by the patient.

We are not aware of any direct empirical evidence that such a nonpharmacological intervention might actually alter reward processing in the brain. Nevertheless, data from studies that have employed traditional CBT strategies to target specific processing styles associated with other psychiatric disorders are beginning to show that nonpharmacological interventions can and sometimes do alter brain functioning. For instance, based on the fact that several studies have demonstrated activation of the insula and ACC in threat processing and symptom provocation in specific phobias, Straube et al. (2006) used fMRI to measure brain activation to spider and control videos in 28 arachnophobics and 14 control subjects. Phobics were randomly assigned to a therapy group (TG) and a waiting-list control group (WG). All phobics were scanned twice, and between scans CBT was given to those in the TG. Results showed that the phobic groups did not differ in brain activation prior to the intervention, and phobics showed greater responses to spider versus control videos in the insula and ACC. CBT strongly reduced phobic symptoms in the TG, while the WG remained behaviorally unchanged. In the second scanning session, a significant reduction of hyperactivity in the insula and ACC was found in the TG compared to the WG. For reasons specific to our model of PG that we will indicate in chapter 8, we suggest there is a strong theoretical motivation for running similar experiments with PG sufferers.

7.6   Classification of Gambling Disorders Revisited

We argued in chapter 6 that the *DSM-IV* PG diagnostic category empirically maps relatively smoothly onto the class of people who exhibit classic patterns of addictive behavior as a result of a specific kind of dysfunction in their dopaminergic reward system and consequent neuroadaptation impairing frontal control circuits. We therefore believe that clarity would be served, especially for clinical and treatment purposes, by replacing the behaviorally derived concept of PG with the neuroscientifically anchored concept of addictive gambling. In the remainder of the book, we will therefore generally use "AG" where formerly, in deference to usage in advance of the new neuroscientific evidence, we have used "PG." This replacement won't be uniform, however. Sometimes we will want to refer to a class of patients from the implied perspective of a clinical community not yet persuaded that gambling addiction is a real scientific phenomenon, or not persuaded that a neuroscientifically derived categorization should trump the traditional view in this instance. We ask the reader to be alert to this slightly subtle referential tactic we will use. We will continue to use "DG" to refer, in propria persona, to the entire class of people—

including AGs as well as non-addicted persons—who demonstrate inconsistent preferences with respect to their gambling behavior, both investing in gambling activity and investing in efforts not to gamble, and who thereby have gambling problems from the perspective of behavioral economics.

The future development of both pharmacological and nonpharmacological treatments for AG necessarily relies on clarifying the uncertainty that exists over basic concepts in the literature of DG. This uncertainty makes it difficult to coordinate on instruments for recruiting and screening research subjects and interpreting research results. As described in chapter 2, to deal with different levels of DG, the psychiatric profession has operationalized the concept of PG but not milder forms of problem gambling that are sometimes thought to be stepping stones to PG. Typically, a person is considered a problem gambler when he or she exhibits one to four of the *DSM-IV* criteria, and a PG when meeting five or more criteria. However, this distinction is at best arbitrary and at worst erroneous, with no empirical evidence supporting differential correlates. Another important issue is whether those who have been traditionally referred to in the psychiatric nomenclature as PGs are genuinely addicted, in a neurochemical sense, or whether common talk of "gambling addiction" should be understood as metaphorical. We have of course defended a strong view on this question in this and the previous chapter.

Based on the conjunction of the BE model of choice over time and the neuroeconomic model of addiction, we propose an operationalization of DG and its subvarieties. With the descriptions of two types of DG (the problem gambler and the AG) we outline several differentiating characteristics and associated treatment and policy implications. Wider scientific implications of the proposal, our primary target in this book, will occupy the next chapter.

7.6.1   Problem Gamblers

A "problem gambler" is a person who (1) gambles often enough to have invested consciously or behaviorally in construction of personal rules to limit their frequency of gambling, or their average amount gambled per session, or both, but for whom (2) these rules are inadequately effective because the person regrets their own gambling behavior on a regular basis, and who (3) does not show the neurochemical signature of neuroadaptation for addiction. Problem gamblers may very well display only one to four diagnostic criteria from *DSM-IV*. Their gambling behavior will be much influenced by the specific gambling environments in which they find themselves. They likely would not exhibit gambling problems if gambling establishments did not exploit the cognitive distortions that attend most everyday human encounters with chance and probability.

Problem gamblers may benefit from at least three intervention approaches. First, traditional CBT interventions that target cognitive distortions or employ response prevention strategies may be beneficial. Second, a principal focus of research that aims at changing problem gamblers' behavior should be the circumstances under which casino and other standard gambling environments interfere with reward bundling. For instance, the price of access to gambling opportunities could be increased for problem gamblers, and the price of opportunities for social interaction could be decreased. Third, problem gamblers may also benefit from interventions from significant others, the implementation of which would be a matter for individuals and thus would not entail significant industrial or regulatory reform. Here, however, the gambling industry may have an interest in participating in and facilitating the operation of an effective intervention system.

7.6.2 Addictive Gamblers

Based on the arguments put forward in this and the previous chapter, most people who have previously been classified in the psychiatric nomenclature as PGs should be referred to as AGs (and the remainder as problem gamblers). While it is likely that such individuals will typically meet more than five criteria on *DSM-IV*, we share the sentiments of Shaffer, Stanton, and Nelson (2006) that future classification of DG subtypes will not depend on the *DSM* classifications. As these authors point out, the diagnosis of AG currently depends on a tautology: the diagnostic inference of a latent state (i.e., addiction) rests upon the putative consequences of that very same latent state (i.e., excessive gambling). By replacing a tautological approach with an approach in which neuroscientific tools are used to uncover the brain mechanisms that distinguish AGs from problem gamblers, clinicians will be able to advance an etiologically based diagnostic classification that is not dependent upon self-report or behavioral observation. One important advantage of, for instance, fMRI and related technology is that they reduce experimenter–subject interactions and thereby minimize subjects' dispositions to sculpt responses to conform to perceived expectations. While it is not yet possible to use fMRI as a diagnostic tool, eventual such development will move us closer to making more reliable clinical diagnoses with clearer treatment indications. Koob (2006) recently reviewed and synthesized the neurobiological bases of addiction with an eye toward diagnostic procedures, and concluded that there is every reason to be optimistic that such procedures will be forthcoming in the near future.

Operationalizing PG as AG, and thus as neurobiologically distinct from problem gambling, also implies a straightforward policy goal: measures should be taken to try to prevent AGs from accessing commercial or other organized gambling environments. We recommend that responsibility to deny AGs access to gaming establishments should be vested in the operators of the establishments. However, the reasonableness of this recommendation is dependent on resources being provided to make AG identification practical. The two prospective scientific means of screening for AG, fMRI and brain fluid examinations, are absurdly expensive procedures for application to mass diagnostics outside self-reporting populations and are not yet sophisticated enough to use as diagnostic tools. Two considerations jointly rescue our policy reflections in this area from futility, however. First, evidence indicates that experienced casino staff are able to detect PG customers with high reliability, and that the requisite level of experience is typically acquired quite quickly. Second, if most PGs were not AGs, then the ability of the studies we reviewed to statistically measure AG in populations drawn using screens that overdiagnose PG would be mysterious. Thus, there are grounds to suppose that casinos are *already* able to identify and screen out AGs, except perhaps AGs in very early stages of morbidity.

The great hope encouraged by developments in the neuroscience of AG is that we will soon be able to exclude AGs from gambling venues in the most benign and welfare-enhancing way of all: by means of a neuropharmacological technology that will reduce or eliminate AGs' interest in gambling in the first place, and their disposition to harm themselves if and when they do find themselves exposed to gambling environments for one reason or another. However, until the neurochemically specified conditions for AG are determined to general satisfaction in the scientific and clinical communities, and then made the basis for sustained epidemiological research, efforts to estimate the costs to the gaming industry of fully, or nearly fully, managing AG are shots in the dark. Though we are sanguine about neuropharmacological research on AG continuing to be well supported, there is need for *integrated* research that includes BE. The recent breakthroughs in understanding addiction in general and AG in particular rest on the conjunction of basic neurochemistry and NE. NE relies heavily on fMRI experiments that in turn require batteries of well-tested behavioral task protocols from BE.

In the next and concluding chapter we will provide a much deeper and more wide-ranging defense of our proposed classification schema and its theoretical underpinnings and implications. On this basis we will then explore general lessons for the integration of BE and NE as frameworks for understanding the reward-seeking behavior of individual human economic agents. Our recommended approach will be critically contrasted with divergent ones proposed by other researchers. In the course of this, the nature of Ross's (2005) framework for the microexplanation of personal economic behavior in the age of cognitive neuroscience will be exemplified in application to the specific empirical phenomenon of DG.

8

The Microexplanation of
Disordered Gambling

8.1   Local Reduction of PG to AG: Philosophical Motivations and Normative Implications

Over the past three chapters, we have argued for the reduction of PG to AG. To make this proposal as explicit as possible: the phenomenon operationalized as PG in *DSM-IV* should be reconceptualized as AG, and theorized according to the I-RISA model (or an improved successor version of it) and the underlying PV model of reward (or an improved successor version of it). In support of the proposal we do not tell a convoluted story of the sort popular in much philosophy of science, according to which the authors of *DSM-IV* always intended "PG" to refer to whatever true "constitutive essence" unites the stereotypical cases, which has turned out empirically to be AG.[1] To the extent that it makes sense in the first place to talk about "intentions" of "authors" of referential conventions that emerge from complex institutional politics and evolving diagnostic practice in clinics and elsewhere over many years, these "intentions" were highly unspecific and should be inferred directly from the general function of *DSM*. That function is to optimally facilitate and standardize clinical reference, diagnosis, and treatment of cases of patients with common symptoms, common etiologies of disturbances, and common response modalities to a common small set of related interventions, with greater weight given to those whose suffering is most severe and chronic. Then, we claim, the empirical evidence strongly suggests that the largest proportion of those "intended" to be diagnosed as PGs by the *DSM* operationalization, including almost all of those whose suffering is severe, chronic, and recalcitrant to low-intensity therapy, are afflicted with neuroadapted hypoactivity of serotonergic circuits that normally inhibit impulsive behavior, and dopaminergic reward circuits that have learned to obsessively pursue and attend to predictors of gambling opportunities. Because of this common condition, almost all PGs are candidates for a common future treatment regimen, identification of which should be (as it fortunately is) the priority in applied research. The priority in basic research on PG should be (as it is) the refinement and generalization of the models that frame AG, so as to improve both predictive power and the depth of our explanation and integration of AG in the wider context of the behavioral and brain sciences. These pragmatic considerations motivate local reduction of PG to AG. Such a reduction need not be (and certainly will not be) what philosophers call "seamless." Those patients that *DSM-IV* "intended" to refer to as PGs who are not AGs should no longer be regarded as PGs, in order to avoid pragmatic confusion. We do not thereby risk misclassifying their essential conditions, because the idea of "essences" is metaphysical pixie dust.

There are objections to the local reduction of PG to AG that are based not on logical or metaphysical convictions but on pragmatic criteria of the kind we endorse in general. Petry (2006), though broadly sympathetic to the conceptualization of PG as AG, and mainly for the reasons we have presented, summarizes the principal worries as follows (though the reconstruction and numbering is ours rather than hers):

1. The classical addictions to drugs involve no phenomenon analogous to "chasing" of losses by PGs. But chasing is cited as a primary motivation for gambling beyond preconceived intended limits by *most* DGs, including most PGs.

2. Harm suffered by PGs involves direct financial losses to an extent not characteristic of classical addictions.

3. Harm suffered by PGs does *not* involve direct general health damage to the extent typical in victims of classical addictions—though, as Petry notes, "global health is poor in gamblers" (p. 157).

4. Classifying PG as AG might increase the stigmatization of PG, and thereby interfere with optimal public health response.

5. Classifying PG as AG might serve as the crucial "wedge" for inflation of the "addiction" concept so that everything some people do to an extent that causes harm is thrown into this basket, thereby obscuring what is distinctive about the classical addictions for no compensating gain in genuine *scientific* unification of phenomena (because the unifying principles are unduly generic).

Objections (1) through (3) have a different logical character from (4) and (5). The first set points to properties that distinguish PG from drug addictions, while the final pair raise normative policy concerns. We will address the disanalogies first, and then, more briefly, consider the policy-related issues.

Disanalogy (2) seems least problematic. Many people who become addicted to cocaine, alcohol, and heroin sacrifice huge proportions of their available budgets in consequence, and regard this as among the worst harms caused (both to themselves and their families) by their dependencies. Even addicts to the least financially damaging of major addictions, nicotine, are often importantly motivated to quit by focus on the monetary opportunity cost of smoking. (Many nicotine addicts are relatively or absolutely poor.) Disanalogy (2) seems most important *in conjunction with* disanalogy (3): it is not obvious that a PG who is rich enough to avoid serious financial harm from gambling has any pressing reason to regard himself or herself as having a problem, whereas a wealthy cocaine addict is still very likely to damage their general health (including social health) even if the financial opportunity cost of their cocaine consumption is trivial.

Our response to these related worries is speculative, but firmly based on the scientific perspective we have defended throughout this book. By the picoeconomic operationalization we have endorsed, the unworried wealthy gambler is not a non-addicted DG: by hypothesis, he or she does not simultaneously invest in both gambling and unsuccessful attempts to stop or cut down. But surely, it might be objected, being unconcerned about his or her gambling losses does not entail that a person's reward system might not be locked onto gambling cues, with cortical inhibition possibly atrophied by neuroadaptation. Thus, it might seem, we must allow that even the wealthy gambler could be an AG, albeit one who does not care about being an AG. Given the most plausible speculative ontogeny of AG, however, it is far from clear that this really makes sense. On the I-RISA/PV model, what draws the reward system to gambling is a person's ability to trigger reliable cues predicting both uncertainty and risk. The wealthy gambler can trigger uncertainty as readily as anyone else. But can she motivate risk so easily? By hypothesis, our concern here is only with the hypothetical gambler who, because of her wealth, isn't bothered by her losses— a wealthy but miserly gambler doesn't raise any special difficulty. If losses are of no importance to a gambler, where is the risk? Something that we have suggested may be a necessary condition for the development of AG may not be a normally possible condition (barring exotic and unusual circumstances) for a gambler who is untroubled by losses. Our hypothesis that PG is AG therefore leads us to predict that there are no PGs who don't care about their losses. If there are nevertheless *regular* gamblers who don't care about their losses, as there appear to be, these might mainly be people responding to boredom-relieving, purely curiosity-stimulated, drives, or people who gamble as part of a larger suite of conspicuous-consumption behaviors. But we are speculating in the absence of empirical data here. If it turns out that people who aren't worried about their gambling losses can become AGs, then either the I-RISA model gives a less complete explanation of AG than we expect, or molar degree of loss aversion doesn't penetrate to mediate reward system response to the extent that emphasis on disanalogy (2) assumes to begin with. Note that it would not be easy to set up rigorous research on significant samples of very wealthy regular gamblers. Observing regular gamblers playing for trivial stakes would not be a helpful approximation, because the activity would almost certainly be found strikingly dull by the subjects.

Petry's disanalogy (1) seems genuine at first glance; there seems to be no counterpart to the gambler's fallacy that applies to drinking, smoking, or snorting cocaine. However, we think the disanalogy does not survive more careful consideration. To explain why, we must first distinguish between two interpretations of loss chasing. The first refers to the explanations of their behavior that DGs often give post hoc to clinicians and researchers. This is the version that tends to be understood as manifestation of a cognitive fallacy. The second idea of loss chasing directs attention to the variety of accounting irrationality—treating gambling units as strings of losses terminating in wins, regardless of closing net balances—identified by Rachlin and described in section 3.4. As we discuss in section 8.5, there is neuroscientific evidence that the pattern Rachlin describes is based on the reward system's natural approach to accounting. In light of the general model of human behavior and its relationship to cognition that has emerged in contemporary psychology, it is very doubtful that people who describe their behavior as loss chasing are reporting an *introspective* discovery they have made about their own brains; there is no plausible access path of this sort. However, they may well be reporting observations they have made about their own *behavior*. Thus, loss chasing is a genuine and recurrent aspect of the way in which the reward system responds to gambling. Understood in this way, however, the intended disanalogy between gambling and drugs collapses. The reward systems of cocaine addicts also account units of consumption by reference to achievements of highs and without regard to costs. In the case of drugs, correlations between costs and frequency of highs will be closer in the short run than with gambling, because of the essential stochastic aspect of the latter. It is possible that DGs sometimes persuade themselves their behavior is rational by listening to their own loss-chasing narratives and then endorsing the gambler's fallacy. Here again, however, it is not obvious that we have a significant disanalogy with drug addiction. Rationalizing self-narratives of various kinds are ubiquitous in addicts.

Loss-chasing narratives, like rationalizations of other addicts, may encourage PGs to remain blind to their problem. This suggests some possible value in including education about the gambler's fallacy in treatment programs—something that is already largely in place wherever evidence-based treatment programs exist to begin with. As discussed in chapter 7, there are widespread doubts in the clinical community about the efficacy of CBT approaches centering on cognitive *content* (as opposed to metacognition). Let us set this aside for the moment, however. If teaching DGs about the independence of probabilities on individual gambles helps *any* DGs reduce the harm they do to themselves, then such teaching should surely be made available, since it is so relatively inexpensive. But this seems to be on all fours with teaching drinkers about the effects of alcohol on their livers and brains, and teaching smokers about the effects of cigarettes on their lungs and hearts.

Disanalogy (3) also seems relevant mainly to treatment strategies rather than to etiology or diagnosis. It may be that vivid physical damage caused by drugs is more salient to addicts than the consequences of PG, and that this makes it easier to convince drug addicts to seek treatment. Petry gives no evidence of this, however, and we are not aware of any. Large financial losses would seem to represent highly visible and salient harms to most people. What may well be true is that, because of the physical health problems associated with drugs, people addicted to them are more likely to be seen by health professionals at earlier stages of their condition than DGs. If this is a fact it is worth noting. However, it does not seem to be a disanalogy so deep as to constitute a serious objection to our proposal.

We find Petry's concern (4) entirely unpersuasive if "stigmatization" is interpreted narrowly and literally. To the extent that (4) is emphasized as a potential problem, it incorporates a distinctively liberal value set. As liberals ourselves, we have no quarrel with that. However, we would then point out that in contemporary liberal societies, unwise *choices* are generally regarded as reflecting badly on people's characters in a way that affliction by diseases is not. We grant that liberals often reason by rationally unratifiable association like all other people, so that even in modern cosmopolitan societies addictions conceived as diseases retain a strong residue of cultural moralization that is not applied to (e.g.) epilepsy. But it hardly seems to make PGs *more* likely to suffer unfair social punishment if their condition is understood to be *less* a function of their autonomous responsibility. Someone might object that if PG is identified with AG it is then more apt to be thought permanent and ineradicable, and thus to disqualify sufferers from some social aspirations. It is true that I-RISA/PV models predict that people who are or who become disposed to an addiction will seldom or never be able to completely reverse the learning undergone by their reward systems, and thus to *some* extent—left entirely quantitatively open—will retain enhanced vulnerability by comparison with randomly drawn comparison samples. However, we question the actual normative seriousness of this. The large modern society *furthest* from achievement of demoralization of behavioral patterns traditionally attributed to standing traits of character has twice elected a self-proclaimed recovered alcoholic president. In any case, since sound policy on all addictions surely counsels efforts at public destigmatization of them, reduction of PG to AG can be argued to have the effect of attaching PG to a trend that is more likely to attenuate than to amplify sufferers' social victimization. Note finally that since, according to our hybrid PE/NE account of DG as a whole (discussed at greater length below), treating a person's AG is only a necessary but not a sufficient condition for treating their DG, and since according to us non-AG DG is a response to cost-benefit incentives, reduction of PG to AG does not imply that any society should necessarily relax emphasis on regulation and normative control of commercial gambling, beyond what it is motivated to do by other policy considerations.

By contrast with concern (4), we view (5) as a potentially serious problem. In chapter 6 we drew attention to "popular polarization between behavioral concepts of addiction, which tend to be a priori liberal about what can and cannot be genuine objects of addiction, and reductionist concepts organized around physiological withdrawal symptoms as the addictive tethers" (p. 161). We pointed out that "[p]romoters and users of the latter concept are often skeptical concerning the appropriateness of regarding anything other than an exogenous chemical as a possible object of addiction. Arguing, as we do, that (1) PG/AG is the basic form of addiction and that (2) addiction should be conceptualized as a neurochemical phenomenon implies direct rejection of the popular disjunction of conceptual alternatives. It thus also invites a casual slide into supposing that anything bearing the behavioral and phenomenological properties that gambling shares with addictive drugs must turn out to be an addiction in the neuroscientific sense that we advocate" (p. 161). We noted that there is limited behavioral evidence, but almost no neuroscientific evidence, for addiction to shopping. The same can be said about addiction to fatty foods, Internet use, and some forms of sexual behavior. However, we then advocated a principle "according to which a variety of impulsivity should be treated as non-addictive until proven (by neuroscience) otherwise" (p. 161). We will now give the argument for this principle, which constitutes our proposal for minimizing the potential harm emphasized by Petry's concern (5). Some principle that limits our proposal's implications for possible inflation and trivialization of the concept of addiction is a necessary part of the case for local reduction of PG to AG, especially since, for reasons we will explain, we think the possible social consequences of this are even more serious than Petry suggests.

Petry's worry about potential stigmatization of addicts can most charitably be read as alluding to a more general concern with the fact that someone's being labeled an "addict" changes their social situation (including their own perception of their social situation). The philosopher Ian Hacking (1999) has investigated the construction of types of people as a basic source of social ontology, which then strongly influences behavior and policy. We suggest that in contemporary democratic societies the disease model of addiction is sufficiently well entrenched that a diagnosis of addiction for a person will typically imply two very general propositions with respect to her legitimate obligations and entitlements:

1. The person is obliged to tolerate a greater level of paternalism with respect to her own behavior from social institutions and authorities than is considered appropriate for fully autonomous adult citizens. In particular, she is expected to cooperate with efforts by others to help her reduce or terminate her addictive consumption.

2. The person is entitled to reduced attribution of personal moral and social responsibility for actions taken when she is in the grip of addiction (*not* understood as equivalent to episodic intoxication).

These two points are related to one another as an *exchange* of social privileges: the addict's entitlement under (2) will impose requirements on others to allow her to "start over"—ideally, to be free from various forms of institutional discrimination—*to the extent that* she fulfills her obligation under (1). An addict who successfully resists treatment may be regarded more appropriately as an object of sadness than of blame (though there is wide variation here), but often people will feel that neglect of such addicts is legitimate because they "can't be helped."

In light of these important social and ethical consequences of applications of the concept of addiction, it is portentous to propose, as we have done, that the basic form of addiction is to something other than a substance. Because the popular philosophy of the person draws a focal "bright line" between endogenous and exogenous causes of behavioral dispositions, it is much easier to contain the application of addiction to substance dependencies, allowing for no so-called "natural" addictions, than to justify extension of addiction to *some* nonsubstance dependencies—such as AG—but not others. Thus, our claim that this bright line will not hold in light of recent neuroscience raises the prospect of a slide into hyper-liberalism with respect to which sorts of molar-scale rewards can be and are addictive to some people. The main problem with such definitional hyper-liberalism is that it in turn threatens medicalization of nonliberal and arbitrary moral preferences. We do not endorse moralization of people's preferences that other people avoid dependence on alcohol, cocaine, heroin, or nicotine (let alone marijuana). We can at least agree, however, that these "bossy" preferences themselves have a strong basis in objective fact: the drugs in question almost always cause serious harm to those who become dependent on them, including by reference to the normative standards of the dependent themselves.[2] By contrast, there is no social consensus, and no prospect of a rationally *justifiable* social consensus, on how much shopping is too much, on how many hours a person ought to spend surfing the Internet or playing online games, or on how much effort, time, and emotional opportunity cost people should devote to various forms of sexual stimulation and gratification. If recognition of gambling addiction leads people to assume that there are also shopping, Internet, and sex addicts, *just because collapse of the bright line around substance addiction leaves no line to be held at all,* there is a real risk of encouraging broadly helpful if sometimes annoying paternalism to slide into moralistic enforcement of popular prejudices against people with minority tastes.

We suggest that sexual behavior (as opposed to, e.g., shopping) is the truly dangerous arena here. In the United States there is a thriving clinical industry built around diagnosing and intervening in so-called "sex addiction." Much of this stems from a series of publications by Patrick Carnes going back to his 1977 book entitled *Don't Call It Love.* Throughout the country there are numerous chapters of Sex Addicts Anonymous, Sexaholics Anonymous, and Sex and Love Addicts Anonymous. (The last name reminds us that Carnes's advertising strategy is not universally imitated by the industry.) For-profit clinics and courses are widespread. In general, sex addiction is constructed by direct analogy with alcoholism and drug addiction as these are represented in 12-step movements, with emphasis on introspectively "discovered" preoccupation, sense of loss of control, and feelings of guilt and shame. Carnes's own "diagnostic criteria" are secrecy of sexual behavior, perception of such behavior as "abusive" or "degrading," perceived use of sex to "avoid painful feelings," and indulgence in sex that is "empty of a caring, committed relationship." The last criterion draws especially clear attention to the fact that the popular sex addiction concept encodes conservative social norms around monogamy and the integration of sex into traditional family structures. According to Carnes, there are 15 million sex addicts in the United States.

There has been almost no systematic social science research on the sex addiction movement, so our outline of its character is based on observations of material found on the ten most frequently visited Web sites devoted to its advertisement. The site www.sexhelp.com provides a "Sexual Addiction Screening Test" for self-assessment. Any two responses of the indicated valence to a short series of yes/no questions "diagnoses" a subject as a sex addict. Possible diagnostic pairs include answering "no" to the question "Do you feel that your sexual behavior is normal?" and "yes" to the question "Do you hide some of your sexual behavior from others?" In light of this, Carnes's figure of 15 million is surprisingly small. According to http://bipolar.about.com/cs/hypersex/a/aa_hypersex.htm/,[3] symptoms of sex addiction include a bizarre mix of socially prohibited (including criminal) behaviors such as rape and pedophilia, non-operationalized quantitative "over-indulgence" in majority behaviors such as masturbation and nonpermanent sexual relationships, "fantasy sex" (with no qualifying restriction as to extent), and "cross-dressing." Inclusion of the final item makes it especially clear that what is being presented by this source as a clinical condition is in fact merely a departure from (vague) culturally inherited and far from universally endorsed normative attitudes. Unsurprisingly, random browsing of postings from self-identified "sex addicts" quickly reveals two recurrent narrative patterns: men whose extramarital affairs have been discovered attribute their behavior to disease, thus applying for entitlement to reduced responsibility, and unmarried women troubled by sexual interests, fantasies, and/or indulged inclinations of which their subcommunities disapprove report relief from guilt and shame following "diagnosis" and "treatment."

There is no neuroscientific evidence for addiction to any form of sexual behavior. Very limited behavioral evidence suggests the existence of nontrivial numbers of people who invest resources in seeking sexual gratification, especially through perusal of pornography and masturbation, and who also invest effort in unsuccessful attempts to reduce or eliminate such consumption and activity (Griffiths 2000). Thus there is *some*—largely anecdotal and impressionistic—reason to believe there are people who are "disordered sexual consumers" in the picoeconomic sense by which we define DG. This is not surprising. Since hyperbolic discounting and at least occasional failures to maintain personal rules are ubiquitous aspects of human life, there are almost certainly disordered consumers of everything anyone consumes, and nontrivial numbers of disordered consumers of everything that is a majority taste. As a near-universal taste, sex and fantasy sex should be anticipated to be prime arenas for intertemporal consumption inconsistencies. This phenomenon might well be economically and socially important, so good research on it should be encouraged.

The question of present concern, however, is whether there is prima facie reason to suspect that some people might be addicted to forms of sexual behavior according to the neuroeconomic model of reward system pathology we have defended in this book. The use of gambling as the template for addiction is particularly helpful for framing this question more precisely. To what extent do various forms of common sexual indulgence resemble gambling with respect to the contingencies that make gambling so readily addictive to many people?

Interpersonal sex has a number of crucial disanalogies with gambling. Typically, an individual does not autonomously control the microcontingencies of reward scheduling in interpersonal sex because they must continuously negotiate these with their partners. Predictor cues for interpersonal sex are often highly unreliable (e.g., flirtation in public), especially as indicators of intervals, or *too* reliable (e.g., commencement of nude foreplay) in relation to any unpredictable variables analogous to gambling payoffs. In general, gambling's pairing of utterly reliable and perfectly manipulable interval predictor cues with entirely unpredictable cash payoffs is reversed where interpersonal sex is concerned; in the case of the latter, hard-to-unilaterally-manage negotiation of strongly variable intervals is coupled with (at least for most males) low-variance hedonic reward. Obviously, this is very far from a knock-down disanalogy, and applies less clearly to most females. The dialectic of the current discussion, however, doesn't call for a knock-down argument if the burden of persuasion lies with the advocate of the *prima facie* plausibility of sex addiction. We will shortly argue that, on public health and ethical grounds, that is where the burden belongs.

First, however, we must concede that even if interpersonal sex does not relevantly resemble gambling in its addiction-inducing properties, there is a much stronger affinity between gambling and use of pornography to facilitate masturbation, especially among males and especially where Internet browsing is concerned. External sources not under the control of the pornography consumer generate images and associated fantasies the seeker cannot precisely predict, but at times and locations and via modes of access that are highly reliable. Consumers can vary sampling frames and so (probably) directly toggle their dopamine circuits, just like drug and gambling addicts and like rats pressing levers in labs. We suggest that males are likely to be more readily drawn into this form of sexual consumption than females simply because male sexual response is more strongly associated with visual cues than female sexual response, but this difference should not be exaggerated when, as here, we are purely speculating. One important *dis*anology between pornography consumption and gambling should be noted: the pornography consumer has almost perfect control over whether and when to masturbate. As noted in chapter 6, the neuroeconomic theory of AG predicts that constant winning would attenuate rather than promote or maintain AG. Thus, it may be important that the pornography consumer is analogous to the gambler who knows he can win any bet he chooses, when he chooses. We would expect such gamblers to be attracted to casinos for the money, but to treat gambling like work rather than as an addictive compulsion.

Let us nevertheless grant that, for all that anecdotal behavioral evidence can tell us, there might well be pornography addicts. We contend that in the absence of neuroscientific evidence for this we should regard all talk of sex addiction with skepticism. Our reasons are rooted in public health and ethical concerns. We argued in chapter 7 that neuropharmacological therapies for addiction will probably appear in the near future. This raises the worry that some people, especially minors—and most particularly female minors—whose sexual interest is found threatening by socially conservative subcommunities and parents, will be inappropriately prescribed anti-addictive drugs when they are not in fact addicted to anything. They might then be expected to show little behavioral modification at normal doses for addictive substance addiction and AG, and this might be expected to provoke resort to elevated dosages. If, as we predict, the new neuropharmacological weapons are dopaminergic agents, the result could be long-term damage to people's motivational systems. (It is important in this connection to point out that, as one of the many respects in which ontogeny does not recapitulate phylogeny, the reward circuit is among the last parts of the human brain to complete its development, usually in a person's early twenties.) We fear that young women would be particularly at risk here for two reasons: (1) traditionalists often believe adolescent male interest in sex to be normal and even healthy (so long as it is heterosexually focused), while adolescent female interest is considered deviant; and (2) some social conservatives might regard compromise of women's motivational systems as a favorable outcome. Young gay people might also be unusually vulnerable to inappropriate neuropharmacological intervention against "sex addiction."

Might this serious concern, then, indeed be a reason for resisting our suggestion to locally reduce PG to AG? Nathan (2005a and elsewhere) has argued that crossing the bright line and allowing application to nonsubstance dependencies, specifically including gambling as the most natural leading candidate, invites populist abuse of the concept. In response, we flag the following considerations. First, the idea of sex addiction is already entrenched and defended by well-funded groups who are strongly invested in maintaining it. Thus, the relevant concern here is with conferring scientific legitimacy on a populist construction, not with perpetuating or amplifying a dangerous idea of marginal currency. Second, pursuit of dopaminergic neuropharmacological thera-pies against addiction will be pursued regardless of definitional scruples among scientists or public health concerns about peripherally influ-enced groups such as hypothetical young people in conservative com-munities. Mounting the strongest possible argument against allowing young people who are receiving behavioral therapy for sexual issues to be prescribed dopaminergic agents requires the premise that there is no sound evidence that they are *in fact* addicted by neuroscientific criteria. This in turn requires the further premise that *true* addiction is a specific, scientifically ratified kind of brain pathology. In response to this point it might be wondered why people who are convinced, on the one hand, that many people are sex addicts, but who do not accept, on the other hand that addiction is a specific brain pathology, would be inclined to turn to neuropharmacology for sex addicts in the first place. However, many such people could and, we think, very likely would, maintain that drugs are often effective as indirect contributing allevia-tors of primarily behavioral conditions. (This general belief is, after all, true.) The best hope for minimizing the kind of harm we fear is, we think, clear maintenance of the view that *if* there turns out to be any genuine form of sex addiction, this is something we must learn from neuroscience; whereas the existence of an industry that presently con-vinces thousands of people each year that they are sex addicts consti-tutes evidence for nothing but the extent of human susceptibility to suggestion.

Let us be clear that we are not arguing that PG should be reduced to AG *because* this will help to protect an unrelated group of hypothetical people from harm. Rather, our contention is that fear of public health damage due to popular inflation of the concept of addiction rests on incomplete consideration of the probable unintended consequences. To pragmatists, gains in scientific prediction and generalization are neces-sary conditions for supporting a local reduction, but in the case of concepts that feature in clinical and public policy these may not be sufficient; welfare consequences should also be considered. We thus think Petry is right to raise concern (5) about the extension of "addic-tion" to cover PG. It is an important part of our answer that we do not *merely* propose that PG be *called* "AG." We propose that PG be reduced to AG *in the specific context of a neuroeconomic theory of addiction*. This limits the conditions for possible inflation of addiction by tethering the concept to specific objectively testable conditions.

We noted above that, despite the worries she rightly raises, Petry appears broadly sympathetic to the policy we suggest. She notes a public health consideration in its favor when she points out that

[i]f pathological gambling were classified along with substance use disorders, the number of criteria needed for a diagnosis might be reduced, thereby perhaps more accurately classifying individuals. Another potential advantage is that a subdiagnostic condition, e.g. gambling abuse [in our terminology, non-addictive DG or "problem gambling"], may be considered. Epidemiological studies indicate that a larger proportion of the population has a sub-threshold condition than those who meet full diagnostic criteria [Shaffer, Hall, and Vender Bilt 1999, Gerstein et al. 1999], and the disorder appears to exist along a continuum [Blanco et al. 2006]. Including less severe forms of disorders in the *DSM* may be appropriate clinically [Kessler et al. 2003]; it may also encourage more research and treatment efforts. Reclassification of the disorders may reduce balkanization of these disorders [i.e., substance addiction and PG] that appear, at least on some levels, to share similar features. (2006, p. 157)

8.2   Local Reduction of PG to AG without "Sundering" of DG

The minority of philosophers of science who promote general reductionism usually take the view that whenever a scientific kind is successfully reduced, this must have one of three implications for the original kind. If the whole of the kind is reduced, but it is regarded as having been crucially defined by reference to relations with similarly higher-level kinds now shown to be superficial, then the original kind should be *eliminated* from science. If the whole of the kind is reduced but its relations with higher-level kinds—presumably now fully explained by the reduction—are still considered essential to its identification, then the original kind should be *identified with* the new kind. Finally, if *part* of the original kind is reduced, then the original kind should be either *sundered* into two new kinds (Kim 1999) or, depending on the fate of attempted reductions of its remaining part(s), eliminated.

If we applied this a priori logic to DG in light of our arguments to this point, then we would be forced to argue that DG should be sundered into two merely superficially related kinds, AG and non-addictive DG or "problem gambling." In that case, if PE is used to model non-addictive DG and NE to model AG, as we have proposed, then it would follow that study of DG did not shed light on the relationship between PE and NE—unless perhaps to suggest, inductively, that phenomena modeled by PE would progressively be sundered through new extensions of NE until PE was entirely "hollowed out" and collapsed, its molar domain shown to be one of merely apparently separate integrity. All finally adequate accounts of individual economic behavior would be NE accounts. As we will see in more detail in the next section, this is the general program for microexplanation in economics currently promoted by a founder of NE, Paul Glimcher. We will complete our statement of why we instead forecast a continuing role for hybrid PE/NE models, such as those favored by Ross (2005), only in the next section, when we consider models of the reward system's role in behavior that differ from the collective construct of Herrnstein, Ainslie, and Rachlin. We will begin the explanation in this section by first sketching our overall high-level model of DG in general.

We begin by echoing the point of Blanco et al. (2006), cited by Petry in the quote on p. 218 above, that DG seems to lie along a continuum of severity moving from non-addictive DG to AG. Why should this be so? A similar fact is not true of all manifestations of consumption impulsivity: virtually all "disordered smokers" and cocaine and heroin abusers are addicts. (The small proportion of "weekend" smokers and less unusual occasional recreational cocaine users don't, in any clear sense, have a substance-related *consumption-impulsivity problem* at all unless their intake is progressively escalating in violation of personal rules.)[4] One of the respects in which AG is the basic or template addiction is that it can be used to exemplify the general, abstract relationship between impulsivity and addiction that is masked by the special properties of most addictive drugs—or so we will argue in this section.

Evenden (1999) documents a variety of specific pathways to and specific kinds of manifestation of impulsivity as identified in personality psychology, psychiatry, BE, and neuropharmacology. The varieties of impulsivity theorized across these disciplines incorporate elements of lack of attentional persistence, failure to reflect before acting, rapid onset of boredom, inability to cope with unforeseen obstacles, disinhibition, preference for SSRs over LLRs, and recurrent preference reversals. Considering only drugs that affect the serotonergic circuit, different drugs influence these distinct factors for impulsivity in various and often opposing ways. With respect to a narrower construct, impulsive substance abuse, Eveden points out a tension in two identified *DSM-IV* criteria: (3) "a great deal of time is spent in activities necessary to obtain the substance (e.g., visiting multiple doctors or driving long distances)" and (4) "the substance use is continued despite knowledge of having a persistent or recurring physical or psychological problem that is likely to have been caused or exacerbated by the substance" (pp. 352–353). He goes on to note:

The strategies which addicts use to cover up their continued abuse to hide it from employers, spouses and treating personnel can also be elaborate and well-planned. Impulsive behavior would be counter-productive. Thus to develop into a disorder which is serious, malignant and difficult to treat, substance abuse disorder must consist of two components—poor impulse control when it comes to assessing the dangers of the substance abuse, coupled to very good impulse control when it comes to feeding and hiding the abuse. (Ibid., p. 353)

In our view, what Evenden should best be understood as drawing attention to here is something to which we alluded in chapter 4, namely, the divergent ontologies of behavioristic and cognitivist mind/brain/ behavioral sciences. The forms of "impulsivity" he lists have, as a whole set, nothing in common aside from being or supporting behavior patterns not ratifiable by (related but distinct) folk standards of rationality and prudence. This is the sort of kind that sound science indeed ought to sunder. We do not favor Evenden's approach of saying that there is a multifactorial but general phenomenon of "impulsive behavior" that attempts to capture and refine all the folk ideas he canvasses. With respect to that target there are merely several phenomena huddling together under a common name, for which no general theory should be expected.

We said in chapter 4 that we would not choose sides in the behavioral versus cognitivist estrangement. Instead we aim to emphasize—and to a modest extent forge—complementarities. We do not attempt this across the whole of the behavioral and cognitive sciences, or with respect to a wide range of phenomena, but concentrate only on our exemplary case, linking PE and NE in a hybrid model of DG. PE of course comes squarely from the behavioral tradition; NE's roots are equally clearly in computational cognitivism. Thus, if we convince the reader that both are best used together to understand DG, a small blow for cosmopolitanism will be struck, which we hope will set a precedent.

We have proposed a PE-based operationalization of impulsivity in a narrower sense than the sprawling target treated by Evenden: as recurrent simultaneous investment in a given type of consumption basket, and in unsuccessful or only incompletely successful efforts to curtail or cease consumption of the basket in question. This pattern applies to a wide range of human and other animal consumption behavior, as lavishly empirically demonstrated over many years by Herrnstein, Ainslie, Rachlin, and others. It applies furthermore to all cases of addiction except the rare instances (at least, rare but in some subpopulations of cigarette smokers and some elderly and/or terminally ill people) of heavy drug users who make no attempts to control their consumption, and who we can accommodate in the model simply by stipulating that *if* they were motivated to reduce their consumption, we would observe at least a period of inconsistent investment. (Phenomenologically, they would experience "inner struggle.") Thus, according to our account, addiction as a neural pathology is one specific form of (severe) consumption impulsivity.

It is useful, indeed important, to apply the PE model of consumption impulsivity to addicts as well as some non-addicts for the following reason. Every person whose budget constraint does not put potential objects of impulsive consumption out of reach (which, if masturbation or fingernail biting can be targets of impulsive consumption, excludes almost no one) has incentive to learn to attach value to personal rules so as to implement bundling. This particularly includes addicts. In addicts, however, bundling will often be ineffective unless neuroadaptations that attenuate serotonergic inhibition are reversed, and/or dopamine concentrations in NAcc are blockaded or relieved. (The latter will be a standard path to the former if the main future pharmacotherapies against addiction are dopaminergic instead of serotonergic or GABAergic.) Addiction distinguishes severely recalcitrant cases of consumption impulsivity, but reversal of addiction cannot generally be expected to be sufficient for preventing consumption impulsivity. Indeed, because the addict's reward system has learned some contingencies that the non-addict's has not, and because this learning is not perfectly reversible, addicts are typically at greater risk of personal-rule collapse than non-addicts. When it is pointed out, as we have done several times in the book, that most DGs "recover" without intervention, the truth to which this refers is that most DGs, including most PGs, are at any given time upholding personal rules that limit indulgence. The key point is that personal-rule maintenance is valuable to people in both addicted and non-addicted situations, at least from the standpoint of utility maximization—the economist's standpoint. For reasons we will discuss shortly, many drugs conceal the continuity between addiction and non-addictive vulnerability to consumption impulsivity because borderline cases tend to collapse into either perfect personal-rule maintenance or addiction. DG, however, is the phenomenon that best exposes the underlying continuity of the mechanisms involved.

Before we address the peculiar properties of drugs by comparison with gambling, we will set our account in the context of an evolutionary hypothesis. This hypothesis is an instance of what people suspicious of adaptationism call a "just-so story." If true, it would explain a number of facts about addiction and consumption impulsivity in humans and other animals, but it is (as far as we know) the only evidence for such explanations. On the other hand, so-called "consilience" (Whewell 1858)—explaining multiple facts by means of single hypotheses—*is* evidence, though never decisive evidence. At the very least, an account of any mental/neural/behavioral disposition so common as consumption impulsivity and addiction must demonstrate its evolutionary plausibility. Thus, late in a book full of more direct forms of evidence, we will allow ourselves to speculate upon history and selection pressures.

Suppose we interpret Herrnstein's work and the tradition it spawned as showing that choice according to the matching law (see chapter 3), and melioration rather than global maximization, are the natural default modes of consumption for cephalic animals. Our phrase "natural default" is intended to allow for the fact that people, at least, can and sometimes do aim to globally maximize—when managing securities portfolios, for example. It seems, however, that this requires special, deliberately constructed and maintained social scaffolding: costly incentives, monitors, and sophisticated technologies for keeping books. Raw brains, stripped of such scaffolding, are hyperbolic discounters that reveal intertemporal preference inconsistency in their consumption. Because of this fact, we don't need to posit any specific reward system pathology to explain a person's mere problem gambling or periodic binges on drugs that impair utility maximization. All we need for that is the fact that the person is rewarded by the gambling experience or high (some people aren't), and that she receives the reward immediately. Then hyperbolic discounting alone will cause her to tend to regret the amounts she gambles except to the extent that she has learned to bundle her future choices with present ones as described in chapter 3. With respect to gambling, as with other legal and accepted addictors (in some societies) such as alcohol or qat, we know that most people successfully learn to bundle. We know this simply because we know that most people nearly always manage to gamble nonproblematically and drink or chew qat (in their respective cultures) moderately. Most of the minority who ingest illegal substances also control their consumption within nonproblem limits (except insofar as habitually breaking the law may constitute a problem in itself). From the policy perspective, societies address mere problem gambling and occasional binge drinking by deciding to what extent they should institute measures that prevent casinos and bars from making it more difficult for customers to bundle, or that force them to help customers bundle a bit better.

What is shown by widespread participation in controlled gambling and drinking is that, at least with respect to these activities and some others, people can marshal resources stronger in effectiveness than the brain processes that naturally dispose them toward myopic melioration. Knowing this opens new questions. Are there opponent brain processes that, in most people, are sufficient by themselves to counteract impulsive dispositions? Or is social and institutional reinforcement of moderation required? *Must* people make reference to socially constructed behavioral bookkeeping strategies, and probable social sanctions based on them, to maintain their personal rules? For example, if Robinson Crusoe had a distillery on his island, and a limitless supply of fermentable material, could he avoid alcoholism? We expect that he could *if* before becoming a castaway he had already been indoctrinated with a set of social norms. We are more doubtful, however, in the case of a feral Crusoe endowed with a cannabis garden.

Even if social scaffolding is necessary for the maintenance of personal rules and control of consumption impulsivity, there must be some brain processes that the scaffolding recruits and through which it operates; social scaffolding, no matter how powerful it might be, is not magical. Let us conjecture, then, that there are two jointly necessary and *usually* jointly sufficient mechanisms for limiting impulsivity in humans: networks of norms and institutions, and frontal circuits that inhibit midbrain mutiny. As we have seen, there is direct evidence for the importance of the latter. Next, note that although laboratory rats have been shown to be capable of bundling in the face of opportunities to impulsively consume food (Ainslie and Monterosso 2003), scientists can bring any rat to addiction to any substance that is a target for addiction in any human. Is this because institutional support is required for bundling choices over addictive substances, or because rat brains do not have adequate natural safeguards against reward system hysteresis?

At this point we do not know the answer to this question. We do know, however, that in general natural selection does not waste resources building organs to support pointless capacities. Until humans developed agriculture, no animals except some social insects could exercise enough control over their own supply schedules to need to control their impulsive dispositions themselves.[5] When a group of elephants comes across fermented marula fruit, each one eats as much of it as he or she can and, if there's enough to go around, all get intoxicated. But however much the elephants would enjoy repeating the experience the next day or the day after, they do not have this option because they cannot cause fermentation to happen or collect and maintain a reliable supply of their drug. Their ecological circumstances thus form a barrier against addiction, and there is no reason why natural selection would have wasted resources equipping them with an inboard one. It must be pointed out that elephants and other animals *do* need to control *some* impulses. A male elephant who attempted indiscriminately to mate with every female on hand would be a social disaster (and therefore of low fitness). If humans control consumption impulsivity by means of a *general* inhibitory mechanism we share with other mammals, then perhaps our special circumstances with respect to control of our supply schedules are of no evolutionary importance; perhaps elephants who could raise marula trees would learn to moderate consumption just in case they could cognitively recognize its potential dangers. However, if we take the point from Evenden that there is no such thing as impulsivity *in general*, then we should also be suspicious of the idea of a generic circuit that inhibits the dopamine reward system as just one aspect of overall prudence enforcement. The limited neuroscientific evidence to date suggests a more dedicated mechanism against reward system hysteresis, one that is thus more likely to have separately evolved and that therefore *might* be specifically adapted to reduce consumption impulsivity and resist addiction.

Since at least the dawn of agriculture, humans have been able to control their supply schedules so as to allow many or most of them to become addicted to consumption targets that (unlike masturbation or fingernail biting, on which they always had the chance to fixate) are dangerous to life and fitness. Archeological evidence indicates that substance abuse has been a problem for some people for at least most of civilized history (Rudgley 1999). Has natural selection responded by evolving a homeostatic neural mechanism that, in most people, blocks consumption of potentially addictive substances beyond a certain threshold? Has this mechanism been supported by social learning that has filled human cultural environments with normative reference points, customs and rituals that allow most people to avoid being enslaved by their own midbrain consumption engines? Were our early agricultural ancestors more threatened by addiction, before the relevant social scaffolding and/or homeostatic mechanisms evolved, than modern people? These are all questions for physical, social, and economic anthropology. At present, we know some things that are relevant to addressing them—for example, that the frontal and prefrontal cortex, the most recent human brain areas to evolve, are responsible for controlling impulsive urges. We don't know whether this is uniquely human equipment, however, or how dependent it is for its effectiveness on social reinforcement.

What about gambling? It might be objected that AG, unlike substance addiction, does not require control over a scarce resource. However, as outlined in chapter 6, the I-RISA/PV model implies that a highly ecologically peculiar degree of control over programming of surprises, at timescales that tap into and manipulate the reward system's expectation windows, is the basis of AG. Indeed, our evolutionary speculations here now suggest that this must also be part of the basis of DG more generally, since DG requires as a minimum condition that a person can deliberately program their environment to provide a dopaminergic cue for risky surprise. It is not impossible that a nonhuman animal could learn to do this; imagine an antelope who discovers that it's fun to hover just on the edge of a lion's capture distance and periodically step over the boundary. Such behavior could even be selected for if it signaled fitness to lions, though there is a fixed lower bound to the level of risk that selection would tolerate as a trade-off.[6]

In any event, our speculations support the following general ideas about the basis of DG and AG. First, the reward system of the cephalic animal is so constructed that a creature with sufficient control of causal contingencies on suitable timescales can discover how to set it into self-amplification. Humans, at least, can achieve such control. Hyperbolic discounting may then lead them to stimulate themselves with gambles to the point where personal rules are required if threats to medium-term utility maximization are to be avoided. Normal brains of (at least) humans are equipped with frontal inhibitory circuits, possibly specifically purpose-adapted, which prevent the reward system from consistently recruiting cortical and mesolimbic control resources so as to crowd out behavior that conflicts with midbrain self-stimulation. These frontal circuits may or may not require support from social reinforcement to function effectively; for what it is worth, we guess that they do, based only on the general induction that socially isolated human brains seem to be about as well adapted for anything as the proverbial fish out of water (Wexler 2006). In any case, the recruitment of these management circuits may be buttressed by conscious processes, and in certain circumstances may require such buttressing. No one knows what, in general, characterizes such circumstances. That is, we do not know which combinations of genetic factors, contingent neural learning, and social-environmental pressures or absences make some people sufficiently vulnerable to DG that they must resort to *conscious* articulation of personal rules to control it. (Note that we do *not*, as behaviorists, assume that personal rules must be consciously rehearsed. They can be implicit in patterns of choice and visible to observation in the breach—e.g., if a person feels uncomfortable and embarrassed when thinking about drinking before lunch.)

We thus predict that DG is an essential part of the causal etiology of AG. In particular, DG is necessary for the neural learning of addiction implemented in early stages by cue sensitization and in later stages by atrophying of serotonergic inhibitory circuits. Furthermore, we predict that AG patients whose neuroadaptations to gambling are reversed will still require behavioral or cognitive behavioral therapy to control DG, which is more dangerous to them than to non-addicts. It is for these reasons that, according to us, AG should be conceptualized as a (particularly problematic) form of DG rather than as an entirely separate phenomenon.

Drug abuse obscures this relationship of continuity between mere impulsivity and addiction to varying degrees in the case of different drugs. Among major drugs of dependence, alcohol obscures it least: many people get into trouble, including serious trouble, on the basis of very occasional and isolated binges. But steady drinking, past a point where it must become problematic, is a necessary part of the etiology of neural alcohol addiction. Nicotine is the drug for which the DG/AG relationship seems least suited as a template. As we have noted, there is no such thing as "problem smoking" short of addiction, and relatively few people who smoke at all are not addicts. However, the peculiarity of smoking here does not seem mysterious to us. Rather, it seems to be mainly explicable by reference to properties of its delivery vehicles. A window is opened here by the recent popularity of social

cigar smoking in communities where cigarette smoking has been stigmatized thanks to public health campaigns and laws. Many occasional
(less than daily) cigar smokers inhale, but such smokers appear to be
at far lower risk of developing nicotine addiction than occasional
cigarette smokers (Gerlach et al. 1998; Rigotti, Lee, and Wheeler 2000).
This is notwithstanding the fact that large cigars are powerful nicotine-
delivery vehicles. Their low level of effectiveness as addiction-
promoters by comparison to cigarettes draws attention to some
unusually insidious properties of cigarettes. Until the widespread
passage in many jurisdictions (at least in wealthy countries) of laws
restricting indoor smoking in public places, inconvenience due to
smoking any given cigarette was minimal, imposing no need to inter-
rupt socializing or other activities. The financial cost of any given
cigarette is trivial to most people's budgets. Furthermore, even for
people for whom the habit of smoking is a significant cost, the decision
to smoke each cigarette draws from an already sunk investment; the
fact that it implies future expenditure will be hyperbolically discounted
by a nonbundling meliorator. Now, cigars are not very costly by comparison with other leading objects of potential addiction. In particular,
cigars, like cigarettes and gambling but unlike alcohol, impose no fear
of loss of social status or productivity due to intoxication. Nevertheless,
the mere switch from the (typically) tiny increment in total nicotine
consumption delivered by a cigarette to the somewhat larger increment
delivered by a cigar makes a dramatic difference to addiction-inducing
power. This leads us to suggest that the tendency of cigarette smoking
behavior to bifurcate into a separating equilibrium of abstinence and
addiction, with near-zero prevalence of non-addicted problem smoking,
results from the fact that the marginal damage each individual cigarette
inflicts on a personal rule in the case of anyone who attempts controlled
smoking is very low. In consequence, people must develop uncharac-
teristically *sophisticated* personal-rule management strategies before
they can learn to control smoking. People who set out to be occasional
cigarette smokers don't generally appreciate this. Thus, there are relatively few such smokers.

In general, PE directs our attention to differences in price variables
when comparing the idiosyncratic properties of different objects of
consumption impulsivity and addiction. If very low marginal cost to
personal-rule assets per unit makes cigarettes unusually addictive,
very *high* marginal unit costs can, perversely, have the same effect. A
person who runs the risk of severe social stigma by buying and using

heroin obtained from a street seller may also be lured by a sunk-cost rationalization pattern, according to which this large *fixed* cost can be justified only by a very high value on the variable benefit—the high— for which the drug is acquired. (We alluded to this earlier in the present chapter when considering analogies in drug addicts to the gambler's fallacy in AGs.)

Gambling, as a model for consumption impulsivity, addiction, and their relationship to one another, is almost ideally free from distorting price discontinuities. Unlike cigarette smokers, gamblers can raise the marginal cost of each gamble without having to manufacture elaborate personal rules: they can simply place larger bets. At the same time, except in class-restricted venues or at exclusive tables in casinos, the gambler does not face the high minimal fixed cost of the heroin user. She can, indeed, control her personal cost scales—total, average, and marginal—as finely as she likes. Again, because of its widespread social acceptance and multimodal availability, alcohol is the major impulsivity target most closely resembling gambling in this respect (though even alcohol, to deliver any observable level of its desired benefits, typically imposes a minimum fixed cost in lost expected productivity). Thus, it is not surprising that problem drinking best resembles DG in its prevalence structure: in any given population, we will find substantially more problem drinkers/gamblers than addicted ones; problem drinking/gambling will be a necessary but usually not sufficient pathway to addictive drinking/gambling; and thus problem and addicted drinking/gambling will demonstrate a wide range of continuum effects despite the fact that addiction is a specific neurochemical pathology while non-addicted recurrent consumption impulsivity is a multifactorial, mainly social syndrome.

Blaszczynski and Nower (2002) argue that there are three distinctive sets of PGs (grouped by clusters of etiologies, typical comorbidities, and typical responsiveness to treatment approaches). The symptoms of the first group are held to be "the consequence, not the cause, of repeated excessive gambling behavior" (p. 492). As far as we can determine, however, repeated gambling is *a* causal factor in *all* DG, including PG/AG. (This applies even to the Parkinson's patients discussed in chapter 7. The fact that dopamine agonists cause them to gamble does not mean that gambling activity is not then part of the cause of the reward system hysteresis which, in them, is particularly quick to be triggered due to the presence of the drug.) We are told that this "behaviorally conditioned" group "reports the least severe gambling and gambling-induced difficulties of any pathological gamblers, and they do not manifest gross signs of major premorbid psychopathology, substance abuse, impulsivity, erratic or disorganized behaviors. . . . Placed at the low end of the pathological dimension, they fluctuate between heavy and problem gambling, demonstrate motivation to enter treatment, comply with instructions and may successfully re-establish controlled levels of gambling post-treatment. It is proposed that counseling and minimal intervention programmes benefit this subgroup" (ibid.). According to our schematic, the group of gamblers thus described are best classified not as PGs, but as non-addicted DGs. To the extent that the *DSM-IV* operationalization classifies them as PGs, it should be changed so that treatment-relevant distinctions are captured. Blaszczynski and Nower's proposed second group are "emotionally vulnerable as a result of psychosocial and biological factors, utilizing gambling primarily to relieve affective states by providing escape or arousal. Once initiated, a habitual pattern of gambling fosters behavioral conditioning in both pathways. However, psychological dysfunction in Pathway 2 gamblers makes this group more resistant to change and necessitates treatment that addresses the underlying vulnerabilities as well as the gambling behavior" (p. 494). On our account, what Blaszczynski and Nower identify here is not a distinct group of gamblers. Rather, in attending to typical specific vulnerabilities in life histories ("history of depression, suicidal attempts and family psychiatric history," p. 493) *in addition to* "biological factors," they provide a partial enumeration of some of the factors that may contribute to DG in general, and sometimes additionally to AG. Finally, their third group consists simply of our AGs, people who have developed neuroadaptation for fixation on gambling. The authors recognize that many of this group probably have native neural dispositions to PG, as a result of which they say that gambling behavior is *not* a cause of this manifestation of PG. But this is a non sequitur. A person with genetic vulnerability to AG who never happens to be exposed to gambling is not a PG; gambling is always *a* causal factor for DG of any form. Blaszczynski and Nower's three-pathways classification, while superficially a challenge to our account, thus represents no challenge that it doesn't readily accommodate. It is of course highly useful to identify, as these authors do, different factors for DG that may be relevant to treatment plans for specific subsets of patients.

This completes our defense of treating AG as a species of DG against those who would urge that, if PG reduces to AG but non-AG DG doesn't reduce, then PG and mere problem gambling should be sundered. This therefore completes *part of* our case for combining PE and NE in the overall account of DG as a general phenomenon. In section 8.4, we turn to a different challenge: the claim that PE accounts are, at best, placeholder models while we wait for NE alone to explain all aspects of impulsivity and addiction, and, at worst, false accounts of the part of DG for which we have not advocated attempted reduction. This challenge can only be clearly formulated, however, following statement of our own unified account. We therefore turn to that first.

8.3 A PE/NE Hybrid Microexplanation of DG

Our conception of DG begins from the PE account of intertemporal preference in general and impulsivity in particular that is due to Herrnstein, Ainslie, and Rachlin. Drawing specifically on Ainslie's account, we understand preference reversal, which is characteristically chronic in DGs, as a consequence of a typical Nash equilibrium in bargaining among subpersonal interests. Myopic behavior at the molar scale, which includes DG in the case of gambling behavior, is the generally expected equilibrium outcome of this bargaining unless short-term interests can be led to attach value to personal rules on consumption scheduling. These rules constitute assets with present value because they license current predictions of improved personal welfare. Thus, if they are broken, their loss is felt in the relatively undiscounted present, and this prospective immediate loss enhances the bargaining power of longer-range interests. This influences distributions of equilibria in subpersonal bargaining games, such that at the molar scale SSRs are more likely to be passed over in preference for LLRs. Thus DG and other impulsive behavioral patterns can be avoided.

We suggest that this account be supplemented by a neuroeconomic model of addiction as follows. To the extent that the dopaminergic reward system controls signals to motor systems without effective prefrontal inhibition, the bargaining power of short-term interests is enhanced. Like all brain regions, the dopamine circuit is evolved to "try to" maximize blood flow to itself. This is in turn correlated with influence over motor output. The reward system bids for control of motor output by firing dopamine forward from VTA. This is an *aspect of*—but not to be identified with—bids by more abstract, molar-scale interests to grab SSRs. A supporting condition for bargaining effectiveness of longer-term interests is inhibition of reward system control by frontal serotonergic circuits. This inhibition is not identical with—is not the reduction of—efforts to change bargaining equilibria so as to maintain personal rules and wait for LLRs. The reason the activity of the inhibitory neural circuit should not be identified with the bargaining activity of a pro-LLR interest is that doing so confuses two different economic agents and two different scales of analysis, the molecular and the molar. The serotonergic circuit is a molecular-scale agent that, like the dopamine system, maximizes its utility function when it maximizes blood flow to itself. As a subpersonal system, it has no access to the molar-scale goals of the whole system (see Ross 2007), even if, at least when the system aims to abstain from SSRs and succeeds in abstaining, it serves these goals. By contrast, the molar-scale interests that bargain for control of the person's consumption schedule in Ainslie's picoeconomic model are time-slices of the whole person, or at least much of the person, not parts of her brain:

[I]nterests are limited in their duration of dominance, but not necessarily in their access to any of the functions that compose the "self" in any of its definit ions. . . . [L]ike parties trying to rule a country, internal interests gain access to most of a person's resources when they prevail. The person who wants to stay up later at night and the person who wants to rest in the morning are indeed entire personalities, in the sense that they have the whole person's psychic apparatus at their disposal; and yet they are clearly in conflict with one another. When an intelligent person is acting in his long-range interest not to smoke, he may use that intelligence to devise better stratagems to precommit his future behavior; but when he acts in his short-range interest to have a cigarette, he can marshall that same intelligence to evade these devices. (Ainslie 1992, p. 94)

The molar-scale interest, which may not but often does consciously entertain personal rules by encoding them in public-language sentences fed by speech-production systems into auditory circuits, mainly represents social pressures conveyed and reinforced by other people and by institutionalized cues for social reward and sanction (Ross 2005).

In our experience, in the face of this sort of picture many people struggle to understand how the molar and the molecular can be distinct without this suggesting some sort of mysterious and anti-scientific dualism. Reductionism is so much easier to grasp that we would welcome it with open arms if only we could believe it were true. But conceptual separation of the molecular and the molar has always been—logically, *must* be—the fundamental idea of behaviorism. Molar interests are not ghosts in the machine. They are not related to molecular processes as either "downstream" or "upstream" elements in causal chains. Rather, molar and molecular processes are simultaneously occurrent, distinct scales of resolution on physical processes in shared substrata, related by mutual feedback. Analogies may be helpful here. A rate of inflation in a macroeconomy is not identical to an aggregation of pricing decisions by all the agents in the economy. If agents did not make pricing decisions there could of course be no inflation rate. But the fact that the inflation rate is x at a given time, and is known to be x, itself influences the pricing decisions that in turn affect the rate. The rate is also driven by causal factors on its own scale, such as changes in interest and exchange rates. To take another example, evolution is not identical to sequences of conceptions of organisms, since evolutionary processes can have properties—e.g., promotion of more or less morphological and ecological complexity—that do not apply to sequences of conceptions. If organisms were not conceived there would be no evolution. But the fact that evolutionary processes of certain sorts are in play is part of the framework for explaining why certain sorts of conceptions happen rather than others. Relationships of this kind are modeled by dynamic systems theory, the general account of how patterns at distinct scales in common physical substrates influence one another by phase shifts that are separately identifiable at each respective scale. In general, macro-scale processes influence micro-scale processes by evolving basins of attraction that constrain degrees of freedom in fluctuations of frequencies in micro-scale parameters, and micro-scale processes in turn influence macro-scale processes by periodically reaching critical masses that break open the boundaries of such basins and thus escape from them. Brin and Stuck (2002) provide an introduction to the relevant mathematics, which are increasingly familiar tools in many fields in the physical, biological, social, and behavioral sciences. Applications to relationships among brains, cognitive dispositions, actions, and environments can be found in work by Kelso (1995), Thelen and Smith (1996), and Port and van Gelder (1998).

The extent to which a dynamic system is controlled by processes on particular scales itself varies. In most complex systems, macro-scale dynamics can collapse under certain conditions, increasing the extent to which the system is controlled by molecular-scale processes. Consider, for example, the probable course of evolution in a lineage if it is shielded from all selection pressure: evolution continues, but is driven mainly by molecular-scale genetic drift. This point is of direct relevance to manifestations of addiction. In general, we suggest, short-term bargaining interests at molar scales will prevail more frequently, all else being equal, the greater the degree of dopaminergic control over motor systems.[7] Long-term interests will prevail more frequently, all else being equal, the greater the degree of frontal and prefrontal control over motor systems. Therefore, a person whose dopamine system has hijacked her brain will tend to act as if she is governed by a dictatorship or by an oligarchy (in the case of a multiply addicted person) of short-range interests. On such occasions, the best hope for the person often lies in recourse to systems that participate in the relevant molar processes but are outside the molecular control circuit—namely, sympathetic friends with the wherewithal to instigate effective treatment intervention.

For addicts, social pressures against impulsive consumption of SSRs may remain as strongly present as before addiction, and if the addict is not neglected by friends, family, and colleagues, may indeed be amplified. This is important to our hopeful remarks in chapter 7 about the potential of metacognitive therapies as complements to drugs in the case of AG, or as therapeutic courses unto themselves for less severe DG. Metacognitive therapy aims to modify cognitive processing, with the aim of thereby causing neuroadaptations, but its levers of control are social-environmental levers. We can also consider the possible value of more conventional cognitive behavioral therapies in this context. Since folk psychology—our everyday theory of our own thought—is a social and normative construction,[8] appeal to an addict's model of their own cognition is in effect appeal to a person's internalization of the normative advice she has picked up from her culture, friends, parents, teachers, counselors and so on over the course of her life. (A danger is that the norms of pushers and bookies may be represented too.) Counselors can then reinforce these influences. However, the addict's normal circuit for inhibiting impulsivity is enfeebled by neuroadaptation caused by persistent dopamine overload in NAcc. Pro-LLR molar interests cannot effectively influence the crucial molecular levers they need to hold the dopamine system—acting, typically, as an agent of the molar interest in SSR consumption—in check. In the limiting case, the dopamine system governs molecular behavior without effective opposition, and in this environment of overwhelming resource strength molar impulsive interests thus have no need to bargain with others. Those rewards the dopamine system has learned to seek and consume most effectively—whiskey in the case of an alcoholic or slot-machine play in the case of an AG—are then consumed uncontrollably. Before (typically imperfect) molar-scale governance by personal rules can again be established, the reward system may need to be fought directly, at the molecular scale, by the agency of other people—hopefully, in the near future, using new drug therapies anticipated by the research we reviewed in chapter 7. If exogenous intervention is effective, this does not imply that the royal road to prudence is then necessarily at hand; it implies, rather, that bargaining between long-range and short-range interests can resume. This is why we do not anticipate relying on neuroscience alone for understanding or treating AG. Addiction, we claim, *has* turned out to be a molecular-scale pathology, to be understood and treated at that scale. But molar DG can persist in the absence of AG, and successful resistance to it in individual cases will generally require measures to be effected at both the molecular and molar scales.

Behaviorism sometimes turns lazy when it is applied as though the molecular scale were relatively unimportant. (In its rhetoric, behaviorism has occasionally turned *insane* by suggesting that the molecular scale is entirely irrelevant.) Though virtual interests, as explained above, are intimately influenced by neural agents, if these interests lose *all* reciprocal influence on *all* neural agents at a given time, they are, at least at that time, *dead*. (Thanks to exogenous influences, especially other people, dead virtual interests *can* in principle be brought back to life, just as software erased from a computer can be reinstalled. This may be true *only* in principle, however.) The cognitivist check on lazy behaviorism insists that molar accounts be grounded in neurocomputational and underlying neurochemical/neurodynamic models of information flow. Attending to the molecular with no regard for the molar leads to behavioral accounts that are at best incomplete; attending to the molar without regard for the molecular leads to pseudo-science that has drifted away from the discipline of measurement. Furthermore, molar-scale accounts are not logically dominant over molecular-scale ones, as behaviorists very often tend to assume. It is not the job of theorists of either scale to sing tunes commissioned by researchers from the other camp. Thus, discoveries in the brain can lead us to revise our views about which molar-scale interests in fact operate to guide behavior. In the study of impulsivity, neuroeconomists have not been shy about promoting such revisions. As we saw in the concluding section of chapter 3, some of these authors challenge the core picoeconomic idea that is also the centerpiece of our hybrid PE/NE model of DG, according to which impulsivity is a discounting phenomenon. We turn to these challenges in the next section.

8.4 Alternative Accounts of Consumption Impulsivity and Confounding of Molar and Molecular Scales

In a 2004 paper, McClure et al. report on an fMRI experiment in which subjects were given choices between SSRs and LLRs. On some choice trials the SSR was available immediately (at the end of the session), while on other trials both rewards were available only after delays. The researchers observed (1) increased activity in "limbic system" (VS and medial OFC) neurons on choices that included an immediate option, relative to choices involving two delayed rewards, (2) increased PFC and lateral OFC activity, relative to rest, on all choices regardless of delay, and (3) increased PFC and lateral OFC activity on choices that included an immediate option when subjects chose the delayed option, relative to when subjects chose the immediate option. Assuming (tendentiously) that longer delays to choice should be indicative of a system controlling less impulsive choice, McClure et al. hypothesize that molar hyperbolic discounting is an abstract description of the aggregated composition of two separate discounting mechanisms lodged in different brain systems. Specifically, they suggest that "short-run impatience is driven by the limbic system, which responds preferentially to immediate rewards and is less sensitive to the value of future rewards, whereas long-run patience is mediated by the lateral prefrontal cortex and associated structures, which are able to evaluate trade-offs between abstract rewards, including rewards in the more distant future" (p. 504). This interpretation exploits earlier modeling work by Laibson (1997), which we introduced in section 3.5, showing how to technically recover *some* of the behavioral data captured in hyperbolic discounting curves by the device of combining two exponential curves of different slopes. As we saw in chapter 3, Laibson calls this "δ-β discounting," where β denotes a steeply sloped family of functions corresponding to one-shot discounting of all delayed prospects, regardless of their delay, and δ denotes a less steeply sloped family corresponding to discounting of delayed prospects proportional to their delay. The hypothesis proposed by McClure et al. to explain their neuroimaging data is that lateral prefrontal areas, which they call the "δ system" after Laibson's model, are active whenever subjects make any decisions. The "β system" (which they equate with the "limbic" system) is active at a level comparable to that of the δ system ("and with a trend toward greater β-system activity" [McClure et al. 2004, p. 505]) when subjects choose earlier options over later ones.

Laibson's original model purporting to explain the "qualitative properties" (i.e., preference reversals) of the hyperbolic curve as a geometric simplification of two exponential curves of different slopes was not empirically motivated to begin with. Rather, its original selling point was that unlike the Herrnstein-Ainslie model, it admits of standard linear programming analysis of demand data as generally used in economics. As such it is, in the first place, a molar rather than a molecular model of behavior. For some modeling contexts, in particular those involving comparative aggregate demand data over periods across which institutional pressures don't bend people to long-run intertemporal consistency, Laibson's model is superior to alternatives and so is just what should be used; questions about its decomposability into individual demand curves, let alone directly neurally instantiated ones, are altogether irrelevant here (as economists Gul and Pesendorfer [forthcoming], despite advocating an alternative molar model of their own, emphasize). However, in proposing to push the Laibson model all the way into the brain, McClure et al. implicitly bid for a radical reduction of the molar to the molecular. The implication is that molar-scale hyperbolic discounting is merely apparent, and should be eliminated as a construct because it is explained away as an artifact of the interactions of the two opponent exponential discounting processes in groups of neurons. Note that the McClure et al. thesis still predicts, but offers an alternative explanation for, consumption impulsivity, preference reversal and the efficacy of reward bundling.

Ainslie and Monterosso (2004) point out that this hypothesis outruns the data obtained by McClure et al. The evidence from an increasing number of studies, some of which we reviewed in chapter 5, indeed suggests that elevated midbrain activity and decreased or impaired prefrontal activity are independently correlated with behavioral impulsivity. As we have seen, this is a crucial aspect of the I-RISA model of addiction, with its emphasis on the limitation of dopamine-circuit control of behavior by serotonin. However, the interpretation of this as indicating two distinct discount rates associated with these opponent processes is a substantial inferential leap. First, it would indeed be open to someone to question—though, for reasons indicated below, we do not—whether the idea of "discounting" should be applied at the molecular scale at all; an across-the-board anti-reductionist might argue that discounting is a fundamentally molar construct. Second, as Glimcher (private correspondence) points out, the assumption that longer delays to choice are diagnostic of a more patient system builds an important aspect of the conclusion into the background assumptions used as premises for it. Third, the apparent simplicity of the model that McClure et al.'s hypothesis would support—which is simply the standard charm of reductionism—trades off against the introduction of new complications in our understanding of the dopamine circuit itself. As Ainslie and Monterosso (2004) object, "[a]lthough the increased activity of . . . lateral prefrontal cortex . . . in response to larger/later selections is an important finding, to accord these areas status as a separate decision-making mechanism would add a complicating factor that would have to be reintegrated with motivation" (p. 423).

McClure et al.'s experimental procedure did not involve comparing the present values of delayed rewards in the *same* brain areas for different delays, nor did they attempt to relate the neural data regarding discounting with behavioral indifference curves; this is what is required to explicitly test their interpretation of their results. Glimcher, Kable, and Louie (2007) have recently reported fMRI data that they interpret as indicating that neurons in midbrain and prefrontal areas in fact implement similar discount functions as one another, irrespective of delay differences. They find, as have others (Hariri et al. 2006), high variability in activation levels in striatum between subjects, which correlate powerfully with variability in molar steepness of discounting. (This degree of behavioral variability had earlier been demonstrated by Simpson and Vuchinich [2000].) However, they find no areas in which activation levels are correlated with steeper or shallower discount functions than those inferred from molar behavior. Glimcher, Kable, and Louie interpret these findings as fatally undermining the McClure et al. hypothesis. We agree. Note that one possible critic of McClure et al. that we considered above, the "across-the-board anti-reductionist" who reserves discounting as a property of molar processes, might add that Glimcher, Kable, and Louie fail to find opponent neural discounting processes because "neural discounting" is a conceptual gaffe to begin with. We would reject this basis for skepticism. Following arguments due to Glimcher (2003) and Ross (2005, forthcoming), there are no persuasive theoretical grounds for denying economic agency to neurons and groups of neurons, and impressive empirical grounds for regarding them as exemplary estimators of utility function maxima (Caplin and Dean 2007). If neurons and groups of neurons are economic agents, and if there is robust correlation between choice-consumption intervals and firing rates in relevant neurons, as Glimcher's team and other researchers (Hariri et al. 2006) find, then discounting should be regarded as a modeling device and an explanatory construct for application at both the molar and molecular scales. Again, we stress: the extent to which reductionism is motivated is an empirical question, not a philosophical one.

Instead of merely casting doubt on the hypothesis that there are distinct δ and β discounting areas in the brain, Glimcher, Kable, and Louie express skepticism about the existence of "separable neural agents that could account for multiple selves that are used to explain hyperbolic-like discounting behavior" (2007, p. 4). In light of the specific phrasing here, an unguarded reader might naturally read this as implied criticism of PE. We therefore reiterate that the multiple selves of the PE model of consumption impulsivity are molar-scale objects, as discussed in the previous section. Evidence that they do not have direct molecular counterparts as McClure et al. suggest is *not* evidence that they don't exist. Note that Glimcher, Kable, and Louie in fact put their negative suggestion more carefully just a few lines later, as follows: "This finding argues strongly against the hypothesis that the sub-personal interests, with different discount functions, are instantiated as discrete neural systems *at the proximal algorithmic level*" (ibid.; emphasis in original). We precisely concur.

Glimcher, Kable, and Louie cautiously suggest that their data might support a molecular-scale account resembling the so-called "temptation" model developed by Gul and Pesendorfer (2001, 2005). This model defines a temptation as a choice option with the property that its presence in the choice set makes an agent worse off, either because this results in her making a worse choice than she would have made in the option's absence, or because to cope with the option the agent must incur a cost of "self-control." Whether or not the hypothesized "force" of self-control is or is not effective in a given instance is exogenous from the point of view of the Gul and Pesendorfer model. Again, this could readily be interpreted as implying controversy with the PE model of consumption impulsivity, due to ambiguity between exogeneity *to the (molar-scale) person* and exogeneity *to a (molecular-level) brain system that the model is taken to represent.* If Gul and Pesendorfer are read as modeling the person, then they will make contrary predictions to Ainslie about slopes of discount curves over bundles that do not include temptations. More subtly, on a reductionist reading of the temptation model, what philosophers call "weakness of will" becomes the function of a hypothetical mechanism within the brain that exerts exogenous influence on choice behavior; failure to bundle would be identified in this context with activity of a mechanism for visceral impulsivity. This leaves no place for a counterpart to the aspect of Ainslie's account that has future-indexed expected utility incorporated into immediately indexed utility as the present value of a personal rule. Thus, as Gul and Pesendorfer (2001) point out, the picoeconomic model admits no role for self-control *in their sense*, that is, as resistance "at the point of choice" (so to speak) to a storm of visceral temptation. In the picoeconomic model, overcoming "weakness of will" is identified with reconfiguration of commodity spaces, with personal rules being added to consumption bundles; in Gul and Pesendorfer's model choice is distinct from the action or failure of willpower, which thus has nothing directly to do with discounting.

This difference is consistent with Gul and Pesendorfer's (forthcoming) general preference for keeping economics and neuroscience cleanly apart at the modeling level. In one sense we share their perspective: according to us, economic models of people (let alone models of aggregates of agents, the objects with which economists do most actual empirical work) are not appropriately interpreted as attempted models of brains. But in another sense we think Gul and Pesendorfer are exactly wrong, since we share the ambition of Glimcher (2003) to model neurons and groups of neurons directly as economic agents, and, in more specific connection with the topic of this book, the ambition of Caplin and Dean (2007) to model the dopamine system as an economic agent.

We thus find *three* general positions in contention here, all quite specific to NE, rather than a simple philosophical tussle along a linear axis over degrees of general reductionism. First, Gul and Pesendorfer resist ascribing utility functions to any subpersonal agents, molar *or* molecular. Next, McClure and co-authors adopt a modeling strategy consistent with composing molar behavior out of choices by neurally distinguishable subpersonal agents, thereby collapsing the molar into the molecular. Finally, Ross's approach agrees that molar differences entail differences in interactive outcomes among neural agents. However, it emphasizes the idea that molar-level objects of choice are individuated on the basis of an agent's ecological—especially its social—context. This leads Ross to doubt that molar-scale economic problems will *generally* strictly decompose into molecular-scale economic problems—for exactly Gul and Pesendorfer's reasons—but, in the absence of a reason for restricting economic agency to people, to allow for, indeed to encourage, such locally reductionist agendas as are empirically motivated. In this framework Glimcher's perspective emerges as a *research program* rather than a philosophical commitment: push as many molar phenomena down into the brain as will fit, that is, push NE as far as it will go.[9] This seems to us to be exactly how a scientist ought to position himself or herself in relation to a conceptual controversy. Scientists should avoid philosophy as much as possible, and wherever in the pursuit of knowledge anyone can do science *instead of* philosophy, they should.

Our claim that DG is a molar-scale phenomenon best modeled by PE, with AG as a severe subvariety that has a molecular-scale neuroeconomic explanation, is thus intended as a strictly empirical hypothesis. We cannot try to furnish positive evidence for the essentially negative claim that non-addictive forms of DG will not each be given neuroeconomic explanations that ultimately render the picoeconomic model redundant, but we have indicated our empirical reasons for betting against such an eventuality. These can be supplemented by induction on the history of science, which is full of successful local reductions but has a poor track record of reducing phenomena that are individuated, as DG is, primarily by reference to environmental variables and social consequences. Because our hypothesis is in this respect negative, it can be verified only by the dedicated pursuit and less-than-complete success of Glimcher's program.

We have now established a general context in which to set comments on three critical rivals to the picoeconomic account of preference reversal, impulsivity, and addiction that were introduced in section 3.5: Loewenstein's "visceral" model (Loewenstein 1999), Read's subadditive model (Read 2001, 2003), and Gul and Pesendorfer's "temptation" model.

Loewenstein's account, according to which addiction consists in aversion to visceral consequences of withdrawal and relapse results from decayed memory of these consequences, only appears as a *rival* to the other models we consider if one attempts to collapse all causal aspects of impulsivity onto a single scale. Behaviorists have never denied the significance of visceral motivations: conditioning work is done, after all, with hungry rats, not satiated ones. The picoeconomic model is committed to no specific molecular mechanism for promoting the bargaining power of short-term interests at the molar scale. We believe that the character of the dopamine system is a significant part of the explanation of this bargaining power, but since we do not promote reduction of short-term molar interests to the molecular scale, we can allow as many other parts to the explanation as science turns out to verify. Hunger for highs, fear of withdrawal in addicts, and decayed memory of past withdrawal pain as a facilitator of relapse might all play supporting roles at *either* the molecular or molar level. That is, visceral states might interact directly with neurotransmitter dynamics in such a way as to strengthen the hand of the dopamine circuit against serotonergic and GABAergic circuits. Alternatively, *perceptions* of visceral states might function on the molar level to enhance the bargaining power of short-range interests. For that matter, visceral states could exert influence along both of these pathways; hunger, for example, surely *is* both a molecular and a molar phenomenon, with different effects in its two guises.[10]

Acknowledging this challenges neither of the core claims defended in this book. First, people will behave with respect to future rewards as if discounting them hyperbolically, and the effective antidote to that must be maintenance of personal rules. Then Loewenstein usefully reminds us that such maintenance might require reminding the recovered but tempted addict that withdrawal was much more unpleasant than she viscerally recalls; perhaps she should be shown a video of her previous suffering. Second, hysteresis of the reward system is the molecular-scale process that explains the phase-shifted character at the molar scale of the transition to addiction. This is something Loewenstein, trying to get visceral forces to carry too much of the explanatory load by themselves, can explain only by appeal to the exogenous chemical effects of drugs. He is thus inclined to doubt the possibility of "true" gambling addiction. We have extensively reviewed the evidence for thinking that such doubt cannot be sustained. Our hunch is that visceral factors will turn out to play interestingly *different* roles in distinct addictions,[11] such that if indeed these roles were the core element of addictive behavior, then we'd be moved away from a unified model of addiction and toward a sundering of the phenomena. Because we are persuaded by the evidence, especially that related to AG, that visceral and other factors contribute to common reward system response patterns in all addicts, we view I-RISA as a general model of addiction. However, we can actually *appeal to* Loewenstein's model in suggesting a possible barrier to unifying non-addictive DG at the molecular level: as with non-addicted heavy drinkers, the visceral urges that send a person who has just broken up with their partner out on a gambling or drinking binge may have nothing molecular in common with those that motivate a bored person or a person celebrating their promotion. But on a molar level, all these bingers may experience similar regrets the next day and attempt to reinstate similar personal rules.

Read's (2001, 2003) subadditive model raises a more direct challenge to PE, and furthermore, one that threatens to generalize. In arguing that impatience and preference reversal are merely apparent phenomena resulting from people's dividing longer delays into subintervals and leaving shorter delays undivided, Read advocates viewing the target phenomena as cognitive *framing* effects rather than consequences of subpersonal bargaining. Even if Read is ultimately not correct, or not completely correct, in positing subadditivity per se as the crucial framing factor for relative impulsivity, the plethora of framing factors that have been forthcoming from cognitive science research over the past thirty years suggest there is no shortage of possible alternatives that might come to be entertained.[12] In this light we can see the Gul and Pesendorfer model as using Loewenstein's ideas to promote such an alternative. According to Gul and Pesendorfer, success or failure in resisting strong visceral temptations determines the frames in which economic behavior will unfold; but then, economic behavior itself, including its discounting aspect, has the same standard model properties in every case.

Our response to suggestions that economically unorthodox discounting be explained as an artifact of framing is somewhat subtle, and rests crucially on earlier arguments given by Ross (2005). As noted on two previous occasions, we share Gul and Pesendorfer's concern that the objectives and point of economic models not be confused with those of cognitive science, even as these disciplines work together to explain transdisciplinary phenomena. If cognitive science could explain all apparent preference reversals by appeal to framing, thereby making it unnecessary to develop specific economic models of reversals like Ainslie's, then such confusion would be nicely blocked. (Gul and

Pesendorfer [2005] go a step further by actually building a model that *externally* defines the conditions under which a framing influence constitutes an item to be put into the "temptation" black box for purposes of economic analysis. It is left to psychology and neuroscience to then shine their lights into the box; the economist, meanwhile, can move on.) On the other hand, Ross (2005) provides an alternative way of blocking the cross-disciplinary muddle. There is no axiom in economic theory that identifies the prototypical economic agent with a whole person. Such an agent can just as well be a cockroach, a rat, a cognitive module—or a subpersonal interest, a neuron, or a neurotransmitter circuit. In picoeconomic models, whole people are *not* paradigmatic economic agents *because* subpersonal interests *are*. That is, the very intertemporal consistency of subpersonal interests playing molar-level bargaining games, and neural systems playing molecular-level games, *predicts* the intertemporal inconsistencies at the personal level that impugn attribution of straightforward economic agency across a person's biography outside of special institutional contexts. Ross appeals to the same modeling methodology favored by Gul and Pesendorfer, standard revealed preference theory, in deriving this result.

Gul and Pesendorfer (forthcoming) reject the possible relevance of Ross's style of analysis by fiat when they say: "That substances addictive for rats are also addictive in humans is not relevant for economics because (standard) economics does not study rats" (p. 23). This amounts to nothing more than a bald assertion that human beings *are so* the paradigmatic economic agents! That economics has historically been applied far more often to *people* than to other animals or to parts of people is, of course, beyond dispute. But what is relevant to Gul and Pesendorfer's negative case, if applied against PE, is whether *whole* people across their entire biographies are the paradigmatic subjects of (standard) economics. As Ross (2005) argues at length, the history of mainstream economics, if one takes the literal mathematics more seriously than the accompanying rhetoric, does not support this claim. The overwhelming majority of economic applications study time slices of people while they are confined within institutional contexts—specific markets—that enforce consistency in revealed preference. Theoretical exercises, such as those of Becker (1976, 1981) (discussed in chapter 3), that insist on lifetime human consistency *across* institutional settings[13] are no more characteristic of "standard" economics[14] than are applications of competitive market models to relationships among animals (which exist in increasing proliferation—see examples in Noë, van

Hoof, and Hammerstein 2001). Gul and Pesendorfer seem to saw off any branch a conceptually conservative economist might want to use to resist Ross's approach when they say that "standard economics . . . tries to evaluate how economic institutions mediate (perhaps psychologically unhealthy) behavior of agents" (forthcoming, p. 3). Just so. Among the fundamental institutions that mediate such behavior are precisely social pressures for maintenance of personal rules, along with institutions aimed at undermining them (including, though not fundamentally, casinos and pubs).

This response to Read and to Gul and Pesendorfer is so far purely defensive, denying their claim that we should prefer framing models to PE for the sake of preventing economics from collapsing into psychology. It does not respond to claims that one or both of their models are empirically superior to Ainslie's. However, *once* the defensive response is on the table, *then* the sharpness of the empirical quarrel begins to dissipate. A person who systematically frames immediate rewards, but not delayed ones, in either more finely divided intervals or as visceral temptations, will tend to make choices that, when placed on indifference curves, yield hyperbolic functions. (Of course, this must be true; if it weren't, then Read and Gul and Pesendorfer would be forced to deny decades of laboratory data.) In that case, the defender of PE as a molar-scale account can accommodate framing accounts in approximately the same way we suggested that she can accommodate visceral accounts. In the case of Gul and Pesendorfer, the reply to Loewenstein now applies exactly. With respect to Read's model the responses are merely similar because cognitive framing, unlike visceral temptation, is itself a molar-scale phenomenon. Molar-scale accounts using the resources of distinct disciplines need not conflict with one another, however. From the perspective of cognitive science, impulsive choice can be modeled as a framing effect, and prudential choice can be modeled as choice in a different frame; from the perspective of economics, the same phenomena can be modeled by reference to discounting and bundling. Read (2001, p. 25) recognizes that Myerson and Green's (1995) adaptation of the standard hyperbolic discounting function to accommodate nonlinear time perception accounts for the data he uses to argue for confirmation of subadditivity theory. As he then points out, this makes *hyperbolic* discounting redundant, since exponential discounting with nonlinear time preference *also* explains the data without requiring recourse to subadditivity.

Thus, adopting the Green and Myerson equation would effectively amount to proposing an alternative framing account emphasizing time perception. What discounting models in general fail to do, Read argues, is explain why some bundles but not others (e.g., those containing gambling and alcohol but not writing paper or petrol, to once again cite Loewenstein's examples) are targets of systematically disordered consumption. Here, Read maintains, we should make recourse to visceral temptations. At *this* point, of course, we can reply to Read on behalf of PE models *exactly* as we did to Loewenstein and to Gul and Pesendorfer.

This might still seem to be a disappointingly tepid response. We normally ask for more in defense of a theory than the claim that it and its alternatives capture data equally well. Should we not, then, aim to identify experiments that would separate the wheat from the chaff? Consider, for example, a study due to Fellows and Farah (2005) that compared four subject groups in a gambling task, and then measured the extent to which they spontaneously set long horizons when asked to imagine specific states of affairs "in the future." The four groups were: (1) subjects with damage to VMPFC, (2) normal controls, (3) subjects with damage to dorsolateral frontal cortex, and (4) subjects with lesions away from the frontal lobes, but of comparable average size to lesions in groups (1) and (3). No differences were found with respect to discounting, or, within group (1), any correlation between k values and sizes of lesions. On future time perspective, group (2) projected longer average futures than groups (3) and (4), and these two groups projected longer average futures than group (1) subjects. Thus VMPFC was implicated in generalized myopic thinking, as in other studies—but the evidence was interpreted by the experimenters as pointing to time-perception framing rather than steep discounting as the relevant explanatory mechanism.

We have indicated the problem with viewing this as evidence bearing on rival *molar-scale* hypotheses, however. The thesis that the person discounts hyperbolically does not entail a claim that impulsivity is necessarily to be explained by the actions of one or more brain systems that also hyperbolically discount (even if, as Glimcher conjectures, brain areas *do* implement their own discounting in their own right). Because molar-scale behavioral phenomena don't reduce to molecular-scale phenomena when we "turn up" the resolving power of our conceptual microscopes (so to speak), there are no molecular facts of the

matter to force choices between framing explanations and picoeconomic ones. It is surely not false to say that people who suffer from
consumption impulsivity disorders should try to change frames.
(Earlier in the history of psychology, we would have said "gestalts.")
Bundling, after all, *is* a kind of framing; as we discussed in chapter 3
in connection with Rachlin's alternative version of Ainslie's narratives
of addiction, the underlying logic is the same. The advantage of emphasizing intertemporal bundling as the mode of framing against consumption impulsivity is that it brings with it recourse to an *economic
rationale*: the nonbundler stands to be money-pumped in institutions
set up to track her preference consistency, such as casinos; the prediction of *intertemporal* inconsistency provides a motivation for putting a
personal rule at stake as an asset in the *present*. Modeling impulsivity
merely as failure to resist visceral temptation, with a model of subadditive discounting to represent this in framing terms, invites no economic elaboration. Perhaps it instead invites Aristotelean elaborations
built around concepts of personal *telos*. We see no reason to scorn the
value of such molar-scale narratives. However, as Ross (2005) shows in
detail, they interfere with rather than abet efforts to integrate cognitive
science and economic theory. (Of course, that is just what Gul and
Pesendorfer might find attractive about them.) If cognitive-science-
based and economic models do not predict rival molecular accounts,
then an argument for *generally* rejecting one kind would require an
argument to the effect that it qualitatively misdescribes behavioral
phenomena at the molar scale. We have reviewed the evidence that
leads us to deny any such contention where DG or addiction are
concerned.

In addition, as we pointed out in connection with our discussion of
Loewenstein's account, emphasis on visceral factors leads naturally to
treating drug dependencies as the central cases of addiction. Continu-
ities and pathway aspects linking non-addictive consumption impulsivity with addiction are thereby lost sight of. Of course, these could
be recovered easily enough in any number of ad hoc ways. But in then
displacing the neuroeconomic model of the dopamine system from
primary focus, in the way that we have shown to be motivated by
attention to AG, the theoretical complementarity of PE and NE as
aspects of a general framework for understanding impulsivity and
addiction together also fades from view. Once again, Gul and Pesendorfer might explicitly welcome this outcome. However, to the extent
that the reader is persuaded by our argument in chapters 5 and 6, she

will have empirical motivations—as opposed to just philosophical ones tied up with concern for the unity of science—for sympathizing with the approach we advocate.

8.5 A Final Illustration

In the previous two sections, we argued that the relationship between molar and molecular factors in behavior is one of mutual feedback between processes operating on distinct scales of resolution on a shared physical substrate (though with somewhat different boundaries, since molar-scale systems extend out into the environment—see Clark 1997). This discussion was highly abstract, and was not applied directly to the details of DG. We therefore close with an illustration of the practical integration of molar-scale picoeconomic and molecular-scale neuroeconomic insights for the understanding of DG dynamics.

Consider Rachlin's molar-scale account of a syndrome he hypothesizes as specifically besetting many DGs, according to which the person compares strings of gambles that end in wins, rather than accounting in terms of constant numbers of gambles or (ideally) simple cash balance sheets. The PV model explains how the dopamine system might plausibly support the kind of habit Rachlin identifies. As a string of gambles unfolds, the gambler will occasionally find that short-run frequencies match the expected convergent frequency of wins and losses; the gambler's fallacy will in these instances seem to be confirmed. We predict that if this was the typical pattern—if the gambler's fallacy wasn't a fallacy!—then most people would find gambling to be dull, and DG would be much less common than it is. But in fact, most of the time the gambler will either be pleasantly surprised by quick wins, or negatively surprised by failures to balance strings of losses with wins as quickly as anticipated. No one's intuitions will find it surprising that events of the first sort encourage further gambling. But in the absence of the neuroeconomic perspective, the idea that losing should attract gamblers to continue should be surprising.[15] The PV model of reward removes the puzzle. When wins fail to come as quickly as expected, dopamine signals are attenuated. The longer the delay to the win, the greater the correction made according to the TD learning algorithm, and hence the stronger the dopamine response from VTA. The enhanced system activity primes motor systems to seek out cues for similar rewards. Then the system learns that it can *create* such cues *by gambling*. At a stroke, we thus account for both the molecular phenomenon of the pathway to neural AG, and the molar phenomenon of loss chasing.

Neural data are consistent with Rachlin's molar-scale hypothesis. Nieuwenhuis et al. (2004) conducted an fMRI experiment in which the possible types of relative monetary prizes available to gambling subjects—large monetary gain, small gain, no gain, large loss, small loss, no loss—and the specific monetary magnitudes at stake were varied independently. They found that subjects' reward-system responses were more sensitive to variations caused by binary context shifts (best versus worst possible prize in a bundle, or winning versus losing) than to variations in available absolute magnitudes. Subjects here were randomly sampled people, not PGs. Gehring and Willoughby (2002) found that randomly drawn subjects in a gambling task not only made riskier choices after losses but also made riskier choices the greater the magnitude of their preceding losses, and that this correlates with activity in VMPFC.

Thus, the brains of normal people attract them not just to gambling but to gambling according to intrinsically dangerous patterns in which losing induces more rather than less attraction—at least, to the reward system taken in isolation. These data by themselves might lead us to wonder why everyone does not succumb to DG. We know independently, however, that most people are not robotic slaves of their reward systems. Most people *notice* when they are drawn to throw important resources away, and stop. As we saw in chapter 6, genetics may turn out to account for a substantial proportion of the people who do *not* stop. But something is still missing at this point. Even genetically vulnerable AGs are not unconscious or generally cognitively incapacitated. Indeed, as we cited Evenden reminding us near the beginning of the present chapter, AGs are typically cunning and resourceful in finding ways to gamble and to conceal their gambling when social forces try to interfere with them. Finally, most AGs *do* eventually recognize that they have a serious problem and make efforts, usually successful following a struggle, to control it. So it seems that when people are hijacked by mutinous reward systems they are not made to walk the plank, but stay on board and, much more often than not, recapture the bridge. NE explains a great deal of how AG begins and develops, and why it features its characteristic patterns while enslavement to gambling is at full roar. Indeed, without the neuroeconomic model, the very existence of *addiction* to gambling is so mysterious that it was widely doubted, notwithstanding many apparently clear behavioral manifestations. In isolation from the complementary molar account of PE, however, NE does not explain the complete phenomenon. A person implements subpersonal economies on at least two scales simultaneously, just as communities of people implement microeconomies and macroeconomies that are intimately related but not by reduction. In making policy for national or regional economies, we would be foolish not to frame and test hypotheses on both scales, as well as trying to model the feedback between them. The same point applies to policies for individual people.

Notes

Chapter 1

1. In this respect too, our philosophical model is Dennett; see Ross 1994.

2. Thus we object when we encounter (for example) Knutson et al. (2007) suggesting that he and his colleagues looked into the brain and discovered that microeconomic consumer theory is not about opportunity cost after all.

Chapter 2

1. We refer here to efficiency with respect to utility rather than public revenues. The idea is that if gamblers behave in a way suggesting that they attach less value to their monetary reserves than other people, then overall disutility from taxes can be reduced by shifting additional burden onto the gamblers.

2. Note that this formulation of Collins's conclusion is ours, not his.

3. That is not, of course, equivalent to actually eliminating it. But almost everyone agrees on what public policy should be when we find it.

4. This committee was charged in 1996 and, in association with the Committee on Law and Justice, reported in 1999.

5. Note that giving greater urgency and higher priority claim on scarce resources to research might actually yield higher human benefits overall, once the long run is considered. But this would involve treating present sufferers as means to be sacrificed on the altar of a greater future good, which is widely deemed incompatible with ethical requirements in circumstances in which the institutions of health research and health service are tightly intertwined. We do not endorse this institutionalization of Kantian over utilitarian metaethics; but it's a policy fact almost everywhere.

6. For examples of this, see Cox, Enns, and Michaud 2004 and Grant et al. 2004.

7. Some research suggests that this would in itself show us that the hypothetical b screen was defective. Toce-Gerstein, Gerstein, and Volberg (2003) compared responses to each *DSM-IV* criterion with overall scores on a *DSM-IV* derived screen, using samples of randomly selected people and people approached on their way to a casino. In both samples, a positive response on criterion (6) was an overwhelmingly reliable predictor of a screen score indicating PG. Unfortunately, the screen used in this study did not

directly probe with respect to criterion (5), which to behavioral economists is the most important one.

8. This would apply to the simplest case where screens rank subjects in the same way.

9. Blaszczynski and Nower maintain that there are three different kinds of pathological gambler, that each kind results from a different psychological process and starting point, and that people suffering from each kind respond best to different sorts of intervention. We'll engage with this thesis at various points in the book.

10. This was the edition of *DSM* that was intermediate between the third and fourth editions.

11. The authors of the present book, with a team of colleagues and students, are currently using both the DIGS and the CGI to screen pathological gamblers for experimental studies in South Africa.

Chapter 3

1. Of course, in any specific study impulsivity will be operationalized more precisely, if only implicitly, by use of a specific measurement scale. Our point here is not to cast doubt on any particular empirical studies, but to make a conceptual point.

2. The most important of Herrnstein's papers are posthumously gathered in Rachlin and Laibson 1997.

3. Matching would also be produced by a maximization choice rule according to which behavior is allocated across the alternatives according to the response distribution (rates of B_1 and B_2) that maximizes global marginal utility ($R_1 + R_2$), rather than according to the response distribution that equalizes the rates of local marginal utility (melioration). Melioration views the organism as continuously choosing between B_1 and B_2 according to which alternative yields the highest local marginal utility (R_1 or R_2). Maximization, on the other hand, views the organism as continuously choosing between different combinations of B_1 and B_2 according to which combination yields the highest global marginal utility ($R_1 + R_2$). To date, it has not been possible to design a critical empirical test between these alternative interpretations of matching, but the weight of the evidence favors melioration (Heyman and Herrnstein 1986; Rachlin, Green, and Tormey 1988).

4. Herrnstein's (1970) seminal theoretical paper on the matching law revolutionized the study of choice in behavioral science. That revolution entailed conceptual and empirical developments that currently are theoretically, methodologically, and quantitatively quite sophisticated (e.g., Grace 1994; Mazur 2001). The complexities and nuances of this current work are beyond our present purpose. Fortunately for this purpose, the basic concepts in the matching law have been more important than the subsequent complexities in extensions to understanding impulsivity and substance abuse. We will therefore focus on the early studies that revealed the basic ideas.

5. This fact can be the basis for a critical point. The economist Ken Binmore has repeatedly argued that behavioral economists often invite unreliable experimental results by paying subjects too little, thus encouraging them to care about variables other than those linked to the money prizes, which are not even within the knowledge of, let alone under the control of, the experimenter. We agree with Binmore that behavioral economists should be strongly attentive to this concern. Fortunately, more and more of them have awoken to it over time.

6. It is important to emphasize that k values vary within individuals under different conditions as well as between individuals. For example, small rewards are discounted more than large rewards (e.g., Green, Myerson, and Macaux 2005), rewards are discounted more than costs (e.g., Murphy, Vuchinich, and Simpson 2001), different rewards are discounted at different rates (e.g., Madden, Bickel, and Jacobs 1999), and discounting increases under conditions of deprivation (e.g., Kirk and Logue 1997).

7. Loewenstein and Prelec (1992) and Myerson and Green (1995) showed, in different ways, that equation 3.3 is a particular instance of a more general family of hyperbolae in which the denominator has a two-parameter exponent representing scaling factors for reward amount and time (the exponent of the denominator of equation 3.3 is 1). Importantly, this family of discount functions lie on a continuum with equations 3.2 and 3.4 at the endpoints. That is, as the scaling factors in the exponent in the denominator get very large, equation 3.3 would converge on equation 3.2 (Laibson 1997). Conversely, as the scaling factors in the exponent in the denominator get very small, equation 3.3 would converge on equation 3.4 (Loewenstein and Prelec 1992). Relevant studies (e.g., Myerson and Green 1995; Simpson and Vuchinich 2000) have found that equation 3.3 with an exponent provides better fits to data from individual participants, as well as it should with an additional free parameter, but the improvement in explained variance was quite small, so there have been no compelling empirical reasons to prefer equation 3.3 with an exponent to equation 3.3 without one. Moreover, every study (e.g., Madden, Bickel, and Jacobs 1999; Vuchinich and Simpson 1998) that has directly compared equation 3.3 to equation 3.4 has found the former to provide a better fit to data from either individual participants or from group averages. Note that any discount function in the family at a point on the continuum away from equation 3.4 would predict preference reversals in intertemporal choice, with those reversals occurring more readily the farther away from equation 3.4 one goes.

8. The main developers of PE, Ainslie, Herrnstein, and Rachlin, label their accounts "theories of addiction." Their use of the term addiction in this context refers generally to excessive consumption. Because we will later argue for a much more specific definition of the term addiction derived from neuroscience, here we use the term "chronic impulsivity" instead of addiction.

9. Construal-level theory (e.g., Liberman and Trope 2003) shares some important similarities with Rachlin's act-pattern theory, insofar as both focus on whether objects are perceived in terms of their more concrete, "lower-level" properties or in terms of their more abstract, "higher-level" properties. If a person is deciding between having a double cheeseburger with fries or a salad for lunch, how those alternative meals are construed may be important. A focus on the meal's concrete properties (i.e., taste, immediate satisfaction) instead of on its abstract properties (i.e., healthfulness) may well contribute to the individual choosing the unhealthy meal, and vice versa.

Chapter 4

1. This paper also showed that substance-dependent subjects did worse at a delayed non-match-to-sample memory task than normal subjects with comparably poor IGT performance. This also suggests that substance dependence, at least in these subjects, is associated with compromised executive cognition.

2. This result may sound surprising, but since the IGT is supposed to measure a kind of "emotional learning," Evans, Kemish, and Turnbull *hypothesized* that more educated

people would decide in more deliberate, and less emotional, ways, and hence do worse.

3. There were three age groups in this study: 9–10 years, 11–13 years, and 14–17 years.

4. Note that the measure of impulsivity here was not behavioral but clinical. Since other work has found a behavioral measure (discounting task) to be a better predictor of gambling severity within a population at a time (Alessi and Petry 2003), it may be that a stronger result would have been found with such a measure.

5. The impulsivity and personality measures used by Hair and Hampson were the Barrett Impulsivity Scale, and the Big Five inventory, both depending on self-report.

6. For a review of the literature on delay and probability discounting, see Green and Myerson 2004.

7. Some studies take considerable care to increase the confidence of subjects that their delayed rewards will be received, for example by giving them preliminary payments by means of a charge card so that by the time of the discounting task they have experienced several successful payments (Kable and Glimcher unpublished).

8. Regular smokers in this study, independent of their answers to the various questions, completed the discounting tasks significantly more quickly than nonsmokers.

9. The mean age of subjects in this study was a little over 20 years.

10. This study also examined discounting for reduced probability—see below for a discussion of this form of discounting.

11. The mean age of subjects in this study was 19.6 years. Note that the (non-PG) gamblers had SOGS scores of 4 or more, whereas control subjects included persons with SOGS scores of zero or 1.

12. Subjects were considered PGs for the Dixon, Marley, and Jacobs study if they had a SOGS score in excess of 4. The mean age of subjects in this study was 40.6 years.

13. This reports preliminary data from a study of gambling severity, delay discounting, probability discounting and other measures. Our preliminary data also suggest that greater gambling severity is associated with decreased sensitivity to risk.

14. The mean age of subjects in this study was 44 years.

15. This paper found that differences in delay discounting predicted SOGS scores 1.4 times as accurately as scores on the Eysenck Impulsivity Scale.

16. Reynolds et al. included multiple behavioral measures: delay discounting, a risk-related task, and a stop and go/no-go task (the latter two both inhibition tasks).

17. Shallice and Burgess's patients showed no deficits in performance at the Wisconsin Card Sorting Task.

18. Ortner, MacDonald, and Olmstead (2003) found that subjects who had consumed alcohol became *less* impulsive than previously.

19. For a review of over 30 laboratory studies on this subject, see Steele and Southwick 1985.

20. A contra-indication is Meier et al. 1996, which found no effect of alcohol administration in response to negative outcomes in a choice task.

Chapter 5

1. Scientists can find the arguments for this in any mainstream undergraduate textbook on the philosophy of mind.

2. We warn the reader that putting things this way is a potentially misleading simplification. The meanings of signals within the brain don't literally have English translations. This is because English is a *public, communal* language that refers to things that people have learned to coordinate on picking out *together*. What's "discussed" inside the brain are things and states of affairs that *parts of the brain* have learned to coordinate on picking out together. A person can't "see inside her head" and register these things consciously, so she can't label them. Thus, types of "brain objects" don't really line up, except (sometimes) very roughly and approximately, with types of "personal objects." Finally, our basis for assigning *any* meanings at all to particular states of (parts of) the brain must be the systematic influences that states of the relevant types have on behavior.

3. When states of affairs are merely *ranked*, this is called "ordinal valuation." When they're ranked *and* scaled with respect to one another—e.g., "This is worth three times what that is worth"—this is called "cardinal valuation." Most of the valuation done by the reward system, the part of the brain that malfunctions in many or most PGs, is cardinal valuation.

4. People sometimes say that "noble" goods like lives and attachments can't be valued in cash currency. This is a comforting sentiment to some, but it isn't true in practice. No one pays infinite amounts for life insurance, and so specific, finite amounts must be worked out. Most people would risk their lives running across a busy freeway for *some or other* amount of money. Of course, the common currency of the brain isn't money. But evidence indicates that the brain codes monetary, social and abstract rewards comparably—as it must if it isn't to be paralyzed when confronted by the need to make trade-offs in the proportions of attention it devotes to each of them.

5. See Brewer and Brown 2003. fMRI measures magnetic field properties that are systematically correlated with different patterns of blood flow in brains. Since we know a lot about the relationships between blood-flow patterns and the ways in which neuronal demands for hemoglobin vary with activity, we can use the blood-flow patterns to make reliable inferences about neural firing rates. In fMRI, these inferences are performed directly by the technology to yield statistical graphs (not, as some people suppose, literal visual images) of neuronal patterns. The fMRI graphs only give us resolution down to the level of *groups* of neurons, but researchers are now discovering forms of statistical inference that (under some conditions) allow the scientist to get from images of groups of neurons to conclusions about single neurons.

6. Positron emission tomography has been around for a bit longer than fMRI and is still the most useful neuroimaging technology for some purposes. Another new approach complementary to fMRI, but limited by its greater degree of invasiveness, is called transcranial magnetic stimulation.

7. The new evidence from Preuschoff, Bossaerts, and Quartz (2006) cited earlier suggests that at this higher level, PV will need to be accompanied by a model of dopaminergic perception of expected reward. One naturally surmises that this is crucial input to computation of reward rate.

256 Notes

8. A motor response is a brain signal ordering some part of the body to do something. (Bodies don't always obey, either because the body is damaged or because some other part of the brain simultaneously has conflicting ideas.)

9. This metaphor should not obscure the fact that the "service" in question may often be quite sophisticated. For example, recent fMRI evidence suggests that the amygdala, a central processing station in the brain for emotions, also plays a role in working memory, a higher cognitive function critical for reasoning and problem solving (Schaefer et al. 2006).

10. Note the implication that our reward system in fact integrates not just two but three separately evolved structures. This doesn't just *add* potential kludges; it *multiplies* their extent and probability, since for every new unit we add to an integrated system, there's a new potential kludge for *each* interface with an existing system.

11. Figure adapted from Laviolette and van der Kooy 2004.

12. Figure adapted from Everitt and Robbins 2005.

13. Figure adapted from "The brain from top to bottom": Canadian Institute of Neurosciences, Mental Health and Addiction (2002).

14. For an early specification of the PV model in application to the dopaminergic system, see Schultz, Dayan, and Montague 1997.

15. "Hedonic pleasure" refers to nice sensations, such as warmth, the texture of fresh bread in the mouth, or tucking the body into a compact, secure space. The point of "hedonic" is to distinguish this sort of pleasure from cognitive pleasure, such as being "pleased" that South Africa has many languages and cultures.

16. A very simple example of this is that many people learn to want—in the sense of behaviorally and neurally treating as rewarding—very hot peppers that are coded by anterior cingulate cortex as aversive.

17. This needs slight qualification, since dopamine also plays a role in identifying potential rewards; these roles are separable, however, so the basic point at issue is not affected.

18. Note that sensitization is, with respect to some purely behavioral indicators, the opposite of "tolerance"—that is, the diminished tendency of a given unit per interval of an addictive target to interfere with capacities for alternative behaviors. See Berke and Hyman 2000.

19. It should also be noted, however, that most adolescents who consume typical addictive targets (including gambling) at rates that would be regarded as indicative of addiction in an adult, smoothly reduce consumption as they acquire adult responsibilities and never show other signs of social or psychological dysfunction associated with the consumption. Consider the stereotypical biography of the heroically beer-drinking American college fraternity boy, for example. This biography doesn't culminate in alcoholism.

20. Stroop tasks measure the difference in how long subjects take to respond to stimuli that they are all supposed to treat in the same way, but which differ in a way chosen by the experimenter. For example, if subjects are asked to read aloud the words presented on a screen, the experimenters will find that subjects take slightly longer to read words associated with suffering than neutral words. Delay in reading is an index of more inter-

nal processing activity having taken place. Data from Stroop tasks can help neuroscientists work out what they are looking for.

21. Early studies of this correlation were cross-sectional, thus not ruling out the possibility that they were merely picking up a selection effect, based on the fact that people who discount less steeply find it easier to quit. More recent prospective studies have confirmed the relationship, however.

22. Recall the earlier point due to Loewenstein.

23. See Chiamulera 2004 for a detailed application of this model to the neural substrates of nicotine addiction and relapse in recovery attempts. In keeping with the reward learning/PV model, Chiamulera refers to cravings as "failed expectations."

Chapter 6

1. Marijuana is the exception that proves the rule here. In many societies, both its financial and legal-risk costs are much lower than those of other illegal drugs. For this reason, popular culture is inclined to doubt that there is such a phenomenon as THC addiction.

2. It might be objected that an argument based, as this one is, on mere rejection of a null hypothesis by significance criteria could not possibly establish that *all* PGs are AGs, yet this is what the reductionist move will have us say. Let us therefore emphasize that our reductionism with respect to this specific case is pragmatic. We recommend that PG be re-operationalized as AG. We do *not* claim, as many philosophers read all reductionist proposals as implying, that PG has turned out to "mean" AG. The strong logical/semantic concept of reduction in analytic philosophy of science is an ascientific fantasy.

3. The implied gender difference here may not amount to anything. The team's female subjects met the significance criterion at $p = .03$, while males were marginal at $p = .09$. Dividing the overall sample in half for gender comparison, of course, also reduces statistical power by half. We thank James MacKillop for bringing this point to our attention.

4. They cite Blum et al. 1995.

5. We again thank James MacKillop.

Chapter 8

1. A fully spelled-out version of the philosophical story to which we allude would have it that, if our proposal warrants acceptance, then "PG" *means* "AG" and always has, including when no one yet thought so because AG, in the specific sense captured by current theory, hadn't yet been conceptualized. Our problem with this story is not that it is counterintuitive, since intuitions are not scientific evidence one way or the other. What is wrong with the story is that it takes the language of science to be governed by logical semantics instead of pragmatics, overemphasizes the significance of meaning in science in the first place, and has the tail (viz., the need for scientists to coordinate in reference and operationalization) wagging the dog (viz., the primary concern of science with prediction and control of actual phenomena).

2. As utilitarians rather than believers in super-instrumental rights, we are not particularly troubled by cases of "happy" alcoholics or smokers who suffer the mild paternalism of social disapproval and diminished grants of autonomy. We think it is reasonable to disapprove of *all* smoking (except perhaps by elderly or terminally ill people) in exactly the same sense that it is reasonable to disapprove of all swimming in crocodile-infested rivers, including by those who are deliberately demonstrating their fearlessness. People who die young of lung cancer and people who are eaten by reptiles impose high costs on others, of which emotional costs are the largest part. We would disapprove of all gambling *if* most gambling led to DG (which it demonstrably and overwhelmingly does not).

3. The Web sites we are describing frequently conflate "sex addiction" with hypersexuality, a condition sometimes genuinely associated with bipolar disorder.

4. Such individuals might, of course, have some *other* problem; the occasional cocaine user might still get arrested, for example. The weekend smoker might trigger lung cancer in herself, or set her clothes on fire, or be spotted by her health insurance agent. If these are risks that the occasional users rationally consider and exponentially discount in their behavior, however, then they are not *consumption-impulsivity* problems.

5. But what *about* social insects? Do invertebrates hyperbolically discount in the first place? If so, are individual ants and wasps vulnerable to impulsivity while colonies control it (as we think is a key part of the story for humans)? These are questions we'd love to see addressed, but on which there has been no research as far as we can determine. Note that squirrels and chickadees hoarding winter food supplies are not, as might initially be supposed, counterexamples to the claim that other nonhuman animals don't need circuits to suppress impulsive consumption. Squirrels and chickadees only cache food when their stomachs are full.

6. Antelopes and other fast herbivores at the peak of health often *do* act boldly, and even "waste" resources leaping into the air, in the presence of predators so as to signal their fitness (Zahavi and Zahavi 1997). However, we are here imagining something more: an antelope who teases the lion without sending any further information, simply because it's exciting. It isn't known whether antelopes are ever tempted to play in this way. Clearly, however, many humans are, as the popularity of risky sports attests.

7. A reader might object that the reward system must surely serve long-term interests too; otherwise, by what means would these interests ever get *their* rewards? In response to this we reiterate Wise's point, cited in chapter 6, that "reward" to the dopamine system and "reward" to the person are not the same thing. In a picoeconomy where long-term interests usually win, the reward system will learn sensitivity to cues for, and disposition to fire dopamine in anticipation of, short-run proxies for LLRs. These proxies should not be confused with the LLRs themselves.

8. We are not claiming here that the disposition to construe the behavior of others in folk-psychological terms is not based on innate dispositions, which it very likely is. But the content of *specific* folk-psychological theories shows wide cross-cultural variation.

9. An analogy for this is: if you've got a very good hammer, try hitting everything with it to see what goes into the wall. That's one way of *discovering* which things are in fact nails.

10. It is hunger-as-molecular-phenomenon that increases mammals' olfactory sensitivity; it is hunger-as-molar-phenomenon that causes people to feel hungry for novel foods while satiated with respect to familiar ones.

11. It might be thought interesting in this connection that Camille et al. (2004) report data which they interpret as suggesting that subjects with lesions to OFC make less advantageous gambling decisions than normal subjects because the former fail to antici-pate and be motivated by the possibility of suffering from regret if they make a risky bet with negative expected return and lose. Unfortunately, we cannot rely on this study, because as Eagleman (2005) shows, there was a discrepancy between the actual expected utilities of the gambles on the one hand, and the expected utilities as the experimenters described them and as they presented them to subjects on the other. See Shiv et al. 2005 (a team that includes Loewenstein), however, for less controversial evidence that bears positively on this hypothesis.

12. For example, Glimcher and Rustichini (2004) suggest that VMPFC attaches so-called "somatic markers"—roughly, emotional biases—to outputs of the reward system that cause most people to fail to behave like expected-utility maximizers, even in the very short run, under certain kinds of situations. They discuss evidence, for example, that most people are averse to losses, in the sense that they'll prefer an expected reward of a given magnitude to another of identical magnitude if the latter has a higher probability of inflicting a loss, and that they'll pay (in expected utility) to avoid ambiguous choices. Glimcher and Rustichini cite observations suggesting that people with damage to pre-frontal brain areas behave *more* like (short-run) expected-utility maximizers in these conditions. See previous note.

13. See Ross 2005 (pp. 148–159) for an argument from within the neoclassical perspective against the practical usefulness of Becker's modeling approach.

14. It might be objected that the model underlying Milton Friedman's permanent-income hypothesis (1957) provides an empirically tested basis for treating whole biographical people as representative economic agents; and if anything can claim to be "standard" economics it is the Friedman model and its extensions. But Friedman's agent is not a whole *de-institutionalized* person; his agent is a limited aspect of a person, namely an investor in money markets, operating under highly explicit institutional settings that happen, in this case, to focus explicitly on trade-offs between long-range returns and short-range consumption. The success of Friedman's model, such as it is, shows some-thing about the effectiveness of institutions in modern economies at encouraging reward bundling.

15. This is probably surprising only on reflection, since the phenomenon of loss chasing is well known to everyone with much experience of gamblers and gambling. In this respect, loss chasing resembles gravity. When Newton incorporated gravity into his universal mechanics, his contemporaries, and Newton himself, were puzzled and trou-bled by it, since it made little sense in a context where a principal working dogma was that bodies could not influence one another at a distance. But over the centuries before Einstein's resolution of the puzzle, everyone got used to gravitational attraction and forgot that they didn't understand it.

References

Agrawal, N. (2004). Neuropsychiatry. *Student British Medical Journal* 12: 110–111.

Ahmed, S. (2004). Addiction as compulsive reward prediction. *Science* 306: 1901–1902.

Ainslie, G. (1975). Specious reward: A behavioral theory of impulsiveness and self-control. *Psychological Bulletin* 82: 463–496.

Ainslie, G. (1992). *Picoeconomics: The Strategic Interaction of Successive Motivational States Within the Person.* Cambridge: Cambridge University Press.

Ainslie, G. (1999). The dangers of willpower. In *Getting Hooked: Rationality and Addiction,* ed. J. Elster and O.-J. Skog, pp. 65–92. Cambridge: Cambridge University Press.

Ainslie, G. (2001). *Breakdown of Will.* Cambridge: Cambridge University Press.

Ainslie, G. (2005). Précis of *Breakdown of Will. Behavioral and Brain Sciences* 28: 635–673.

Ainslie, G., and V. Haendel (1983). The motives of the will. In *Etiology Aspects of Alcohol and Drug Abuse,* ed. E. Gottheil, K. Druley, T. Skodola, and H. Waxman, pp. 119–140. Springfield, Ill.: Charles C. Thomas.

Ainslie, G., and J. Monterosso (2003). Building blocks of self-control: Increased tolerance for delay with bundled rewards. *Journal of the Experimental Analysis of Behavior* 79: 37–48.

Ainslie, G., and J. Monterosso (2004). A marketplace in the brain? *Science* 306: 421–423.

Akers, R. (1991). Addiction: The troublesome concept. *Journal of Drug Issues* 21: 777–793.

Alessi, S., and N. Petry (2003). Pathological gambling severity is associated with impulsivity in a delay discounting procedure. *Behavioural Processes* 64: 345–354.

American Psychiatric Association (1952). *Diagnostic and Statistical Manual of Mental Disorders.* Washington, D.C.: American Psychiatric Association.

American Psychiatric Association (1968). *Diagnostic and Statistical Manual of Mental Disorders,* 2nd edn. Washington, D.C.: American Psychiatric Association.

American Psychiatric Association (1980). *Diagnostic and Statistical Manual of Mental Disorders,* 3rd edn. Washington, D.C.: American Psychiatric Association.

American Psychiatric Association (1987). *Diagnostic and Statistical Manual of Mental Disorders,* 3rd edn. (revised). Washington, D.C.: American Psychiatric Association.

American Psychiatric Association (2000). *Diagnostic and Statistical Manual of Mental Disorders*, 4th edn. Washington, D.C.: American Psychiatric Association.

Amit, D. (1989). *Modeling Brain Function*. Cambridge: Cambridge University Press.

Andreoli, M., M. Tessari, M. Pilla, E. Valerio, J. Hagen, and C. Heidbreder (2003). Selective antagonism at D3 receptors prevents nicotine-triggered relapse to nicotine-seeking behavior. *Neuropsychopharmacology* 28: 1272–1280.

Babor, T. F. (1990). Social, scientific, and medical issues in the definition of alcohol and drug dependence. In *The Nature of Drug Dependence*, ed. G. Edwards and M. Lader, pp. 19–36. Oxford: Oxford University Press.

Baik, J., R. Picetti, A. Saiardi, G. Thirlet, A. Dierich, A. Depaulis, M. Le Meur, and E. Borrelli (1995). Parkinson-like locomotor impairment in mice lacking dopamine D2 receptors. *Nature* 377: 424–428.

Baird, J. R. (1998). Promoting willingness and ability to learn: A focus on ignorance. *Reflect* 4: 21–26.

Bargh, J. (1990). Auto-motives: Preconscious determinants of social interaction. In *Handbook of Motivation and Cognition*, vol. 2, ed. T. Higgins and R. Sorrentino, pp. 93–130. New York: Guilford.

Bargh, J. (1992). Being unaware of the stimulus vs. unaware of its interpretation: Why subliminality per se does matter to social psychology. In *Perception without Awareness*, ed. R. Bornstein and T. Pittman, pp. 236–255. New York: Guilford.

Baron, E., and M. Dickerson (1999). Alcohol consumption and self-control of gambling behaviour. *Journal of Gambling Studies* 15: 3–15.

Baunez, C., C. Dias, M. Cador, and M. Amalric (2005). The subthalamic nucleus exerts opposite control on cocaine and "natural" rewards. *Nature Neuroscience* 8: 484–489.

Bechara, A., and E. Martin (2004). Impaired decision making related to working memory deficits in individuals with substance addictions. *Neuropsychology* 18: 152–162.

Bechara, A., A. R. Damasio, H. Damasio, and S. Anderson (1994). Insensitivity to future consequences following damage to human prefrontal cortex. *Cognition* 50: 7–15.

Bechara, A., H. Damasio, D. Tranel, and A. R. Damosio (1997). Deciding advantageously before knowing the advantageous strategy. *Science* 275: 1293–1295.

Bechara, A., H. Damasio, D. Tranel, and A. R. Damasio (2005). The Iowa Gambling Task and the somatic marker hypothesis: Some questions and answers. *Trends in Cognitive Sciences* 9: 159–162.

Bechara, A., D. Tranel, and H. Damasio (2000). Characterization of the decision-making impairment of patients with bilateral lesions of the ventromedial prefrontal cortex. *Brain* 123: 2189–2202.

Becker, G. (1976). *The Economic Approach to Human Behavior*. Chicago: University of Chicago Press.

Becker, G. (1981). *A Treatise on the Family*. Cambridge, Mass.: Harvard University Press.

Becker, G., and K. Murphy (1988). A theory of rational addiction. *Journal of Political Economy* 96: 675–700.

Bergh, C., T. Eklund, P. Sodersten, and C. Nordin (1997). Altered dopamine function in pathological gambling. *Psychological Medicine* 27: 473–475.

Berke, J., and S. Hyman (2000). Addiction, dopamine, and the molecular mechanisms of memory. *Neuron* 25: 515–532.

Berns, G. (2005). *Satisfaction*. New York: Henry Holt.

Berns, G., S. McClure, G. Pagnoni, and P. R. Montague (2001). Predictability modulates human brain response to reward. *Journal of Neuroscience* 21: 2793–2798.

Berridge, K., and T. Robinson (1998). What is the role of dopamine in reward: Hedonic impact, reward learning, or incentive salience? *Brain Research Reviews* 28: 309–369.

Berridge, K., and E. Valenstein (1991). What psychological process mediates feeding evoked by electrical stimulation of the lateral hypothalamus? *Behavioral Neuroscience* 105: 3–14.

Bickel, W., R. DeGrandpre, and S. Higgins (1993). Behavioral economics: A novel experimental approach to the study of drug dependence. *Drug and Alcohol Dependence* 33: 173 192.

Bickel, W., R. DeGrandpre, S. Higgins, and J. Hughes (1990). Behavioral economics of drug self-administration: I. Functional equivalence of response requirement and drug dose. *Life Sciences* 47: 1501–1510.

Bickel, W., R. DeGrandpre, J. Hughes, and S. Higgins (1991). Behavioral economics of drug self-administration: II. A unit-price analysis of cigarette smoking. *Journal of the Experimental Analysis of Behavior* 55: 145–154.

Bickel, W., and M. Johnson (2003). Delay discounting: A fundamental behavioral process of drug dependence. In *Time and Decision: Economic and Psychological Perspectives on Intertemporal Choice*, ed. G. Loewenstein, D. Read, and R. Baumeister, pp. 419–440. New York: Russel Sage Foundation.

Bickel, W., G. Madden, and N. Petry (1998). The price of change: The behavioral economics of drug dependence. *Behavior Therapy* 29: 545–565.

Bickel, W., and L. Marsch (2001). Toward a behavioral economic understanding of drug dependence: Delay discounting processes. *Addiction* 96: 73–86.

Bickel, W., A. Odum, and G. Madden (1999). Impulsivity and cigarette smoking: Delay discounting in current, never, and ex-smokers. *Psychopharmacology* 146: 447–454.

Billieux, J., M. Van der Linden, and G. Ceschi (2007). Which dimensions of impulsivity are related to cigarette craving? *Addictive Behaviors* 32: 1189–1199.

Bishop, M., and J. Trout (2004). *Epistemology and the Psychology of Human Judgment*. Oxford: Oxford University Press.

Bizot, J.-C., C. Le Bihan, A. Puech, M. Hamon, and M.-H. Thiébot (1999). Serotonin and tolerance to delay of reward in rats. *Psychopharmacology* 146: 400–412.

Bjork, K., B. Knutson, G. Fong, D. Caggiano, S. Bennett, and D. Hommer (2004). Incentive-elicited brain activation in adults: Similarities and differences from young adults. *Journal of Neuroscience* 24: 1793–1802.

Black, D. W. (2004). An open-label trial of bupropion in the treatment of pathological gambling. *Journal of Clinical Psychiatry* 24: 108–110.

Blair, R. (2001). Neurocognitive models of aggression, the antisocial personality disorders, and psychopathy. *Journal of Neurology and Neurosurgical Psychiatry* 71: 727–731.

Blair, R. (2003). Neurobiological basis of psychopathy. *British Journal of Psychiatry* 182: 5–7.

Blair, R., K. Peschardt, S. Budhani, D. Mitchell, and D. Pine (2006). The development of psychopathy. *Journal of Child Psychology and Psychiatry* 47: 262–275.

Blanco, C., D. Hasin, N. Petry, F. Stinson, and B. Grant (2006). Sex differences in subclinical and *DSM-IV* pathological gambling: Results from the National Epidemiologic Survey on Alcohol and Related Conditions. *Psychological Medicine* 36: 943–953.

Blanco, C., A. Ibáñez, C.-R. Blanco-Jerez, E. Baca-Garcia, and J. Sáiz-Ruiz (2001). Plasma testosterone and pathological gambling. *Psychiatry Research* 105: 117–121.

Blanco, C., E. Petkova, A. Ibáñez, and J. Saiz-Ruiz (2002). A pilot placebo-controlled study of fluvoxamine for pathological gambling. *Annals of Clinical Psychiatry* 14: 9–15.

Blaszczynski, A. (2005). Conceptual and methodological issues in treatment outcome research. *Journal of Gambling Studies* 21: 5–11.

Blaszczynski, A., and L. Nower (2002). A pathways model of problem and pathological gambling. *Addiction* 97: 487–499.

Blaszczynski, A., Z. Steel, and N. McConaghy (1997). Impulsivity in pathological gambling: The antisocial impulsivist. *Addiction* 92: 75–87.

Blum, K., E. Braverman, J. Holder, J. F. Lubar, V. Monastra, D. Miller, J. O. Lubar, T. Chen, and D. Comings (2000). Reward deficiency syndrome: A biogenetic model for the diagnosis and treatment of impulsive, addictive and compulsive behaviors. *Journal of Psychoactive Drugs* 32: 1–112.

Blum, K., P. Sheridan, R. Wood, E. Braverman, T. Chen, and D. Comings (1995). Dopamine D2 receptor gene variants: Associative and linkage studies in impulsive-addictive-compulsive behavior. *Pharmacogenetics* 5: 121–141.

Bohus, M., C. Schmahl, and K. Lieb (2004). New developments in the neurobiology of borderline personality disorder. *Current Psychiatry Reports* 6: 43–50.

Bossaerts, P., and C. Plott (2004). Basic principles of asset pricing theory: Evidence from large-scale experimental financial markets. *Review of Finance* 8: 135–169.

Boulenguez, P., J. Rawlins, J. Chauveau, M. Joseph, S. Mitchell, and J. Gray (1996). Modulation of dopamine release in the nucleus accumbens by $5-HT_{1B}$ agonists: Involvement of the hippocampo-accumbens pathway. *Neuropharmacology* 35: 1521–1529.

Boyer, M., and M. Dickerson (2003). Attentional bias and addictive behaviour: Automaticity in a gambling-specific modified Stroop task. *Addiction* 98: 61–70.

Brand, M., E. Kalbe, K. Labudda, E. Fujiwara, J. Kessler, and H. Markowitsch (2005). Decision-making impairments in patients with pathological gambling. *Psychiatry Research* 133: 91–99.

Breiter, H., I. Aharon, D. Kahneman, A. Dale, and P. Shizgal (2001). Functional imaging of neural responses to expectancy and experience of monetary gains and losses. *Neuron* 30: 619–639.

Brewer, T., and J. Brown (2003). Principles of pleasure prediction: Specifying the neural dynamics of human reward learning. *Neuron* 38: 150–152.

Brin, M., and G. Stuck (2002). *Introduction to Dynamical Systems.* Cambridge: Cambridge University Press.

Bunzeck, N., and E. Düzel (2006). Absolute coding of stimulus novelty in the human substantia nigra/VTA. *Neuron* 51: 369–379.

Camerer, C., G. Loewenstein, and M. Rabin, eds. (2003). *Advances in Behavioral Economics.* Princeton: Princeton University Press.

Camille, N., G. Coricelli, J. Sallet, P. Pradet-Diehl, J.-R. Duhamel, and A. Stigu (2004). The involvement of the orbitofrontal cortex in the experience of regret. *Science* 304: 1167–1170.

Canadian Institute of Neurosciences, Mental Health and Addiction (2002). The brain from top to bottom. Http://www.thebrain.mcgill.ca/flash/i/i_03/i_03_cl/i_03_cl_que/i_03_cl_que.html/.

Caplin, A., and M. Dean (2007). The neuroeconomic theory of learning. *American Economic Review* 97: 148–152.

Carnes, P. (1977). *Don't Call It Love.* New York: Random House.

Carroll, M. (1996). Reducing drug abuse by enriching the environment with alternative non-drug reinforcers. In *Advances in Behavioral Economics: Vol. 3. Substance Use and Abuse,* ed. L. Green and J. Kagel, pp. 37–68. Norwood, N.J.: Ablex.

Catania, A. (1963). Concurrent performances: A baseline for the study of reinforcement magnitude. *Journal of the Experimental Analysis of Behavior* 6: 299–300.

Cavedini, P., G. Riboldi, R. Keller, A. D'Annucci, and L. Bellodi (2002). Frontal lobe dysfunction in pathological gambling patients. *Biological Psychiatry* 51: 334–341.

Chaloupka, F. (1991). Rational addictive behavior and cigarette smoking. *Journal of Political Economy* 99: 722–742.

Chaloupka, F., M. Grossman, and J. Tauras (1999). The demand for cocaine and marijuana by youth. In *The Economic Analysis of Substance Use and Abuse: An Integration of Econometric and Behavioral Economic Perspectives,* ed. F. Chaloupka, W. Bickel, M. Grossman, and H. Saffer, pp. 133–156. Chicago: University of Chicago Press.

Chambers, R. A., and M. Potenza (2003). Neurodevelopment, impulsivity and adolescent gambling. *Journal of Gambling Studies* 19: 53–84.

Chambers, R. A., J. Taylor, and M. Potenza (2003). Developmental neurocircuitry of motivation in adolescence: A critical period of addiction vulnerability. *American Journal of Psychiatry* 160: 1041–1052.

Chao, L., and R. Knight (1995). Human prefrontal lesions increase distractibility to irrelevant sensory inputs. *Neuroreport* 6: 1605–1610.

Chapman, G. (1996a). Expectations and preferences for sequences of health and money. *Organizational Behavior and Human Decision Processes* 67: 59–75.

Chapman, G. (1996b). Temporal discounting and utility for health and money. *Journal of Experimental Psychology: Learning, Memory, and Cognition* 22: 771–791.

Chiamulera, C. (2004). Cue reactivity in nicotine and tobacco dependence: A "multiple-action" model of nicotine as a primary reinforcement and as an enhancer of the effects of smoking-associated stimuli. *Brain Research Reviews* 48: 74–97.

Chiu, Y.-C., C.-H. Lin, J.-T. Huang, S. Lin, P.-L. Lee, and J.-C. Hsie (2005). Immediate gain is long-term loss: Are there foresighted decision makers in the Iowa Gambling Task? Presentation at the third meeting of the Society for Neuroeconomics, Kiawah Island, September 2005.

Chung, S., and R. Herrnstein (1967). Choice and delay of reinforcement. *Journal of the Experimental Analysis of Behavior* 10: 67–74.

Churchland, P., and T. Sejnowski (1992). *The Computational Brain*. Cambridge, Mass.: MIT Press.

Clark, A. (1997). *Being There*. Cambridge, Mass.: MIT Press.

Cleckley, H. (1941). *The Mask of Sanity*. St. Louis: Mosby.

Collins, P. (2003). *Gambling and the Public Interest*. Westport, Conn.: Praeger.

Comings, D., R. Rosenthal, and H. Lesieur (1996). A study of the dopamine D2 receptor gene in pathological gambling. *Pharmacogenetics* 6: 223–234.

Committee on the Social and Economic Impact of Pathological Gambling (1999). *Pathological Gambling: A Critical Review*. Washington, D.C.: National Academy Press.

Cox, B., M. Enns, and V. Michaud (2004). Comparisons between the South Oaks Gambling Screen and a *DSM-IV*-based interview in a community survey of problem gambling. *Canadian Journal of Psychiatry* 49: 258–264.

Cox, W., J. Fadardi, and E. Pothos (2006). The addiction-Stroop test: Theoretical considerations and procedural recommendations. *Psychological Bulletin* 132: 443–476.

Crockford, D., and N. el-Guebaly (1998a). Psychiatric comorbidity in pathological gambling. A critical review. *Canadian Journal of Psychiatry* 43: 43–50.

Crockford, D., and N. el-Guebaly (1998b). Naltrexone in the treatment of pathological gambling and alcohol dependence. *Canadian Journal of Psychiatry* 43: 86.

Crockford, D., B. Goodyear, J. Edwards, J. Quickfall, and N. el-Guebaly (2005). Cue-induced brain activity in pathological gamblers. *Biological Psychiatry* 58: 787–795.

Cubitt, R., and R. Sugden (2001). On money pumps. *Games and Economic Behavior* 37: 121–160.

Cunningham-Williams, R., L. Cottler, W. Compton, and E. Spitznagel (1998). Taking chances: Problem gambling and mental health disorders—Results from the St. Louis Epidemiological Catchment Area (ECA) study. *American Journal of Public Health* 88: 1093–1096.

Dannon, N., K. Lowengrub, Y. Gonopolski, E. Musin, and M. Kotler (2005a). Topiramate versus fluvoxamine in the treatment of pathological gambling: A randomized, blind-rater comparison study. *Clinical Neuropharmacology* 28: 6–10.

Dannon, N., K. Lowengrub, E. Musin, Y. Gonopolski, and M. Kotler (2005b). Sustained-release bupropion versus naltrexone in the treatment of pathological gambling: A preliminary blind-rater study. *Journal of Clinical Psychopharmacology* 25: 593–596.

Dannon, P., K. Lowengrub, M. Sasson, B. Shalgi, L. Tuson, Y. Saphir, and M. Kotler (2004). Comorbid psychiatric diagnoses in kleptomania and pathological gambling: A preliminary comparison study. *European Psychiatry* 19: 299–302.

Daw, N. (2003). Reinforcement learning models of the dopamine system and their behavioral implications. Doctoral dissertation, Carnegie Mellon University, Pittsburgh.

Dayan, P., and J. Williams (2006). Putting the computation back into computational modeling of psychiatric disorders. *Pharmacopsychiatry* 39: 50–51.

De la Gandara, J. J. (1999). Fluoxetine: Open-trial in pathological gambling. Presented at the 152nd Annual Meeting of the American Psychiatric Association, May 16–21. Washington, D.C. (abstract).

De Wit, H., J. Flory, A. Acheson, M. McCloskey, and S. Manuck (2007). IQ and nonplanning impulsivity are independently associated with delay discounting in middle-aged adults. *Personality and Individual Differences* 42: 111–121.

DeGrandpre, R., W. Bickel, J. Hughes, and S. Higgins (1992). Behavioral economics of drug self-administration: III. A reanalysis of the nicotine regulation hypothesis. *Psychopharmacology* 108: 1–10.

Dehaene, S., M. Kerszberg, and J.-P. Changeux (1998). A neuronal model of a global workspace in effortful cognitive tasks. *Proceedings of the National Academy of Sciences USA* 95: 14529–14534.

Dell'Osso, B., A. Allen, and E. Hollander (2005). Comorbidity issues in the pharmacological treatment of pathological gambling: A critical review. *Clinical Practice and Epidemiology in Mental Health* 1: 21.

Denburg, N., D. Tranel, and A. Bechara (2005). The ability to decide advantageously declines prematurely in some normal older persons. *Neuropsychologia* 43: 1099–1106.

Dennett, D. (1969). *Content and Consciousness*. London: Routledge and Kegan Paul.

Dennett, D. (1991). *Consciousness Explained*. Boston: Little, Brown.

Dias, R., T. Robbins, and A. Roberts (1996). Primate analogue of the Wisconsin Card Sorting Test: Effects of excitotoxic lesions of the prefrontal cortex in the marmoset. *Behavioral Neuroscience* 110: 872–886.

Dickerson, E., and E. Baron (2000). Contemporary issues and future directions for research into pathological gambling. *Addiction* 95: 1145–1159.

Dixon, M., J. Marley, and E. Jacobs (2003). Delay discounting by pathological gamblers. *Journal of Applied Behavior Analysis* 36: 449–458.

Dodd, M., K. Klos, J. Bower, Y. Geda, K. Josephs, and E. Ahlskog (2005). Pathological gambling caused by drugs used to treat Parkinson disease. *Archives of Neurology* 62: 1–5.

Dom, G., B. De Wilde, W. Hulstijn, and B. Sabbe (2007). Dimensions of impulsive behaviour in abstinent alcoholics. *Personality and Individual Differences* 42: 465–476.

Dorris, M., and P. Glimcher (2004). Activity in posterior parietal cortex is correlated with the relative subjective desirability of action. *Neuron* 44: 365–378.

Du, W., L. Green, and J. Myerson (2002). Cross-cultural comparisons of discounting delayed and probabilistic rewards. *Psychological Record* 52: 479–492.

Dumont, E., G. Mark, S. Mader, and J. Williams (2005). Self-administration enhances excitatory synaptic transmission in the bed nucleus of the stria terminalis. *Nature Neuroscience* 8: 413–414.

Durstewitz, D., M. Kelc, and O. Güntürkün (1999). A neurocomputational theory of the dopaminergic modulation of working memory functions. *Journal of Neuroscience* 19: 2807–2822.

Eagleman, D. (2005). Comment on "The involvement of the orbitofrontal cortex in the experience of regret." *Science* 308: 1260b.

Echeburúa, E., C. Baez, and J. Fernandez-Montalvo (1996). Comparative effectiveness of three therapeutic modalities in the psychological treatment of pathological gambling: Long-term outcome. *Behavioral and Cognitive Psychotherapy* 24: 51–72.

Edelman, G. (1987). *Neural Darwinism*. New York: Basic Books.

Eisen, S., N. Lin, M. Lyons, J. Scherrer, K. Griffith, W. True, J. Goldberg, and M. Tsuang (1998). Familial influences on gambling behavior: An analysis of 3359 twin pairs. *Addiction* 93: 1375–1384.

Evans, C., K. Kemish, and O. Turnbull (2004). Paradoxical effects of education on the Iowa Gambling Task. *Brain and Cognition* 54: 240–244.

Evenden, J. (1999). Varieties of impulsivity. *Psychopharmacology* 146: 348–361.

Everitt, B., A. Dickinson, and T. Robbins (2001). The neuropsychological basis of addictive behavior. *Brain Research Reviews* 36: 129–138.

Everitt, B., and T. Robbins (2005). Neural systems of reinforcement for drug addiction: From actions to habit to compulsion. *Nature Neuroscience* 8: 1481–1489.

Eysenck, S. B. G., and H. J. Eysenck (1978). Impulsiveness and venturesomeness: Their position in a dimensional system of personality description. *Psychological Reports* 43: 1247–1255.

Feigelman, W., P. Kleinman, H. Lesieur, R. Millman, and M. Lesser (1995). Pathological gambling among methadone patients. *Drug and Alcohol Dependence* 39: 75–81.

Fellows, L., and M. Farah (2005). Dissociable elements of human foresight: A role for the ventromedial frontal lobes in framing the future, but not in discounting future rewards. *Neuropsychologia* 43: 1214–1221.

Ferris, J., and H. Wynne (2001a). The Canadian Problem Gambling Index Draft User Manual. Http://www.ccsa.ca/NR/rdonlyres/4F76DA2F-8304-4E5E-8B02-187C0F8FA40B/0/ccsa0093812001.pdf.

Ferris, J., and H. Wynne (2001b). The Canadian Problem Gambling Index: Final Report. Http://www.ccsa.ca/NR/rdonlyres/58BD1AA0-047A-41EC-906E-87F8FF46C91B/0/ccsa0088052001.pdf.

Field, M., B. Eastwood, B. Bradley, and K. Mogg (2006). Selective processing of cannabis cues in regular cannabis users. *Drug and Alcohol Dependence* 85: 75–82.

Flavell, J. H. (1979). Metacognition and cognitive monitoring: A new area of cognitive-developmental inquiry. *American Psychologist* 34: 906–911.

Fonagy, P., G. Gergely, E. Jurist, and M. Target (2002). *Affect Regulation, Mentalization, and the Development of Self.* New York: Other Press.

Forzano, L., and A. Logue (1992). Self-control in adult humans: Comparison of qualitatively different reinforcers. *Learning and Motivation* 25: 65–82.

Frank, R. (1992). Frames of reference and the intertemporal wage profile. In *Choice Over Time*, ed. G. Loewenstein and J. Elster, pp. 265–284. New York: Russel Sage Foundation.

Frederick, S., G. Loewenstein, and T. O'Donoghue (2003). Time discounting and time preference: A critical review. In *Time and Decision: Economic and Psychological Perspectives on Intertemporal Choice*, ed. G. Loewenstein, D. Read, and R. Baumeister, pp. 13–88. New York: Russel Sage Foundation

Friedman, M. (1957). *A Theory of the Consumption Function.* Princeton: Princeton University Press.

Fuster, J. (2004). Upper processing stages of the perception–action cycle. *Trends in Cognitive Sciences* 8: 143–145.

Gaboury, A., R. Ladouceur, G. Beauvais, L. Marchand, and Y. Martineau (1988). Cognitive and behavioral dimensions in regular and occasional blackjack players. *International Journal of Psychology* 23: 283–291.

Galanter, M., ed. (1997). *Recent Developments in Alcoholism, Vol. 13. Alcohol and Violence: Epidemiology, Neurobiology, Psychology, Family Issues.* New York: Plenum Press.

Gallistel, C. (1990). *The Organization of Learning.* Cambridge, Mass.: MIT Press.

Gallistel, C., and J. Gibbon (2000). Time, rate and conditioning. *Psychological Review* 107: 289–344.

Garavan, H., and J. Stout (2005). Neurocognitive insights into substance abuse. *Trends in Cognitive Sciences* 9: 195–201.

Garavan, H., J. Pankiewicz, A. Bloom, J. Cho, L. Sperry, T. Ross, B. Salmeron, R. Risinger, D. Kelley, and E. Stein (2000). Cue-induced cocaine craving: Neuroanatomical specificity for drug users and drug stimuli. *American Journal of Psychiatry* 157: 1789–1798.

Gehring, W., and A. Willoughby (2002). The medial frontal cortex and the rapid processing of monetary gains and losses. *Science* 295: 2279–2282.

Gerlach, K., K. Cummings, A. Hyland, E. Gilpin, M. Johnson, and J. Pierce (1998). *Cigars: Health Effects and Trends.* Http://cancercontrol.cancer.gov/tcrb/monographs/9/m9_2 .pdf/.

Gerstein, D., R. Volberg, M. Toce, R. Harwood, E. Christiansen, and J. Hoffman (1999). *Gambling Impact and Behavior Study.* Report to the National Gambling Impact Study Commission. Chicago: National Opinion Research Center.

Gibbon, J. (1977). Scalar expectancy theory and Weber's Law in animal timing. *Psychological Review* 84: 279–335.

Giordano, L., W. Bickel, G. Loewenstein, E. Jacobs, L. Marsch, and G. Badger (2002). Mild opioid deprivation increases the degree that opioid-dependent outpatients discount delayed heroin and money. *Psychopharmacology* 163: 174–182.

Glicksohn, J., R. Naor-Ziv, and R. Leshem (2007). Impulsive decision-making: Learning to gamble wisely? *Cognition* 105: 195–205.

Glimcher, P. (2003). *Decisions, Uncertainty, and the Brain*. Cambridge, Mass.: MIT Press.

Glimcher, P., J. Kable, and K. Louie (2007). Neuroeconomic studies of impulsivity: Now or just as soon as possible? *American Economic Review* 97: 142–147.

Glimcher, P., and B. Lau (2005). Rethinking the thalamus. *Nature Neuroscience* 8: 983–984.

Glimcher, P., and A. Rustichini (2004). Neuroeconomics: The consilience of brain and decision. *Science* 306: 447–452.

Goldman-Rakic, P. (1992). Working memory and the mind. *Scientific American* 267: 110–117.

Goldstein, R., and N. Volkow (2002). Drug addiction and its underlying neurobiological basis: Neuroimaging evidence for the involvement of the prefrontal cortex. *American Journal of Psychiatry* 159: 1642–1652.

Gosling, S., and S. Vazire (2002). Are we barking up the right tree? Evaluating a comparative approach to personality. *Journal of Research in Personality* 36: 607–614.

Goudriaan, A., J. Oosterlaan, E. De Beurs, and W. Van den Brink (2004a). Decision making in pathological gambling: A comparison between pathological gamblers, alcohol dependents, persons with Tourette syndrome, and normal controls. *Cognitive Brain Research* 23: 137–151.

Goudriaan, A., J. Oosterlaan, E. De Beurs, and W. Van den Brink (2004b). Pathological gambling: A comprehensive review of biobehavioral findings. *Neuroscience and Biobehavioral Reviews* 28: 123–141.

Grace, R. (1994). A contextual model of concurrent chains choice. *Journal of the Experimental Analysis of Behavior* 61: 113–129.

Graham, K. (1980). Theories of intoxicated aggression. *Canadian Journal of Behavior Science* 12: 141–158.

Granfield, R., and W. Cloud (2001). Social context and "natural recovery": The role of social capital in the resolution of drug-associated problems. *Substance Use and Misuse* 36: 1543–1570.

Grant, J., S. Kim, and M. Potenza (2003). Advances in the pharmacological treatment of pathological gambling. *Journal of Gambling Studies* 19: 85–109.

Grant, J., S. Kim, M. Potenza, and C. Blanco (2003). Paroxetine treatment of pathological gambling: A multi-centre randomized controlled trial. *International Clinical Psychopharmacology* 18: 243–249.

Grant, J., M. Steinberg, S. Kim, B. Rounsaville, and M. Potenza (2004). Preliminary validity and reliability testing of a structured clinical interview for pathological gambling. *Psychiatry Research* 128: 79–88.

Grant, J. E., and M. Potenza (2006). Escitalopram treatment of pathological gambling with co-occurring anxiety: An open-label pilot study with double-blind discontinuation. *International Clinical Psychopharmacology* 21: 203–209.

Grant, J. E., M. Potenza, E. Hollander, R. Cunningham-Williams, T. Nurminen, G. Smits, and A. Kallio (2006). Multicenter investigation of the opioid antagonist Nalmefene in the treatment of pathological gambling. *American Journal of Psychiatry* 163: 303–312.

Gray, P. (2004). Evolutionary and cross-cultural perspectives on gambling. *Journal of Gambling Studies* 20: 347–371.

Green, L., and D. Holt (2003). Economic and biological influences on key pecking and treadle pressing in pigeons. *Journal of the Experimental Analysis of Behavior* 80: 43–58.

Green, L., A. Fry, and J. Myerson (1994). Discounting of delayed rewards: A life-span comparison. *Psychological Science* 5: 33–36.

Green, L., and J. Myerson (2004). A discounting framework for choice with delayed and probabilistic rewards. *Psychological Bulletin* 130: 769–792.

Green, L., J. Myerson, and E. Macaux (2005). Temporal discounting when the choice is between two delayed rewards. *Journal of Experimental Psychology: Learning, Memory, and Cognition* 31: 1121–1133.

Green, L., J. Myerson, and E. McFadden (1997). Rate of temporal discounting decreases with amount of reward. *Memory and Cognition* 25: 715–723.

Green, L., J. Myerson, and P. Ostaszewski (1999). Amount of reward has opposite effects on the discounting of delayed and probabilistic outcomes. *Journal of Experimental Psychology: Learning, Memory, and Cognition* 25: 418–427.

Green, L., and H. Rachlin (1975). Economic and biological influences on the pigeon's key peck. *Journal of the Experimental Analysis of Behavior* 23: 55–62.

Griffiths, M. (1994). The role of cognitive bias and skill in fruit machine playing. *British Journal of Psychology* 85: 365–372.

Griffiths, M. (2000). Excessive Internet use: Implications for sexual behavior. *Cyberpsychological Behavior* 3: 537–552.

Grosset, K. A., G. Macphee, G. Pal, D. Stewart, A. Watt, J. Davie, and D. G. Grosset (2006). Problematic gambling on dopamine agonists: Not such a rarity. *Movement Disorders* 21: 2206–2208.

Gul, F., and W. Pesendorfer (2001). Temptation and self control. *Econometrica* 69: 1403–1436.

Gul, F., and W. Pesendorfer (2005). The simple theory of temptation and self-control. Http://www.princeton.edu/~pesendor/finite.pdf/.

Gul, F., and W. Pesendorfer (forthcoming). The case for mindless economics. In *The Handbook of Economic Methodologies*, vol. 1, ed. A. Caplin and A. Schotter. Oxford: Oxford University Press.

Gulledge, A., and D. Jaffe (2001). Multiple effects of dopamine on layer V pyramidal cell excitability in rat prefrontal cortex. *Journal of Neurophysiology* 86: 586–595.

Hacking, I. (1999). *The Social Construction of What?* Cambridge, Mass.: Harvard University Press.

Hair, P., and S. Hampson (2006). The role of impulsivity in predicting maladaptive behaviour among female students. *Personality and Individual Differences* 40: 943–952.

Haller, R., and H. Hinterhuber (1994). Treatment of pathological gambling with carbamazepine. *Pharmacopsychiatry* 27: 129.

Halpern-Felsher, B., S. Millstein, and J. Ellen (1996). Relationship of alcohol use and risky sexual behavior: A review and analysis of findings. *Journal of Adolescent Health* 19: 331–336.

Hardoon, K., H. Baboushkin, J. Derevensky, and R. Gupta (2001). Underlying cognitions in the selection of lottery tickets. *Journal of Clinical Psychology* 57: 749–763.

Hare, R. (1991). *The Hare Psychopathy Checklist-Revised Manual*. Toronto: Multi-Health Systems.

Harinder, A., P. Sokoloff, and R. J. Beninger (2002). A dopamine D3 receptor partial agonist blocks the expression of conditioned activity. *Learning and Memory* 13: 1–4.

Hariri, A., S. Brown, D. Williamson, J. Flory, H. de Wit, and S. Manuck (2006). Preference for immediate over delayed rewards is associated with magnitude of ventral striatal activity. *Journal of Neuroscience* 26: 13213–13217.

Harmsen, H., G. Bischof, A. Brooks, F. Hohagen, and H.-J. Rumpf (2005). The relationship between impaired decision-making, sensation seeking and readiness to change in cigarette smokers. *Addictive Behaviors* 31: 581–592.

Hayes, S. C., K. Strosahl, and K. G. Wilson (1999). *Acceptance and Commitment Therapy: An Experiential Approach to Behavior Change*. New York: Guilford.

Henningfield, J., C. Cohen, and W. Pickworth (1993). Psychopharmacology of nicotine. In *Nicotine Addiction: Principles and Management*, ed. C. Orleans and J. Slade, pp. 24–45. New York: Oxford University Press.

Henningfield, J., L. Schuh, and M. Jarvik (1995). Pathophysiology of tobacco dependence. In *Psychopharmacology: The Fourth Generation of Progress*, ed. F. Bloom and D. Kupfer, pp. 1715–1729. New York: Raven Press.

Herrnstein, R. (1961). Relative and absolute strength of response as a function of frequency of reinforcement. *Journal of the Experimental Analysis of Behavior* 4: 267–272.

Herrnstein, R. (1970). On the law of effect. *Journal of the Experimental Analysis of Behavior* 13: 243–266.

Herrnstein, R. (1997). *The Matching Law: Papers in Psychology and Economics by Richard Herrnstein*. Ed. H. Rachlin and D. Laibson. Cambridge, Mass.: Harvard University Press.

Herrnstein, R. (1982). Melioration as behavioral dynamism. In *Quantitative Analyses of Behavior, Vol. II: Matching and Maximizing Accounts*, ed. M. Commons, R. Herrnstein, and H. Rachlin, pp. 433–458. Cambridge, Mass.: Ballinger. Reprinted in Rachlin and Laibson 1997, pp. 74–99.

Herrnstein, R., and D. Prelec (1992). A theory of addiction. In *Choice Over Time*, ed. G. Loewenstein and J. Elster, pp. 331–360. New York: Russell Sage Foundation.

Hester, R., V. Dixon, and H. Garavan (2006). A consistent attentional bias for drug-related material in active cocaine users across word and picture versions of the emotional Stroop task. *Drug and Alcohol Dependence* 81: 251–257.

Heyman, G. (1996). Resolving the contradictions of addiction. *Behavioral and Brain Sciences* 19: 561–610.

Heyman, G. (1998). On "the science of substance abuse." *Science* 280: 807–808.

Heyman, G., and R. Herrnstein (1986). More on concurrent ratio-interval schedules: A replication and review. *Journal of the Experimental Analysis of Behavior* 46: 331–351.

Higgins, S., S. Heil, and J. Lussier (2004). Clinical implications of reinforcement as a determinant of substance use disorders. *Annual Reviews of Psychology* 55: 431–461.

Hoch, S., and G. Loewenstein (1991). Time-inconsistent preferences and consumer self-control. *Journal of Consumer Research* 17: 492–507.

Hodgins, C., K. Makarchuk, N. el-Guebaly, and N. Peden (2002). Why problem gamblers quit gambling: A comparison of methods and samples. *Addiction Research and Theory* 10: 203–218.

Hollander, E., C. DeCaria, J. Finkell, T. Begaz, C. Wong, and C. Cartwright (2000). A randomized double-blind fluvoxamine/placebo crossover trial in pathologic gambling. *Biological Psychiatry* 47: 813–817.

Hollander, E., C. DeCaria, E. Mari, C. Wong, S. Mosovich, R. Grossman, and T. Begaz (1998). Short-term single-blind fluvoxamine treatment of pathological gambling. *American Journal of Psychiatry* 155: 1781–1783.

Hollander, E., M. Frenkel, C. DeCaria, S. Trungold, and D. J. Stein (1992). Treatment of pathological gambling with clomipramine. *American Journal of Psychiatry* 149: 710–711.

Hollander, E., S. Pallanti, A. Allen, E. Sood, and N. Baldini-Rossi (2005a). Does sustained-release lithium reduce impulsive gambling and affective instability versus placebo in pathological gamblers with bipolar spectrum disorders? *American Journal of Psychiatry* 162: 137–145.

Hollander, E., E. Sood, S. Pallanti, N. Baldini-Rossi, and B. Baker (2005b). Pharmacological treatments of pathological gambling. *Journal of Gambling Studies* 21: 99–108.

Holt, D., L. Green, and J. Myerson (2003). Is discounting impulsive? Evidence from temporal and probability discounting in gambling and non-gambling college students. *Behavioural Processes* 64: 355–367.

Hooper, C., M. Luciana, H. Conklin, and R. Yarger (2004). Adolescents' performance on the Iowa Gambling Task: Implications for the development of decision making and ventromedial prefrontal cortex. *Developmental Psychology* 40: 1148–1158.

Horn, N., M. Dolan, R. Elliott, J. Deakin, and P. Woodruff (2003). Response inhibition and impulsivity: An fMRI study. *Neuropsychologia* 41: 1959–1966.

Houston, A., A. Kacelnik, and J. McNamara (1982). Some learning rules for acquiring information. In *Functional Ontogeny*, ed. D. McFarland, pp. 140–191. Boston: Pitman.

Ibáñez, A., C. Blanco, I. Perez de Castro, J. Fernandez-Piqueras, and J. Sáiz-Ruiz (2003). Genetics of pathological gambling. *Journal of Gambling Studies* 19: 11–22.

Ichikawa, J., and H. Meltzer (1995). Effect of antidepressants on striatal and accumbens extracellular dopamine levels. *European Journal of Pharmacology* 281: 255–261.

Jaroni, J., S. Wright, C. Lerman, and L. Epstein (2004). Relationship between education and delay discounting in smokers. *Addictive Behaviors* 29: 1171–1175.

Kable, J., and P. Glimcher (unpublished). Matching mental and neural representations of value during intemporal choice. Http://www.cns.nyu.edu/events/neuroecon/ KableGlimcher.pdf/.

Kagel, J., and A. Roth, eds. (1995). *The Handbook of Behavioral Economics*. Princeton: Princeton University Press.

Kahneman, D., and A. Tversky (1979). Prospect theory: An analysis of decision under risk. *Econometrica* 47: 263–269.

Kalenscher, T., S. Windmann, B. Diekamp, J. Rose, O. Güntürkün, and M. Colombo (2005). Single units in the pigeon brain integrate reward amount and time-to-reward in an impulsive control task. *Current Biology* 15: 594–602.

Kalivas, P., N. Volkow, and J. Seamans (2005). Unmanageable motivation in addiction: A pathology in prefrontal-accumbens glutamate transmission. *Neuron* 45: 647–650.

Kelley, A. (2004). Memory and addiction: Shared neural circuitry and molecular mechanisms. *Neuron* 44: 161–179.

Kelso, S. (1995). *Dynamic Patterns*. Cambridge, Mass.: MIT Press.

Kerr, A., and P. Zelazo (2004). Development of "hot" executive function: The children's gambling task. *Brain and Cognition* 55: 148–157.

Kertzman, S., K. Lowengrub, A. Aizer, Z. Nahum, M. Kotler, and P. Dannon (2005). Stroop performance in pathological gamblers. *Psychiatry Research* 142: 1–10.

Kessler, R., K. Merikanagas, P. Berglund, W. Eaton, D. Koretz, and E. Walters (2003). Mild disorders should not be eliminated from the *DSM-IV*. *Archives of General Psychiatry* 60: 1117–1122.

Kim, J. (1999). *Mind in a Physical World*. Cambridge, Mass.: MIT Press.

Kim, S., and J. Grant (2001a). An open naltrexone treatment study of pathological gambling disorder. *International Clinical Psychopharmacology* 16: 285–289.

Kim, S., and J. Grant (2001b). The psychopharmacology of pathological gambling. *Seminars in Clinical Neuropsychiatry* 6: 184–194.

Kim, S., J. Grant, D. Adson, and R. Remmel (2001). Double-blind naltrexone and placebo comparison study in the treatment of pathological gambling. *Biological Psychiatry* 49: 914–921.

Kim, S., J. Grant, D. Adson, Y. Shin, and R. Zaninelli (2002). A double-blind, placebo-controlled study of the efficacy and safety of paroxetine in the treatment of pathological gambling. *Journal of Clinical Psychiatry* 63: 501–507.

Kim, S., J. Grant, G. Yoon, K. Williams, and R. Remmel (2006). Safety of high-dose naltrexone treatment: Hepatic transaminase profiles among outpatients. *Clinical Neuropharmacology* 29: 77–79.

Kirby, K. (1997). Bidding on the future: Evidence against normative discounting of delayed rewards. *Journal of Experimental Psychology: General* 126: 54–70.

Kirby, K., and B. Guastello (2001). Making choices in anticipation of similar future choices can increase self-control. *Journal of Experimental Psychology: Applied* 7: 154–164.

Kirby, K., and R. Herrnstein (1995). Preference reversals due to myopic discounting of delayed rewards. *Psychological Science* 6: 83–89.

Kirby, K., and N. Petry (2004). Heroin and cocaine abusers have higher discount rates for delayed rewards than alcoholics or non-drug-using controls. *Addiction* 99: 461–471.

Kirby K., N. Petry, and W. Bickel (1999). Heroin addicts discount delayed rewards at higher rates than non-drug using controls. *Journal of Experimental Psychology: General Processes* 128: 78–87.

Kirby, K., G. Winston, and M. Santiesteban (2005). Impatience and grades: Delay-discount rates correlate negatively with college GPA. *Learning and Individual Differences* 15: 213–222.

Kirk, J., and A. Logue (1997). Effects of deprivation level on humans' self-control for food reinforcers. *Appetite* 28: 215–226.

Kischka, U., T. Kammer, S. Maier, M. Weisbrod, M. Thimm, and M. Spitzer (1996). Dopaminergic modulation of semantic network activation. *Neuropsychologia* 34: 1107–1113.

Knight, R., and M. Grabowecky (1995). Escape from linear time: Prefrontal cortex and conscious experience. In *The Cognitive Neurosciences*, ed. M. Gazzaniga, pp. 1357–1371. Cambridge, Mass.: MIT Press.

Knutson, B., C. Adams, G. Fong, and D. Hommer (2001). Anticipation of increasing monetary reward selectively recruits nucleus accumbens. *Journal of Neuroscience* 21: RC159.

Knutson, B., S. Rick, G. Wimmer, D. Prelec, and G. Loewenstein (2007). Neural predictors of purchases. *Neuron* 53: 147–156.

Koechlin, E., C. Ody, and F. Kouneiher (2003). The architecture of cognitive control in the human prefrontal cortex. *Science* 302: 1181–1185.

Koepp, M., R. Gunn, A. Lawrence, V. Cunningham, A. Dagher, T. Jones, D. Brooks, C. Bench, and P. Grasby (1998). Evidence for striatal dopamine release during a video game. *Nature* 393: 266–268.

Kollins, S. (2003). Delay discounting is associated with substance use in college students. *Addictive Behaviors* 28: 1167–1173.

Koob, G. (2006). The neurobiology of addiction: A neuroadaptational view relevant for diagnosis. *Addiction* 101 (suppl. 1): 23–30.

Koob, G., and M. Le Moal (2000). Drug addiction, dysregulation of reward and allostasis. *Neuropsychopharmacology* 24: 1–129.

Koob, G., P. Paolo Sanna, and F. Bloom (1998). Neuroscience of addiction. *Neuron* 21: 467–476.

Krishnan-Sarin, S., B. Reynolds, A. Duhig, A. Smith, T. Liss, A. McFetridge, D. Cavallo, K. Carroll, and M. Potenza (2007). Behavioral impulsivity predicts treatment outcome in a smoking cessation program for adolescent smokers. *Drug and Alcohol Dependence* 88: 79–82.

Kudadjie-Gyamfi, E., and H. Rachlin (1996). Temporal patterning in choice among delayed outcomes. *Organizational Behavior and Human Decision Processes* 65: 61–67.

Kyngdon, A., and M. Dickerson (1999). An experimental study of the effect of prior alcohol consumption on a simulated gambling activity. *Addiction* 94: 697–707.

Laakso, A., A. Mohn, R. Gainetdinov, and M. Caron (2002). Experimental genetic approaches to addiction. *Neuron* 36: 213–228.

Ladd, G., and N. Petry (2002). Gender differences among pathological gamblers seeking treatment. *Experimental and Clinical Psychopharmacology* 10: 302–309.

Ladd, G., and N. Petry (2003). A comparison of pathological gamblers with and without substance abuse treatment histories. *Experimental and Clinical Psychopharmacology* 11: 202–209.

Ladouceur, R., J. Boisvert, and J. Dumont (1994). Cognitive-behavioral treatment for adolescent pathological gamblers. *Behavior Modification* 18: 230–242.

Ladouceur, R., C. Sylvain, C. Boutin, S. Lachance, C. Doucet, and J. Leblond (2003). Group therapy for pathological gamblers: A cognitive approach. *Behavior Research and Therapy* 41: 587–596.

Ladouceur, R., C. Sylvain, C. Boutin, S. Lachance, C. Doucet, J. Leblond, and C. Jacques (2001). Cognitive treatment of pathological gambling. *Journal of Nervous and Mental Disease* 189: 774–780.

Ladouceur, R., C. Sylvain, H. Letarte, I. Giroux, and C. Jacques (1998). Cognitive treatment of pathological gamblers. *Behavior Research and Therapy* 36: 1111–1119.

Ladyman, J., and D. Ross (2007). *Every Thing Must Go: Metaphysics Naturalised.* Oxford: Oxford University Press.

Laibson, D. (1997). Golden eggs and hyperbolic discounting. *Quarterly Journal of Economics* 112: 443–477.

Laibson, D. (1998). Life-cycle consumption and hyperbolic discount functions. *European Economic Review* 42: 861–871.

Laibson, D., A. Repetto, and J. Tobacman (1998). Self-control and saving for retirement. *Brookings Papers on Economic Activity* 1: 91–196.

Lau, M., R. Pihl, and J. Peterson (1995). Provocation, acute alcohol intoxication, cognitive performance, and aggression. *Journal of Abnormal Psychology* 104: 150–155.

Laviolette, S., and D. van der Kooy (2004). The neurobiology of nicotine addiction: Bridging the gap from molecules to behaviour. *Nature Reviews Neuroscience* 5: 55–65.

Lejoyeux, M., J. Ades, V. Tassein, and J. Solomon (1996). Phenomenology and psychopathology of uncontrolled buying. *American Journal of Psychiatry* 153: 1524–1529.

Lesieur, H. (1987). Gambling, pathological gambling and crime. In *The Handbook of Pathological Gambling*, ed. T. Galski, pp. 89–110. Springfield: Charles H. Thomas.

Lesieur, H., and S. Blume (1987). The South Oaks Gambling Screen (The SOGS): A new instrument for the identification of problem gamblers. *American Journal of Psychiatry* 144: 1184–1188.

Leung, S.-F., and C. Phelps (1993). "My kingdom for a drink . . . ?" A review of the estimates of the price sensitivity of demand for alcoholic beverages. In *Economics and the Prevention of Alcohol-Related Problems*, ed. M. Hilton and G. Bloss, pp. 1–31. Rockville, Maryland: National Institute on Alcohol Abuse and Alcoholism Research Monograph No. 25. NIH Pub. No. 93–3513.

Levine, H. (1978). The discovery of addiction: Changing conceptions of habitual drunkenness in America. *Journal of Studies on Alcohol* 39: 143–174.

Liberman, N., and Y. Trope (2003). Construal level theory of intertemporal judgment and decision. In *Time and Decision: Economic and Psychological Perspectives on Intertemporal Choice*, ed. G. Loewenstein, D. Read, and K. Baumeister, pp. 245–276. New York: Russel Sage Foundation.

Lindsley, O. R., B. F. Skinner, and H. C. Solomon (1953). *Studies in Behavior Therapy. Status Report 1*. Waltham, Mass.: Metropolitan State Hospital.

Loewenstein, G. (1996). Out of control: Visceral influences on behavior. *Organizational Behavior and Human Decision Processes* 65: 272–292.

Loewenstein, G. (1999). A visceral account of addiction. In *Getting Hooked: Rationality and Addiction*, ed. J. Elster and O.-J. Skog, pp. 235–264. Cambridge, Mass.: Cambridge University Press.

Loewenstein, G., and D. Prelec (1992). Anomalies in intertemporal choice: Evidence and an interpretation. *Quarterly Journal of Economics* 107: 573–597.

Loewenstein, G., and D. Prelec (1993). Preferences for sequences of outcomes. *Psychological Review* 100: 91–108.

Logue, A., G. King, A. Chavarro, and J. Volpe (1990). Matching and maximizing in a self-control paradigm using human subjects. *Learning and Motivation* 21: 340–368.

Logue, A., and T. Peña-Correal (1985). The effect of food deprivation on self-control. *Behavioural Processes* 10: 355–368.

Logue, A., T. Peña-Correal, M. Rodriguez, and E. Kabela (1986). Self-control in adult humans: Variation in positive reinforcer amount and delay. *Journal of the Experimental Analysis of Behavior* 46: 159–173.

MacKillop, J., E. Anderson, B. Castelda, R. Mattson, and P. J. Donovick (2006). Divergent validity of measures of cognitive distortions, impulsivity, and time perspective in pathological gambling. *Journal of Gambling Studies* 22: 339–354.

Madden, G., W. Bickel, and E. Jacobs (1999). Discounting of delayed rewards in opioid-dependent outpatients: Exponential or hyperbolic discounting functions. *Experimental and Clinical Psychopharmacology* 7: 284–293.

Madden, G., N. Petry, G. Badger, and W. Bickel (1997). Impulsive and self-control choices in opioid-dependent subjects and non-drug using controls: Drug and monetary rewards. *Experimental and Clinical Psychopharmacology* 5: 256–262.

Mahoney, M. J. (1974). *Cognition and Behavior Modification*. Cambridge, Mass.: Ballinger.

Maia, T., and J. McClelland (2004). A reexamination of the evidence for the somatic marker hypothesis: What participants really know in the Iowa Gambling Task. *Proceedings of the National Academy of Sciences* 101: 16075–16080.

Mandler, M. (1999). *Dilemmas in Economic Theory*. Oxford: Oxford University Press.

Marks, I. (1990). Behavioural (non-chemical) addictions. *British Journal of Addictions* 85: 1389–1394.

Martin-Soelch, C., K. Leenders, A. Chevally, J. Missimer, G. Künig, S. Magyar, A. Milno, and W. Schultz (2001). Reward mechanisms in the brain and their role in dependence: Evidence from neurophysiological and neuroimaging studies. *Brain Research Reviews* 36: 139–149.

May, J. C., M. Delgado, R. Dahl, V. A. Stenger, N. Ryan, J. Fiez, and C. Carter (2004). Event-related functional magnetic resonance imaging of reward-related brain circuitry in children and adolescents. *Biological Psychiatry* 55: 359–366.

Mazur, J. (1987). An adjusting procedure for studying delayed reinforcement. In *Quantitative Analysis of Behavior Vol. 5: The Effect of Delay and of Intervening Events on Reinforcement Value*, ed. M. Commons, J. Mazur, J. Nevin, and H. Rachlin, pp. 55–73. Hillsdale, N.J.: Lawrence Erlbaum.

Mazur, J. (2001). Hyperbolic value addition and general models of animal choice. *Psychological Review* 108: 96–112.

McCarthy, G., A. Blamire, A. Puce, A. Nobre, G. Bloch, H. Fahmeed, P. Goldman-Rakic, and R. Shulman (1994). Functional magnetic resonance imaging of human prefrontal cortex activation during a spatial working memory task. *Proceedings of the National Academy of Sciences* 91: 8690–8694.

McClure, S., G. Berns, and R. Montague (2003). Temporal prediction errors in a passive learning task activate human striatum. *Neuron* 38: 339–346.

McClure, S., N. Daw, and R. Montague (2003). A computational substrate for incentive salience. *Trends in Neuroscience* 26: 423–428.

McClure, S., D. Laibson, G. Loewenstein, and J. Cohen (2004). Separate neural systems value immediate and delayed monetary rewards. *Science* 306: 503–507.

McConaghy, N., M. Armstrong, A. Blaszczynski, and C. Allcock (1983). Controlled comparison of aversive therapy and imaginal desensitization in compulsive gambling. *British Journal of Psychiatry* 142: 366–372.

McConaghy, N., M. Armstrong, A. Blaszczynski, and C. Allcock (1988). Behavior completion versus stimulus control in compulsive gambling: Implications for behavioral assessment. *Behavior Modification* 12: 371–384.

McConaghy, N., A. Blaszczynski, and A. Frankova (1991). Comparisons of imaginal desensitization with other behavioral treatment of pathological gambling: A two- to nine-year follow-up. *British Journal of Psychiatry* 159: 390–393.

McCulloch, W., and W. Pitts (1943). A logical calculus of the ideas immanent in nervous activity. *Bulletin of Mathematical Biophysics* 5: 115–133.

Meichenbaum, D. (1977). *Cognitive-Behavior Modification*. New York: Plenum Publishing.

Meier, S., T. Brigham, D. Ward, F. Meyers, and L. Warren (1996). Effects of blood alcohol concentrations on negative punishment: implications for decision making. *Journal of Studies on Alcohol* 57: 85–96.

Meyer, G., J. Schwertfeger, M. Exton, O. Janssen, W. Knapp, M. Stadler, M. Schledowski, and T. Krüger (2004). Neuroendocrine response to casino gambling in problem gamblers. *Psychoneuroendocrinology* 29: 1272–1280.

Miller, E. (2000). The prefrontal cortex and cognitive control. *Nature Reviews Neuroscience* 1: 59–65.

Miller, E., and J. Cohen (2001). An integrative theory of prefrontal cortex function. *Annual Review of Neuroscience* 24: 167–202.

Milner, B. (1963). Effects of different brain lesions on card sorting. *Archives of Neurology* 9: 90–100.

Mintzer, M., and L. Stitzer (2002). Cognitive impairment in methadone maintenance patients. *Drug and Alcohol Dependence* 67: 41–51.

Mirenowicz, J., and W. Schultz (1996). Preferential activation of midbrain dopamine neurons by appetitive rather than aversive stimuli. *Nature* 379: 449–451.

Mitchell, S. (1999). Measures of impulsivity in cigarette smokers and non-smokers. *Psychopharmacology* 146: 455–464.

Montague, P. R. (2006). *Why Choose This Book?* New York: Dutton.

Montague, P. R., and G. Berns (2002). Neural economics and the biological substrates of valuation. *Neuron* 36: 265–284.

Montague, P. R., P. Dayan, and T. Sejnowski (1996). A framework for mesencephalic dopamine systems based on predictive Hebbian learning. *Journal of Neuroscience* 16: 1936–1947.

Montague, P. R., B. King-Cassas, and J. Cohen (2006). Imaging valuation models in human choice. *Annual Review of Neuroscience* 29: 417–448.

Monterosso, J., and G. Ainslie (1999). Beyond discounting: Possible experimental models of impulse control. *Psychopharmacology* 146: 339–347.

Monterosso, J., R. Ehrman, K. Napier, C. O'Brien, and A. Childress (2001). Three decision-making tasks in cocaine-dependent patients: Do they measure the same construct? *Addiction* 96: 1825–1837.

Moskowitz, J. (1980). Lithium and lady luck: Use of lithium carbonate in compulsive gambling. *New York State Journal of Medicine* 80: 785–788.

Müller, A., H. Reinecker, C. Jacobi, L. Reisch, and M. de Zwaan (2004). Pathologisches Kaufen: Eine Literaturübersicht. *Pathologische Praxis* 31: 1–10.

Murphy, J., C. Correia, S. Colby, and R. Vuchinich (2005). Using behavioral theories of choice to predict drinking outcomes following a brief intervention. *Experimental and Clinical Psychopharmacology* 13: 93–101.

Murphy, J., R. Vuchinich, and C. Simpson (2001). Delayed reward and cost discounting. *The Psychological Record* 51: 571–588.

Murrell, B., D. Spurrett, A. Hofmeyr, S. Dellis, P. Schwardman, C. Sharp, J. Rousseau, R. Vuchinich, and D. Ross (2006). Problem gambling severity and disposition to bundle rewards in South African gamblers. Poster presentation at the 7th annual National Center for Responsible Gambling Conference on Gambling and Addiction, Las Vegas, November 12–14, 2005.

Myerson, J., and L. Green (1995). Discounting of delayed rewards: Models of individual choice. *Journal of the Experimental Analysis of Behavior* 64: 263–276.

Nakahara, H., H. Itoh, R. Kawagoe, Y. Takikawa, and O. Hikosaka (2004). Dopamine neurons can represent context-dependent prediction error. *Neuron* 41: 269–280.

Nasqvi, N., D. Rudrauf, H. Damasio, and A. Bechara (2007). Damage to the insula disrupts addiction to cigarette smoking. *Science* 315: 531–534.

Nathan, P. (2005a). Commentary. *Journal of Gambling Studies* 21: 355–361.

Nathan, P. (2005b). Methodological problems in research on treatments for pathological gambling. *Journal of Gambling Studies* 21: 109–114.

National Gambling Impact Study Commission (1999). *National Gambling Impact Study Commission Final Report.* Http://govinfo.library.unt.edu/ngisc/reports/finrpt.html/.

Navarick, D. (1982). Negative reinforcement and choice in humans. *Learning and Motivation* 13: 361–377.

Navarick, D. (1986). Human impulsivity and choice: A challenge to traditional operant methodology. *Psychological Record* 36: 343–356.

Neville, M., E. Johnstone, and R. Walton (2004). Identification and characterization of ANKK1: A novel kinase gene closely linked to DRD2 on chromosome band 11q23.1. *Human Mutation* 23: 540–545.

Niesink, R., R. Jaspers, L. Kornet, and J. van Ree, eds. (1999). *Drugs of Abuse and Addiction: Neurobehavioral Toxicology.* Boca Raton, Fla.: CRC Press.

Nieuwenhuis, S., D. Heslenfeld, N. Alting von Geusau, R. Mars, C. Holroyd, and N. Yeung (2004). Activity in human reward-sensitive brain areas is strongly context dependent. *NeuroImage* 25: 1302–1309.

Noë, R., J. van Hoof, and P. Hammerstein, eds. (2001). *Economics in Nature.* Cambridge: Cambridge University Press.

Nordin, C., and T. Eklundh (1999). Altered CSF 5-H1AA disposition in pathological male gamblers. *CNS Spectrums* 4: 25–33.

O'Donoghue, T., and M. Rabin (1999). Incentives for procrastinators. *Quarterly Journal of Economics* 114: 769–816.

Odum, A., G. Madden, G. Badger, and W. Bickel (2000). Needle sharing in opioid-dependent outpatients: Psychological processes underlying risk. *Drug and Alcohol Dependence* 60: 259–266.

Orsini, C., G. Koob, and L. Pulvirenti (2001). Dopamine partial agonist reverses amphetamine withdrawal in rats. *Neuropsychopharmacology* 25: 789–792.

References

Ortner, C., T. MacDonald, and M. Olmstead (2003). Alcohol intoxication reduce. impulsivity in the delay-discounting paradigm. *Alcohol and Alcoholism* 38: 151–156.

Ostaszewski, P., L. Green, and J. Myerson (1998) Effects of inflation on the subjective value of delayed and probabilistic rewards. *Psychonomic Bulletin and Review* 5: 324–333.

Pallanti, S., L. Quercioli, E. Sood, and E. Hollander (2002). Lithium and valproate treatment of pathological gambling: A randomized single-blind study. *Journal of Clinical Psychiatry* 63: 559–564.

Pallesen, S., M. Mitsem, G. Kvale, B. H. Johnsen, and H. Molde (2005). Outcome of psychological treatments of pathological gambling: A review and meta-analysis. *Addiction* 100: 1412–1422.

Patak, M., and B. Reynolds (2007). Question-based assessments of delay discounting: Do respondents spontaneously incorporate uncertainty into their valuations for delayed rewards? *Addictive Behaviors* 32: 351–357.

Patrick, C., J. Curtin, and A. Tellegen (2002). Development and validation of a brief form of the multidimensional personality questionnaire. *Psychological Assessment* 14: 150–163.

Patton, J., M. Stanford, and E. Barratt (1995). Factor structure of the Barratt impulsiveness scale. *Journal of Clinical Psychology* 51: 768–774.

Perez de Castro, I., A. Ibáñez, P. Torres, J. Sáiz-Ruiz, and J. Fernandez-Piqueras (1997). Genetic association study between pathological gambling and a functional DNA polymorphism at the D4 receptor. *Pharmacogenetics* 7: 345–348.

Perry, J., E. Larson, J. German, G. Madden, and M. Carroll (2005). Impulsivity (delay discounting) as a predictor of acquisition of IV cocaine self-administration in female rats. *Psychopharmacology* 178: 193–201.

Petry, N. (2000). Gambling problems in substance abusers are associated with increased sexual risk behaviors. *Addiction* 95: 1089–1100.

Petry, N. (2001a). Pathological gamblers, with and without substance abuse disorders, discount delayed rewards at high rates. *Journal of Abnormal Psychology* 110: 482–487.

Petry, N. (2001b). Substance abuse, pathological gambling, and impulsiveness. *Drug and Alcohol Dependence* 63: 29–38.

Petry, N. (2001c) Delay discounting of money and alcohol in actively using alcoholics, currently abstinent alcoholics, and controls. *Psychopharmacology* 154: 243–250.

Petry, N. (2005). *Pathological Gambling: Etiology, Comorbidity and Treatment*. Washington, D.C.: American Psychological Association.

Petry, N. (2006). Should the scope of addictive behaviours be broadened to include pathological gambling? *Addiction* 101 (suppl.): 152–160.

Petry, N., and T. Casarella (1999). Excessive discounting of delayed rewards in substance abusers with gambling problems. *Drug and Alcohol Dependence* 56: 25–32.

Petry, N., and C. Oncken (2002). Cigarette smoking is associated with increased severity of gambling problems in treatment-seeking gamblers. *Addiction* 97: 745–753.

...etry, N., and R. Pietrzak (2004). Comorbidity of substance use and gambling dis-
orders. In *Dual Diagnosis and Psychiatric Treatment: Substance Abuse and Comorbid Disorders*, 2nd edn., ed. H. R. Kranzler and J. A. Tinsley, pp. 437–459. New York: Marcel Dekker.

Phelps, E., and R. Pollack (1968). On second-best national saving and game equilibrium growth. *Review of Economic Studies* 35: 201–208.

Pilla, M., S. Perachon, F. Sautel, F. Garrido, A. Mann, C. Wemuth, J. Schwartz, B. Everitt, and P. Sokoloff (1999). Selective inhibition of cocaine-seeking behaviour by a partial dopamine D3 receptor agonist. *Nature* 400: 371–375.

Pochon, J., R. Levy, P. Fossati, S. Lehericy, J. Poline, B. Pillon, D. Le Bihan, and B. Dubois (2002). The neural system that bridges reward and cognition in humans: An fMRI study. *PNAS* 99: 5669–5674.

Port, R., and T. van Gelder (1998). *Mind as Motion: Explorations in the Dynamics of Cognition*. Cambridge, Mass.: MIT Press.

Goudri, M. (2006). Should addictive disorders include non-substance-related conditions? *Addiction* 101 (suppl.): 142–151.

Potenza, M., and R. A. Chambers (2001). Schizophrenia and pathological gambling. *American Journal of Psychiatry* 158: 497–498.

Potenza, M., C. Gottschalk, P. Skudlarski, R. Fulbright, C. Lacadie, M. Wilber, M. Steinberg, B. Rounsaville, T. Kosten, J. Gore, R. Constable, and B. Wexler (2004). Neuroimaging studies of behavioral and drug addictions: Gambling urges in pathological gambling and cocaine cravings in cocaine dependence. New York: American Psychiatric Association.

Potenza, M., H.-C. Leung, H. Blumberg, B. Peterson, R. Fulbright, C. Lacadie, P. Skudlarski, and J. Gore (2003a). An fMRI Stroop task study of ventromedial prefrontal cortical function in pathological gamblers. *American Journal of Psychiatry* 160: 1990–1994.

Potenza, M., M. Steinberg, P. Skudlarski, R. Fulbright, C. Lacadie, M. Wilber, B. Rounsaville, J. Gore, and B. Wexler (2003b). Gambling urges in pathological gambling. A functional magnetic resonance imaging study. *Archives of General Psychiatry* 60: 828–836.

Potenza, M., H. Xian, K. Shah, J. Scherrer, and S. Eisen (2005). Shared genetic contributions to pathological gambling and major depression in men. *Archives of General Psychiatry* 62: 1015–1021.

Poulos, C., J. Parker, and D. Le (1998). Increased impulsivity after injected alcohol predicts later alcohol consumption in rats: Evidence for "loss-of-control drinking" and marked individual differences. *Behavioral Neuroscience* 112: 1247–1257.

Preuschoff, K., P. Bossaerts, and S. Quartz (2006). Neural differentiation of expected reward and risk in human subcortical structures. *Neuron* 51: 381–390.

Pulvirenti, L., and G. Koob (1994). Dopamine receptor agonists, partial agonists and psychostimulant addiction. *Trends in Pharmacological Science* 15: 374–379.

Rachlin, H. (1987). Animal choice and human choice. In *Advances in Behavioral Economics*, vol. 1, ed. L. Green and J. Kagel, pp. 48–64. Norwood, N.J.: Ablex.

References

Rachlin, H. (1990). Why do people gamble and keep gambling despite heavy losses? *Psychological Science* 1: 294–297.

Rachlin, H. (1995). Self-control: Beyond commitment. *Behavioral and Brain Sciences* 18: 109–159.

Rachlin, H. (1996). Can we leave cognition to cognitive psychologists? Comments on an article by George Loewenstein. *Organizational Behavior and Human Decision Processes* 65: 296–299.

Rachlin, H. (1997). Four teleological theories of addiction. *Psychonomic Bulletin and Review* 4: 462–473.

Rachlin, H. (2000). *The Science of Self-Control.* Cambridge, Mass.: Harvard University Press.

Rachlin, H., and L. Green (1972). Commitment, choice, and self-control. *Journal of the Experimental Analysis of Behavior* 17: 15–22.

Rachlin, H., L. Green, and B. Tormey (1988). Is there a decisive test between matching and maximization? *Journal of the Experimental Analysis of Behavior* 50: 113–123.

Rachlin, H., A. Logue, J. Gibbon, and M. Frankel (1986). Cognition and behavior in studies of choice. *Psychological Review* 93: 33–45.

Rachlin, H., A. Raineri, and D. Cross (1991). Subjective probability and delay. *Journal of the Experimental Analysis of Behavior* 55: 233–244.

Rachlin, H., E. Siegel, and D. Cross (1994). Lotteries and the time horizon. *Psychological Science* 5: 390–393.

Read, D. (2001). Is time-discounting hyperbolic or subadditive? *Journal of Risk and Uncertainty* 23: 5–32.

Read, D. (2003). Subadditive intertemporal choice. In *Time and Decision: Economic and Psychological Perspectives on Intertemporal Choice*, ed. G. Loewenstein, D. Read, and R. Baumeister, pp. 301–322. New York: Russel Sage Foundation.

Redish, A. (2004). Addiction as a computational process gone awry. *Science* 306: 1944–1947.

Regard, M., D. Knoch, E. Guetling, and T. Landis (2003). Brain damage and addictive behavior: A neuropsychological and electroencephalogram investigation with pathological gamblers. *Cognitive Behavioral Neurology* 16: 47–53.

Rescorla, R., and A. Wagner (1972). A theory of Pavolvian conditioning: Variations in the effectiveness of reinforcement and nonreinforcement. In *Classical Conditioning II: Current Research and Theory*, ed. A. Black and W. Prokasy, pp. 64–99. New York: Appleton Century Crofts.

Reuter, J., T. Raedler, M. Rose, I. Hand, J. Gläscher, and C. Büchel (2005). Pathological gambling is linked to reduced activation of the mesolimbic reward system. *Nature Neuroscience* 8: 147–148.

Reynolds, B., A. Ortengren, J. Richards, and H. de Wit (2006). Dimensions of impulsive behavior: Personality and behavioral measures. *Personality and Individual Differences* 40: 305–315.

ςynolds, B., J. Richards, and H. de Wit (2006). Acute-alcohol effects on the Experiential ϶iscounting Task (EDT) and a question-based measure of delay discounting. *Pharmacol-ogy, Biochemistry and Behavior* 83: 194–202.

Reynolds, B., J. Richards, K. Horn, and K. Karraker (2004). Delay discounting and probability discounting as related to cigarette smoking status in adults. *Behavioural Processes* 65: 35–42.

Reynolds, B., and R. Schiffbauer (2004). Measuring state changes in human delay discounting: An experiential discounting task. *Behavioral Processes* 67: 343–356.

Rice, D. (1999). Economic costs of substance abuse. *Proceedings of the Association of American Physicians* 111: 119–125.

Richards, J., L. Zhang, S. Mitchell, and H. de Wit (1999). Delay or probability discounting as a model of impulsive behavior: Effect of alcohol. *Journal for the Experimental Analysis of Behavior* 71: 121–143.

Rigotti, N., J. E. Lee, and H. Wheeler (2000). US college students' use of tobacco products. *Journal of the American Medical Association* 284: 699–705.

Rilling, J., A. Glenn, M. Jairam, G. Pagnoni, D. Goldsmith, H. Elfenbein, and S. Lilienfeld (2007). Neural correlates of social cooperation and non-cooperation as a function of psychopathy. *Biological Psychiatry* 61: 1260–1271.

Robins, L., B. Locke, and D. Regier (1991). An overview of psychiatric disorders in America. In *Psychiatric Disorders in America: The Epidemiologic Catchment Area Study*, ed. L. Robins and D. Regier, pp. 328–366. New York: Free Press.

Robinson, I., G. Gorny, E. Milton, and B. Kolb (2001). Cocaine self-administration alters the morphology dendrites and dendritic spines in the nucleus accumbens and neurocortex. *Synapse* 39: 257–266.

Rogers, R., B. Everitt, A. Baldacchino, A. Blackshaw, R. Swainson, K. Wynne, N. Baker, J. Hunter, T. Carthy, E. Booker, M. London, J. Deakin, B. Sahakian, and T. Robbins (1999). Dissociable deficits in the decision-making cognition of chronic amphetamine abusers, opiate abusers, patients with focal damage to prefrontal cortex, and tryptophan-depleted normal volunteers: Evidence for monomaminergic mechanisms. *Neuropsychopharmacology* 20: 322–339.

Rosenkrantz, J., and A. Grace (2001). Dopamine attenuates prefrontal cortical suppression of sensory inputs to the basolateral amygdala of rats. *Journal of Neuroscience* 21: 4090–4103.

Ross, D. (1994). Dennett's conceptual reform. *Behavior and Philosophy* 22: 41–52.

Ross, D. (2005). *Economic Theory and Cognitive Science, Vol. 1: Microexplanation*. Cambridge, Mass.: MIT Press.

Ross, D. (2007). The economics of the sub-personal: Two research programs. In *Economics and the Mind*, ed. B. Montero and M. White, pp. 41–57. London: Routledge.

Ross, D. (forthcoming). Integrating the dynamics of multi-scale economic agency. In *The Oxford Handbook of Philosophy of Economic Science*, ed. H. Kincaid and D. Ross. Oxford: Oxford University Press.

References

Rotheram-Fuller, E., S. Shoptaw, S. Berman, and E. London (2004). Impaired performar in a test of decision-making by opiate-dependent tobacco smokers. *Drug and Alcoh Dependence* 73: 79–86.

Rougier, N., D. Noelle, T. Braver, J. Cohen, and R. O'Reilly (2005). Prefrontal cortex and flexible cognitive control: Rules without symbols. *Proceedings of the National Academy of Sciences USA* 102: 7338–7343.

Rousseau, F., R. Vallerand, C. Ratelle, G. Mageau, and P. Provencher (2002). Passion and gambling: On the validation of the Gambling Passion Scale (GPS). *Journal of Gambling Studies* 18: 45–66.

Roy, A., B. Adinoff, L. Roehrich, D. Lamparski, R. Custer, V. Lorenz, M. Barbaccia, A. Guidotti, E. Costa, and M. Linnoila (1988). Pathological gambling: A psychobiological study. *Archives of General Psychiatry* 45: 369–373.

Rudgley, R. (1999). *The Lost Civilizations of the Stone Age*. New York: Free Press.

Rugle, L., and L. Melamed (1993). Neuropsychological assessment of attention problems in pathological gamblers. *Journal of Nervous and Mental Diseases* 181: 107–112.

Saiz-Ruiz, J., C. Blanco, A. Ibáñez, X. Masramon, M. Gomez, M. Madrigal, and T. Diez (2005). Sertraline treatment of pathological gambling: A pilot study. *Journal of Clinical Psychiatry* 66: 28–33.

Samuelson, P. (1937). A note on the measurement of utility. *Review of Economic Studies* 4: 155–161.

Sanabria, F., and P. Killeen (2005). Freud meets Skinner: Hyperbolic curves, elliptical theories, and Ainslie interests. *Behavioral and Brain Sciences* 28: 660–661.

Sarbin, T. (1968). Ontology recapitulates philology: The mythic nature of anxiety. *American Psychologist* 23: 411–418.

Schaefer, A., T. Braver, J. Reynolds, G. Burgess, T. Yarkoni, and J. Gray (2006). Individual differences in amygdala activity predict response speed during working memory. *Journal of Neuroscience* 26: 10120–10128.

Schelling, T. (1960). *The Strategy of Conflict*. Cambridge, Mass.: Harvard University Press.

Schelling, T. (1978). Economics, or the art of self-management. *American Economic Review* 68: 290–294.

Schelling, T. (1980). The intimate contest for self-command. *Public Interest* 60: 94–118.

Schelling, T. (1984). Self-command in practice, in policy, and in a theory of rational choice. *American Economic Review* 74: 1–11.

Schroeder, T. (2004). *Three Faces of Desire*. Oxford: Oxford University Press.

Schultz, W. (2002). Getting formal with dopamine and reward. *Neuron* 36: 241–263.

Schultz, W., P. Dayan, and P. R. Montague (1997). A neural substrate of prediction and reward. *Science* 275: 1593–1599.

Seamans, J., and C. Yang (2004). The principal features and mechanisms of dopamine modulation in the prefrontal cortex. *Progress in Neurobiology* 74: 1–57.

References

...fer, H., M. Hall, and J. Vander Bilt (1999). Estimating the prevalence of disordered ...mbling behavior in the United States and Canada: A research synthesis. *American* *urnal of Public Health* 89: 1369–1376.

Shaffer, H., M. Stanton, and S. Nelson (2006). Trends in gambling studies research: Quantifying, categorizing, and describing citations. *Journal of Gambling Studies* 22: 427–442.

Shallice, T., and P. Burgess (1991). Deficits in strategy application following frontal lobe deficits in man. *Brain* 114: 727–741.

Sharp, C., and P. Fonagy (forthcoming). The parent's capacity to treat the child as a psychological agent: Constructs, measures and implications for developmental psychopathology. *Social Development.*

Sharpe, L. (2002). A reformulated cognitive-behavioral model of problem gambling: A biopsychosocial perspective. *Clinical Psychology Review* 22: 1–25.

Shimamura, A. (2000). The role of the prefrontal cortex in dynamic filtering. *Psychobiology* 28: 207–218.

Shinohara, K., A. Yanigasawa, Y. Kagota, A. Gomi, K. Nemoto, E. Moriya, E. Furusawa, K. Furuya, and K. Teresawa (1999). Physiological changes in Pachinko players: Beta-endorphin, catecholamines, immune system substances and heart rate. *Applied Human Sciences* 18: 37–42.

Shiv, B., G. Loewenstein, A. Bechara, H. Damasio, and A. Damasio (2005). Investment behavior and the negative side of emotion. *Psychological Science* 16: 435–439.

Siegel, E., and H. Rachlin (1996). Soft commitment: Self-control achieved through response persistence. *Journal of the Experimental Analysis of Behavior* 64: 117–128.

Simpson, C., and R. Vuchinich (2000). Reliability of a measure of temporal discounting. *Psychological Record* 50: 3–16.

Slutske, W. (2006). Natural recovery and treatment-seeking in pathological gambling: Results from two US national surveys. *American Journal of Psychiatry* 163: 297–302.

Slutske, W., S. Eisen, W. True, M. Lyons, J. Goldberg, and M. Tsuang (2000). Common genetic vulnerability for pathological gambling and alcohol dependence in men. *Archives Of General Psychiatry* 57: 666–673.

Spear, L. P. (2000). The adolescent brain and age-related behavioral manifestations. *Neuroscience and Biobehavioral Reviews* 24: 417–463.

Steel, Z., and A. Blaszczynski (1998). Impulsivity, personality disorders and pathological gambling severity. *Addiction* 93: 895–905.

Steele, C., and L. Southwick (1985). Alcohol and social behavior I: The psychology of drunken excess. *Journal of Personality and Social Psychology* 48: 18–34.

Steenbergh, T., A. Meyers, R. May, and J. Whelan (2002). Development and validation of the Gamblers' Beliefs Questionnaire. *Psychology of Addictive Behaviors* 16: 143–149.

Steketee, J. (2002). Neurotransmitter systems of the medial prefrontal cortex: Potential role in sensitization to psychostimulants. *Brain Research Reviews* 42: 203–228.

References

Stephens, D., and D. Anderson (2001). The adaptive value of preference for immediac When short-sighted rules have far-sighted consequences. *Behavioral Ecology* 12: 330 339.

Stephens, D., B. Kerr, and E. Fernandez-Juricic (2004). Impulsiveness without discounting: The ecological rationality hypothesis. *Proceedings of the Royal Society of London (B)* 271: 2459–2465.

Sterelny, K. (2003). *Thought in a Hostile World.* Oxford: Blackwell.

Stewart, S., L. McWilliams, J. Blackburn, and R. Klein (2002). A laboratory-based investigation of relations among video lottery terminal (VLT) play, negative mood, and alcohol consumption in regular VLT players. *Addictive Behaviors* 27: 819–835.

Stojanov, W., F. Karayanidis, P. Johnston, A. Bailey, V. Carr, and U. Schall (2003). Disrupted sensory gating in pathological gambling. *Biological Psychiatry* 54: 474–484.

Straube, T., M. Glauer, S. Dilger, H. Mentzel, and W. Miltner (2006). Effects of cognitive-behavioral therapy on brain activation in specific phobia. *Neuroimage* 29: 125–135.

Sutton, R., and A. Bartow (1998). *Reinforcement Learning: An Introduction.* Cambridge, Mass.: MIT Press.

Tamminga, C., and E. Nestler (2006). Pathological gambling: Focusing on the addiction, not the activity. *American Journal of Psychiatry* 163: 180–181.

Thelen, E., and L. Smith (1996). *A Dynamic Systems Approach to the Development of Cognition and Action.* Cambridge, Mass.: MIT Press.

Tobler, P., C. Fiorello, and W. Schultz (2005). Adaptive coding of reward value by dopamine neurons. *Science* 307: 1642–1645.

Toce-Gerstein, M., D. Gerstein, and R. Volberg (2003). A hierarchy of gambling disorders in the community. *Addiction* 98: 1661–1672.

Toneatto, T., and R. Ladouceur (2003). Treatment of pathological gambling: A critical review of the literature. *Psychology of Addictive Behaviors* 17: 284–292.

Tucker, J., R. Vuchinich, B. Black, and P. Rippens (2006). Significance of a behavioral economic index of reward value in predicting drinking problem resolution. *Journal of Consulting and Clinical Psychology* 74: 317–326.

Tucker, J., R. Vuchinich, and P. Rippens (2002a). Environmental contexts surrounding resolution of drinking problems among problem drinkers with different help-seeking experiences. *Journal of Studies on Alcohol* 63: 334–341.

Tucker, J., R. Vuchinich, and P. Rippens (2002b). Predicting natural resolutions of alcohol-related problems: A prospective behavioral economic analysis. *Experimental and Clinical Psychopharmacology* 10: 248–257.

Tulving, E. (1972). Episodic and semantic memory. In *Organization of Memory*, ed. E. Tulving and W. Donaldson, pp. 381–403. New York: Academic Press.

US Department of Health and Human Services (1988). *The Health Consequences of Smoking: Nicotine Addiction.* A report of the Surgeon General. Washington, D.C.: US Government Printing Office.

Van Fraassen, B. (1980). *The Scientific Image.* Oxford: Oxford University Press.

n Honk, J., D. Schutter, E. Hermans, P. Putman, A. Tuiten, and H. Koppeschaar (2004). estosterone shifts the balance between sensitivity for punishment and reward in healthy young women. *Psychoneuroendocrinology* 29: 937–943.

Vitaro, F., L. Arseneault, E. Richard, and R. Tremblay (1999). Impulsivity predicts problem gambling in low SES adolescent males. *Addiction* 94: 565–575.

Vuchinich, R. (1999), Behavioral economics as a framework for organizing the expanded range of substance abuse interventions. In *Changing Addictive Behavior: Bridging Clinical and Public Health Strategies*, ed. J. Tucker, D. Donovan and G. Marlatt, pp. 191–218. New York: Guilford.

Vuchinich, R., and N. Heather, eds. (2003). *Choice, Behavioral Economics, and Addiction*. Oxford: Pergamon/Elsevier.

Vuchinich, R., and C. Simpson (1998). Hyperbolic temporal discounting in social drinkers and problem drinkers. *Experimental and Clinical Psychopharmacology* 6: 292–305.

Vuchinich, R., and J. Tucker (1996). Alcoholic relapse, life events, and behavioral theories of choice: A prospective analysis. *Experimental and Clinical Psychopharmacology* 4: 19–28.

Wager, T., J. Rilling, E. Smith, A. Sokolik, K. Casey, R. Davidson, S. Kosslyn, R. Rose, and J. Cohen (2004). Placebo-induced changes in fMRI in the anticipation and experience of pain. *Science* 303: 1162–1167.

Warner, J. (1994). Resolv'd to drink no more: Addiction as a preindustrial construct. *Journal of Studies on Alcohol* 55: 685–691.

Wells, A. (2000). *Emotional Disorders and Metacognition: Innovative Cognitive Therapy*. Chichester: John Wiley.

Wells, A., and C. Purdon (1999). Metacognition and cognitive-behaviour therapy: A special issue. *Clinical Psychology and Psychotherapy* 6: 71–72.

Wexler, B. (2006). *Brain and Culture*. Cambridge, Mass.: MIT Press.

Whewell, W. (1858). *Novum Organon Renovatum*. London: Parker and Son.

Whiteside, S., and D. Lynam (2001). The five-factor model and impulsivity: Using a structural model of personality to understand impulsivity. *Personality and Individual Differences* 30: 669–689.

Whiteside, S., D. Lynam, J. Miller, and S. Reynolds (2005). Validation of the UPPS impulsive behavior scale: A four-factor model of impulsivity. *European Journal of Personality* 19: 559–574.

Whitlow, C., A. Liguori, L. Livengood, S. Hart, B. Mussat-Whitlow, C. Lamborna, P. Laurienti, and L. Porrino (2004). Long-term heavy marijuana users make costly decisions on a gambling task. *Drug and Alcohol Dependence* 76: 107–111.

Williams, J., and P. Dayan (2005). Dopamine, learning, and impulsivity: A biological account of attention-deficit/hyperactivity disorder. *Journal of Child and Adolescent Psychopharmacology* 15: 160–179.

Williams, J., and E. Taylor (2004). Dopamine appetite and cognitive impairment in attention deficit/hyperactivity disorder. *Neural Plasticity* 11: 114–132.

Wilson, M., and M. Daly (2003). Do pretty women inspire men to discount the future? *Proceedings of the Royal Society of London* 271: S177–179.

Winkielman, P., K. Berridge, and J. Wilbarger (2005). Unconscious affective reactions to masked happy versus angry faces influence consumption behavior and judgments of value. *Personality and Social Psychology Bulletin* 31: 121–135.

Winters, K., S. Specker, and R. Stinchfield (2002). Measuring pathological gambling with the Diagnostic Interview for Gambling Severity (DIGS). In *The Downside: Problem and Pathological Gambling*, ed. J. Marotta, J. Cornelius, and W. Eadington, pp. 143–148. Reno: Institute for the Study of Gambling and Commercial Gaming, University of Nevada.

Winters, K., R. Stinchfield, and J. Fulkerson (1990). Adolescent gambling behavior in Minnesota: Benchmark. *Report to the Department of Human Services Mental Health Division*. Duluth: Center for Addiction Studies, University of Minnesota.

Wise, R. (2000). Addiction becomes a brain disease. *Neuron* 26: 27–33.

Wise, R. (2002). Brain reward circuitry: Insights from unsensed incentives. *Neuron* 36: 229–240.

Wolpe, J. (1952). Objective psychotherapy of the neuroses. *South African Medical Journal* 26: 825–829.

World Health Organization (1957). *WHO Expert Committee on Addiction-Producing Drugs. Technical Report Series No. 116*. Geneva: World Health Organization.

World Health Organization (1982). *Sixth Review of Psychoactive Substances for International Control*. Geneva: World Health Organization.

Yang, C., J. Seamans, and N. Gorelova (1999). Developing a neuronal model for the pathophysiology of schizophrenia based on the nature of electrophysiological actions of dopamine in the prefrontal cortex. *Neuropsychopharmacology* 21: 161–194.

Zack, M., and C. Poulos (2004). Amphetamine primes motivation to gamble and gambling-related semantic networks in problem gamblers. *Neuropsychopharmacology* 29: 195–207.

Zahavi, A., and A. Zahavi (1997). *The Handicap Principle*. Oxford: Oxford University Press.

Zajonc, R. (1980). Feeling and thinking: Preferences need no inferences. *American Psychologist* 35: 151–175.

Zajonc, R. (1984). On the primacy of affect. *American Psychologist* 39: 117–123.

Zimmerman, M., R. Breen, and M. Posternak (2002). An open-label study of citalopram in the treatment of pathological gambling. *Journal of Clinical Psychiatry* 63: 44–48.

Zink, C., G. Pagnoni, M. Martin-Skurski, J. Chappelow, and G. Berns (2004). Human striatal responses to monetary reward depend on saliency. *Neuron* 42: 509–717.

Index

Index